In my field, athletes are always looking to gain a competitive edge. In the past, clinicians who worked with these athletes relied on incomplete methodologies. Now, Dr. Yun-tao Ma provides the clinician with a detailed reference manual demonstrating advanced dry needling techniques which enhance the neuromuscular, musculoskeletal and physiological systems of the elite, professional and recreational athlete.

Medical doctors, doctors of chiropractic, physical therapists, and acupuncturists aspiring to achieve optimal balance and maximize athletic performance will find that Dr. Ma's book provides a simple, detailed and proven process for detecting and correcting soft tissue dysfunction, preventing chronic sports injuries and maintaining homeostasis by utilizing advanced dry needling techniques to de-stress the musculoskeletal system.

It will teach you the science and provide the "how to" for you to increase microcirculation and reduce cellular aging in the athlete. Not only does it provide valuable practical information and techniques, but the book gives the clinician the effective tools to use for assessing, analyzing and evaluating the autonomic nervous system. It merges Eastern philosophy and Western philosophy to create wholeness for the advancement of sports medicine.

After 10 years of working as a personal performance enhancement doctor, Dr. Ma's course and book taught me one new modality that may add years to the career and life of my athletes. What you will learn in this section alone makes the book priceless. Dr. Ma gets the nervous system firing, the clinician excited and makes the athlete say "Wow!" after receiving his advanced dry needling therapy.

Dr. Clayton Gibson, III, MSA, DC, CCSP, CCEP, RTP, CSCS, CNT, FIAMA
Board Certified Chiropractic Sports Physician
Personal Physician to Numerous Elite, Olympic and Professional Athletes (NFL, NBA, MLB, USATF and NCAA)
Chief Functional Integrative Sports Performance Officer at Vitality Health Care, Inc.
Atlanta, Georgia

Presently we have a great confusion of various ideas regarding dry needling. Dr. Yun-tao Ma's book is destined to play a truly integrating role, explaining the mechanism of dry needling, offering a system for practical application and clarifying misunderstandings. Current myofascial trigger point approach focuses on localized or regionalized symptoms. Integrative systemic dry needling pays attention to both regionalized symptoms and their pathological influence over the entire musculoskeletal system. This approach can be successfully used for both treating and preventing myofascial symptoms, facilitating physical movement of both athletes and nonathlete patients.

Peter Lundgren, Physiotherapist
Director, AKNA Institute
Tyreso, Sweden

The concept of Dr. Ma's book is fantastic for physicians and other medical professionals, providing detailed practical procedures for treatment and prevention of sports and nonsports injuries using dry needling modality. Dr. Ma's fundamental approach to applying dry needling for sports medicine can be successfully used for helping athletes to achieve a peak performance, preventing soft tissue injuries, and facilitating rehabilitation after injuries or surgeries.

The de-stress treatment developed by Dr. Ma is a breakthrough in preventing and treating difficult conditions like overtraining syndrome and delayed onset of muscle soreness. Dr. Ma's concept of pain management for sports injuries focusing on functional restoration is especially valuable to athletes and their team doctors. The clinical techniques presented in this book are clear, simple and effective. I would recommend this book to all my colleagues and medical professionals whose clinical practice involves sports medicine and pain management.

Randall L. Snook, MD
CEO and Founder
Advanced Integrative Medicine
Denver, Colorado

Pain management and trauma rehabilitation is especially challenging when treating veterans and active duty personnel given the traumas experienced during combat. Dr. Yun-tao Ma's textbook provides an excellent alternative and augmentation to standard pain medicine approaches.

Jeffrey L. Hunter, DC, DO, FAAFP
Clinical Assistant Professor
Department of Family Medicine
College of Medicine
Ohio State University
Columbus, Ohio

The dry needling technique as described in Dr. Yun-tao Ma's textbook has proven to be one of the most profoundly beneficial treatments I have ever offered to my patients. This approach is unsurpassed for facilitating recovery from acute injury. It is even more valuable in assisting an athlete in restoring high performance abilities after months or years of experiencing subtle chronic injuries that have been masked by compensation. Dr. Ma's assessment and dry needling treatment protocols are pragmatic and designed to easily be incorporated into a modern clinic.

Mark A. Kestner, DC, FIAMA, CCSP, CSCS
Kestner Chiropractic & Acupuncture Center
Murfreesboro, Tennessee

What an exciting resource! This textbook will revolutionize our profession. Athletes are constantly looking for ways they can get an edge and perform at their best, especially when rehabilitating from an injury. Dr. Yun-tao Ma blends his many years of experience with his rich scientific background in bringing his unique system of integrative systemic dry needling to the sports world. Whether treating an acute sprain or strain, joint edema, delayed onset muscle soreness, or overtraining syndrome, I am thrilled to have this new tool to utilize in getting the elite and recreational athletes I treat back to competition quicker than ever.

Robert Ohashi PT, DPT, OCS, ATC, CSCS
Physical Therapist for elite athletes
Athletes' Performance Company
Phoenix, Arizona

Integrative systemic dry needling has brought a whole new dimension to physical therapy. Dr. Yun-tao Ma's virtually painless dry needling techniques described in this book allow for dynamic treatment of the body as a whole. I am amazed at the body's reaction to Dr. Ma's dry needling: the rapid reduction of pain, edema, and muscle spasm, which in turn restores proper postural alignment, enhancing total body function.

Janine K. Rodriguez, PT
Physical therapist with 25 years of clinical experience
Colorado Springs, Colorado

Dr. Ma's approach to dry needling is an integrative and systematic methodology specifically designed for medical/healthcare professionals. He is a true master with an ability to convey his extensive knowledge in a clear, concise, and enthusiastic manner. His latest book reveals an in-depth understanding into various sports-related injuries and treatment for athletes, which has helped me to attain optimal results with my patients.

Laina Eskin, PT
10 years of experience in dry needling
Vail, Colorado

This is the most important book written to modernize acupuncture in the 21st century. Dr. Yun-tao Ma brings this field to the next level by incorporating dry needling into acupuncture. I believe dry needling is a modality necessary for any acupuncturist who wants to successfully practice in the modern world.

Jai H. Sue, LAc
Hackensack University Medical Center
Westwood, New Jersey

A brilliant insight into the world of biomedical dry needling. Conventional pain concepts focus on neurological processes. Dr. Ma's integrative systemic dry needling technique treats both neurological dysfunction and pathohistological abnormalities of soft tissues, the main causes of soft tissue pain. His approach aims at tissue healing, providing pain relief without any side-effects. His new concept and approach greatly improve quality of clinical pain management, especially for athletes who suffer from overtraining and various injuries.

Lorenzo Gonzalez, PT, DPT, OSC, MS, LAT
Team Physical Therapist
2008 USA Olympic Silver Medal Women's Foil and Men's Sabre Fencing Teams
International Faculty Member
Hamilton, Ontario, Canada

BIOMEDICAL ACUPUNCTURE for SPORTS and TRAUMA REHABILITATION

Dry Needling Techniques

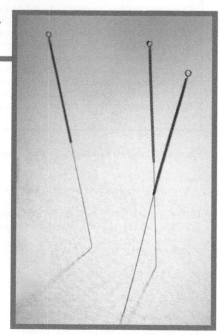

Yun-tao Ma, PhD, LAc

Director and Founder
Biomedical Acupuncture Institute and
American Dry Needling Institute
Boulder, Colorado
Visiting Professor, Medical Faculty
Paris XI (Orsay) University
Paris, France

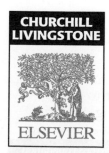

CHURCHILL
LIVINGSTONE

ELSEVIER

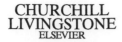

3251 Riverport Lane
St. Louis, Missouri 63043

Biomedical Acupuncture for Sports and Trauma Rehabilitation: ISBN: 978-1-4377-0927-8
Dry Needling Techniques

Notice

Knowledge and best practice in this field are constantly changing. As new research and experience broaden our knowledge, changes in practice, treatment and drug therapy may become necessary or appropriate. Readers are advised to check the most current information provided (i) on procedures featured or (ii) by the manufacturer of each product to be administered, to verify the recommended dose or formula, the method and duration of administration, and contraindications. It is the responsibility of the practitioner, relying on their own experience and knowledge of the patient, to make diagnoses, to determine dosages and the best treatment for each individual patient, and to take all appropriate safety precautions. To the fullest extent of the law, neither the Publisher nor the Author assumes any liability for any injury and/or damage to persons or property arising out of or related to any use of the material contained in this book.

The Publisher

Library of Congress Cataloging-in-Publication Data

Ma, Yun-tao.
    Biomedical acupuncture for sports and trauma rehabilitation : dry needling techniques / Yun-tao Ma.
        p. ; cm.
    ISBN 978-1-4377-0927-8 (hardcover : alk. paper) 1. Sports injuries–Patients–Rehabilitation. 2. Acupuncture.
    I. Title. [DNLM: 1. Athletic Injuries–therapy. 2. Acupuncture Therapy. 3. Sports Medicine–methods.
    QT 261 M111b 2011]
    RD97.M3 2011
    617.1'027–dc22   2010000460

Vice President and Publisher: Linda Duncan
Senior Editor: Kellie White
Developmental Editor: Kelly Milford
Publishing Services Manager: Catherine Jackson
Associate Project Manager: Jennifer Boudreau
Book Designer: Margaret Reid

Disease is a drama in two acts. The first one happens in the gloomy silence of the tissues, with the stage lights off. The pain or other symptoms only arrive in Act Two.
~R. Leriche, MD, French surgeon and author of
La Phylosophie de la Chirurgie (1955)

For Mila, Katrine, and Anton.
With love,
Yun-tao Ma

Foreword

Finally! A definitive text on dry needling in the sports environment has arrived. Until now I have found no meaningful information in print or on the Internet that deals exclusively with the use of dry needling in the treatment and management of athletes.

The use of dry needling in sporting clubs is not new. However, it has been my experience and observation that needling is used simply as an adjunct to traditional treatment techniques and is therefore restricted to the release of trigger points.

Working with elite athletes on a daily basis I am constantly looking for techniques that will give us an advantage in reducing recovery time and returning the athlete to competition. We are under pressure to return athletes to competition as soon as possible. While I was achieving good results incorporating dry needling with the management of injuries, it was not until I had contact with Dr. Ma, and started using the correct techniques, that I noted the recovery time for contusions, strains, and sprains was nothing less than amazing.

This book presents information that will aid in the prevention of injury by detailing needling techniques to facilitate maximal recovery from training and competition, delayed onset muscle soreness and overtraining syndrome. Prevention is always far better then cure, but traditionally we have looked to our strength and conditioning and skills coaches to build "bullet proof" athletes.

By providing regular de-stressing treatments as detailed in this book you can substantially improve physical performance and give your athletes the edge over their competitors.

This is a truly exciting text and a must-have for anyone working with athletes and sporting teams.

Tim Cooper
Physical therapist for the Australian Rules football teams and other elite athletes
Queensland, Australia

Foreword

Dr. Ma takes our understanding of dry needling to a new level by explaining the comprehensive biological and physiological processes involved with using needles.

Dry needling research has traditionally focused on treating local pathology and the local effects. Advancing the use of dry needling from a focus on local responses allows the practitioner to apply this intervention with a better understanding of all of the potential systemic effects including those on the central nervous system.

Biomedical acupuncture combines the research on dry needling with the worldwide research that explains the effects of this intervention from a modern scientific perspective, giving us a more comprehensive understanding of its effects.

Using the research foundation compiled in this book and the clinical insights in treating patients and athletes, the use of needles as a treatment modality can be studied with a solid scientific foundation, enhancing our understanding of this valuable intervention.

In our physical therapy clinics, many athletes request a comprehensive dry needling intervention as developed by Dr. Ma and presented in this book, noting improvement in flexibility and faster recovery. For the athlete, dry needling may be considered a "total body" intervention to enhance performance and maintain function after training and competition.

Herbert L. Silver, PT, ECS, OCS
Senior Clinician and President
Velocity Spine and
Sports Physical Therapy
Atlanta, Georgia

Foreword

Foreword

Dr. Ma, after 40 years of clinical experience and extensive research in the fields of neuroscience and pain at National Institute of Health (NIH), University of Maryland, and the University of Iowa, has formulated a unique approach that addresses both local and systemic effects of dry needling for normalizing myofascial and soft tissue function, regulating body homeostasis, preventing injuries, treating movement dysfunctions, and enhancing athletic performance beyond conventional methods.

Integrative systemic dry needling (ISDN) is an indispensible modality that is easy to learn and can be effectively applied by many clinical practitioners involved in preventing and treating sport injuries, chronic pain, and movement dysfunctions with predictable prognosis in athletes, military personnel and individuals involved in heavy labor work.

Dr. Ma defines a new meaning for dry needling and provides a simple but comprehensive and thorough rationale and explanation of the mechanism of effects of integrative systemic dry needling on psychological, behavioral and physical aspects of the athlete's performance. He provides ample functional and practical implications for using ISDN in any clinical setting.

M. Reza Nourbakhsh, PT, PhD, OCS
Professor, Department of Physical Therapy
North Georgia College and State University
Dahlonega, Georgia

Preface

BACKGROUND

Dry needling acupuncture is a new medical modality for treating patients with soft tissue pain and sports injuries.

Sports are specialized, skilled activities requiring actions that are highly coordinated among different body systems. The nerves, muscles, and skeletal system must cooperate in elaborate patterns of activity according to a precise timing sequence. If a muscle cannot conform to the current timing and pattern, the coordination is broken and the speed and precision of the performance will be impaired, possibly resulting in injury.

In clinical terms, optimal performance is dynamic and *needs continuous maintenance.* Many factors, especially overtraining, can obstruct the achievement of optimal performance. Sports scientists, doctors, coaches, and athletes are always seeking more effective procedures for treating intrinsic muscular fatigue and other problems, and now dry needling acupuncture offers a solution.

The use of needling to improve performance in sport and to treat related problems and injuries is not new. In ancient China, all Kung Fu masters were also masters of acupuncture. Today, although clinical successes in treating athletes with needling therapy are reported from time to time, the full potential of dry needling in sports medicine has not been recognized for at least three reasons.

First, the majority of practitioners do not understand the physiological mechanisms of dry needling, and so their practice is mostly empirical, based on their personal clinical experience.

Second, although empirical practice can produce good results—sometimes even apparent miracles—in most cases the results are not as good as they could be. For example delayed onset muscle soreness (DOMS) and insufficient recovery between training sessions and competition are common problems in most active athletes, and many athletes never take the time for complete regeneration and repair. This makes them prone to injury, impairs their performance, and may ultimately shorten their sports career. It is my belief that dry needling is the most effective therapy yet discovered for helping athletes to recover completely from those conditions, as long as the practitioners know the underlying mechanisms of needling and understand how to use the needles correctly. This especially true in athletes who do not show any physical signs of pathology, but are affected by deep physiological stress which can lead to future injury or premature tissue degeneration.

Finally, many practitioners only concentrate on needling trigger points, when research tells us there are at least three other types of myofascial conditions affecting athletes, each requiring a different needling technique.

This book provides a thorough and complete explanation of how to treat soft tissue dysfunction and prevent the development of chronic injuries in sports training and exercise, and it includes specific needling procedures for achieving maximal recovery from training and competition, DOMS, and overtraining syndrome. Athletes can substantially improve their physical performance through regular use of the de-stressing therapy introduced in this book, and they can also achieve complete recovery from intrinsic fatigue, overtraining, and musculoskeletal stress, while increasing the integration of all their physiological systems.

It should be emphasized that *the modern modality known as dry needling acupuncture does not share any common foundation with traditional Chinese acupuncture,* which is based on ancient Chinese philosophical and cultural concepts. The term *acupuncture* is used here in the sense of its original Latin roots: *acus* (needle) and *punctura* (puncture or piercing).

In recent years the unique efficacy of dry needling therapy has been recognized by an increasing number of medical doctors, physical therapists, chiropractors, occupational therapists, and others, who have appreciated its value and incorporated it into their clinical practices. "Dry" as opposed to "wet" needling is defined by Drs. Janet G. Travell and David G. Simons as "needling the soft tissue without injection of any liquid substance to treat human pathology" in their classic text, *Myofascial Pain and Dysfunction: The Trigger Point Manual.*

They also state: "In comparative studies, dry needling was found to be as effective as injecting an anesthetic solution such as procaine or lidocaine in terms of immediate inactivation of the trigger point".[1] Their ground-breaking work and other innovative needling methods such as the approach of Dr. C. Chan Gunn, which is known as Intramuscular Stimulation (IMS), have laid the foundation of what is now known as the new modality of dry needling acupuncture.

Clinically, soft tissue pain is an aspect of soft tissue dysfunction and may include myofascial pain, other musculoskeletal pain, fibromyalgia, and other soft tissue pathology. Soft tissue injury is present in most types of sports injury. Dry needling acupuncture is a very effective modality for treating acute and chronic soft tissue damage. An additional clinical benefit of dry needling is that it is effective in preventing the chronic injuries which result from repetitive overuse of muscles as is commonly seen in sports and physical exercise.

Dry needling acupuncture is a unified system which successfully combines both systemic and analytical approaches. Practitioners should not treat local symptoms only, but also need to restore the systemic homeostasis of their patients.

In contrast to wet needling, the clinical procedure of dry needling acupuncture emphasizes more tissue healing than pain relief, a more systemic approach than treatment of local pathology, and both post-injury treatment and pre-injury prevention.

A brief history of dry needling acupuncture

Like any medical procedure, dry needling acupuncture has gone through a period of development and may now be considered to be reaching its maturity. Dry needling as a medical technique has been observed in various human civilizations for over two millennia. From historical literature, we know that it appeared in Egypt, Greece, India, Japan, and China. The Chinese, as we know, systematically preserved this technique, developed its medical value, and formulated the well-known acupuncture of traditional Chinese medicine (TCM), widely acknowledged as one of the great inheritances of Chinese civilization.

Modern dry needling started in the 1930s in England and developed to maturity in the United States (see Chapter 10). Travell and Simons did comprehensive clinical research that led them to define and locate most of the important trigger points of skeletal muscles in the human body. They also noticed the relationship between trigger points and internal visceral pathology.[1] From the beginning they noticed that trigger points affect the posture and biomechanical balance of the musculoskeletal system. Other clinicians contributed different dry needling techniques, such as the Intramuscular Stimulation technique developed by Dr. C. Chan Gunn.[2] These researchers created the foundation of the analytical approach in dry needling therapy. Then came the synthetic approach.

Dr. Ronald Melzack found that more than 70% of the classic meridian acupoints corresponded to commonly used trigger points.[3] Then the discovery of homeostatic trigger points by Dr. H.C. Dung, Professor of Anatomy at the University of Texas Health Science Center at San Antonio, advanced our understanding of the connection between homeostatic trigger points and the principle of the central innervation of trigger points (see Chapters 7 and 8). Travell herself paid attention to Dung's work (personal communications between Travell and Dung in 1984 and between Dr. Dung and myself).

With 40 years of clinical experience and medical training, I found that both the analytical and synthetic approaches could be organically integrated into a new modality—modern dry-needling therapy. Working in the neuroscience program of the National Institutes of Health and in the physical therapy department of the University of Iowa, I did research on pain relief and the neuropharmacology of the central nervous system, kinesiology, cognitive neural science, and neurology. I was able to incorporate all these fields into dry needling therapy.

For the last 10 years, my colleagues in the U.S., China, Germany, Brazil and other countries and I have used dry needling acupuncture to treat thousands of patients, including elite athletes. All this research and clinical experience has helped to develop the practice of dry needling into its current form.

As with any modern medical technique, our current knowledge is built on the past. We constantly evolve new wisdom and demolish old dogma. We forge new perspectives in our practice and continually redefine our goals. This dynamic process advances our knowledge and prevents stasis, and in this way dry needling acupuncture will continue to grow.

CONCEPTUAL APPROACH

Lesion mechanisms of dry needling

Understanding the basic physiological mechanisms of dry needling is of the most fundamental importance to the practitioner. These mechanisms underlie the actual process of stimulation by needles, and how such stimulation brings about therapeutic effects.

Needling is both a physical disturbance to soft tissue and a minute biological traumatic inoculation into soft tissue. The physical movement and manipulation of the needles in deep tissues increases the tension of the muscle fibers and connective tissue and creates the effect of mechanical signal transduction, which leads to self-healing.

A minute traumatic lesion and the lesion-induced inflammation remain in the tissue when the needle is removed. The diameter of a skeletal muscle fiber is 50 μm and the average diameter of the dry needles used in clinical practice is about 250 μm (gauges 32-36). Therefore if a needle is inserted into a muscle, perpendicularly to the fibers and to a depth of 1 cm, it may break at least 1,000 muscle fibers. If the needle is inserted deeper into the muscle, with manipulation, tens of thousands of muscle fibers as well as some capillaries and nerve endings may be broken or injured by it.

The brain identifies the traumatic lesion in the soft tissue and directs biological systems, including the cardiovascular, immune and endocrine systems, to replace the damaged tissue with the same type of fresh tissue within a few days. In this way self-healing starts in the needling location. In addition to this local healing effect, the lesion induces systemic effects to restore homeostasis through a number of reflex processes at different levels of the central nervous system.

It should be emphasized that dry needling, as a nonpharmaceutical modality, promotes self-healing by reducing the mechanical and biological stress of the body. Some patients with soft-tissue pain will achieve self-healing without any medical intervention after a sufficient period of time. Nevertheless, dry needling accelerates this self-healing process and reduces unnecessary suffering. This acceleration also helps to prevent the development of chronic pathology. Without this understanding there is a potential for confusion. For example, a recent study showed that in the first 10 weeks of treatment, a needling-treated group experienced a much higher level of improvement (4.4 points) than a group treated with conventional methods (2.1 points). After 52 weeks, however, there was little difference between the group treated with needling and the control group.[8] This result is objective and can be correctly interpreted if the physiological nature of needling therapy is understood: both groups achieved self-healing by the end of the research period (52 weeks), but the group treated with needling suffered much less and had less potential for developing chronic pain than the control group. This is the clinical value of dry needling therapy.

Dry needling is a specific therapy for restoring soft-tissue dysfunction

Dry needling creates minute lesions in specific areas of soft tissue to normalize the soft tissue dysfunction without the involvement of any pharmacological process. By its physiological nature, dry needling is a specific therapy for myofascial pain and other soft-tissue dysfunction. Muscle accounts for 50% of human body mass, and so most human pathological conditions involve soft tissue dysfunction, whether in the case of physical injuries such as muscles damaged by overuse in daily life or in sporting activity, or in cases like Parkinson's disease, drug addiction, stroke, or cancer.

Of all the types of soft tissue dysfunction, pain is the most common neurological disorder, at any given time affecting about 35% of the North American and European population. More than $100 billion is spent every year for pain management. Recent studies suggest that more than 6 in every 10 adults over the age of 30 experience chronic pain. Expenditure on the relief of back and neck pain alone has risen to more than $80 billion per year in the United States, a dramatic increase over the past 8 years. In addition to the lost productivity of employees who can no longer work because of pain, an estimated $64 billion per year is lost due to the reduced performance of workers who continue to work while in pain.[4]

Dry needling as a specific soft tissue therapy is a valuable modality which has few or no side-effects if practiced properly. Several evidence-based studies show that needling is more effective than conventional therapy for back pain.[5,6] This is because dry needling therapy emphasizes and promotes the healing of tissue, with pain relief as a result or positive "side effect."

In sports medicine, it is not uncommon for injured athletes, both professional and amateur, to be permanently disabled due to their treatment's focus on pain relief rather than on restoring optimum function.

A systemic approach is necessary in dry-needling acupuncture

Clinical observation and evidence-based research reveal that an injury produces both local symptoms and systemic dysfunction, especially in active athletes.[7] Systemic dysfunction will continue if treatment is directed only at local symptoms. For example, knee pain can affect how the muscles are used to control the gait of the other leg, the movement of both feet and the hips, the spinal balance from the sacral to the cervical regions, and the functioning of the neck and even the eye muscles. The patient may not consciously realize this chain of dysfunction in their body, but an experienced clinician can easily recognize the interrelationship and identify the systemic dysfunction. The patient's brain, specifically the hypothalamus, will also subconsciously register this systemic dysfunction.

The interrelationship between local pathology and systemic dysfunction is felt in both the central and peripheral nervous system and in the musculoskeletal system. Visceral physiology can be affected as well. For example, a sensitized trigger point on the iliotibial band, related to lower limb dysfunction, will increase the sensitivity of trigger points on the pectoralis major muscle. Both local symptoms and systemic dysfunction should therefore be treated at the same time to achieve restoration of homeostasis. *This systemic approach is essential in the treatment of athletes to rehabilitate the current injury as well as to prevent injury in the future.*

This systemic chain reaction of local symptoms is registered in the nervous and musculoskeletal systems, and will affect physiologic homeostasis which is regulated by the hypothalamus. The integrative neuromuscular acu-reflex point system (INMARPS) introduced in this book is a way of tracking the degree of both physical and physiological homeostasis, thus providing a map for restoring homeostasis to the system.

Four types of myofascial pain and their different pathology

The majority of clinical pain is myofascial. It has been reported that 85% of back pain and 54.6% of chronic headache and neck pain is myofascial pain.[8] We currently categorize myofascial pain into four types:

1. Trigger points
2. Muscle spasm
3. Muscle tension
4. Muscle deficiency

Each type of myofascial pain requires a different dry needling technique and will follow its own healing pattern. Unfortunately many clinicians are trained to concentrate on trigger points to the exclusion of the other types of myofascial pain. Such narrow emphasis is contrary to the clinical realities and reflects a lack of understanding of the pathophysiolology of myofascial pain.[9]

Myofascial pain includes various types of soft tissue dysfunction. An analysis of such soft tissue pain involves at least the following types of pathology:

1. Tissue inflammation
2. Tissue contracture

3. Microcirculatory deficiency, which includes blood and lymphatic circulation, ischemia and/or edema
4. Trophic deficiency, including tissue degeneration
5. Tissue adhesion
6. Scarring of tissue
7. Biomechanical imbalance of the musculo-skeletal system, including improper posture.

Soft tissue pain, especially chronic pain, always involves all these dysfunctions and clinicians should treat all of them to achieve the optimum level of pain relief and recovery of tissue function. For example, when a joint is out of alignment, it causes both the attached and opposing muscle groups to be shortened or lengthened, which compromises the surrounding neuromuscular structures and connective tissues. Muscle spasm, muscle tension, and increased sympathetic output ensue, resulting in soft tissue pain, and the development of trigger points, edema, ischemia, and tissue degeneration. If the condition continues to the point of becoming chronic, tissue adhesion and the formation of scar tissue will occur and central sensitization will follow.

Myofascial trigger points are small, circumscribed, hyperirritable foci in muscles and fascia, often found within a firm or taut band of skeletal muscles.[10] Trigger points may also occur in ligaments, tendons, joint capsules, skin and periosteum. They have been described as tender nodes of degenerated tissue that can cause local and radiating or referred pain. The extent of the area of referred pain has been defined as the zone of reference. Please note that referred pain patterns do not correspond to dermatomal, myotomal or sclerotomal patterns and that the patterns of referred pain from a particular trigger point are not always the same. Myofascial pain symptoms presented by a patient may include pain, muscle weakness, decreased joint motion, and paresthesia, as well as autonomic symptoms like sweating, lacrimation, localized vasoconstriction, and pilomotor activity.

Trigger points show dynamic features. They can be asymptomatic (latent) or symptomatic (active). Primary trigger points develop independently and are not related to trigger-point activity elsewhere.

Secondary trigger points develop in neighboring and anatagonistic muscles as the result of stress and muscle spasm. Satellite trigger points appear in the area of referred pain as the result of persistent resting motor unit activity.

Muscle spasm is the involuntary contraction of muscle caused by acute or chronic trauma, excessive tension, or visceral disorder. An untreated spasm will lead to decreased blood flow in the muscle and edema in the tissue, which initiates a vicious cycle of more muscle spasm and pain.

Muscle tension is defined by Hans Kraus as "a prolonged contraction of a muscle or muscle groups beyond functional or postural need."[11] Muscle tension may have postural, emotional, or situational causes. Improper posture or a negative emotional experience (e.g., unresolved anger or psychological stress) can cause muscle tension and result in muscle pain.

Muscles are considered deficient when they are weak or stiff and proper posture and muscle function cannot be maintained. Muscle deficiencies can be a source of pain and make a person prone to injury. The fact that weakened abdominal muscles can cause back pain is a typical example of this *causal connection*.

Clinicians should keep in mind that chronic pain may involve all types of soft tissue dysfunction and varied techniques should be incorporated to achieve maximal healing and restoration of function. There is considerable clinical evidence that focusing only on pain and ignoring the healing of soft tissue can be disastrous for athletes.

The unique efficacy of dry-needling acupuncture in sports medicine

Some athletes resort to drugs to achieve better performance, and they risk paying a high price for this in the future. Anabolic steroids greatly increase the risk of cardiovascular damage, heart attack, and stroke, because they cause hypertension, a decrease in high-density blood lipoproteins, and an increase in low-density lipoproteins. The consumption of male sex hormones by male athletes can decrease testicular function, causing both lowered sperm formation and a reduction in the natural secretion of testosterone. The use of amphetamines and cocaine ultimately leads to a deterioration of performance. Some athletes have died during athletic events because of the interaction between such drugs and the norepinephrine and epinephrine which are naturally released by the sympathetic nervous system during high levels of activity. Under these circumstances, one cause of death is over-excitation of the heart leading to ventricular fibrillation, which is lethal within seconds.

Dry needling therapy can be seen as a safe means of enhancing performance. Dry needling reduces mechanical and intrinsic stress in the musculoskeletal system. This increases the efficiency of energy consumption and will therefore increase the endurance of the musculoskeletal system, improving physical performance. In addition, regular dry needling as a "maintenance" factor improves recovery and regeneration from the damage caused by training and competition, enabling the athlete to recover faster and continue training at a higher level, thereby also potentially increasing performance.

The difference between dry needling and wet needling therapy

Dry and wet needling share many common mechanisms, but there are significant differences between the two modalities. Dry needling can be used alone or in combination with wet needling to treat soft tissue pain, and when they are used together dry needling is a very good adjunct procedure to wet needling therapy. Dry needles inoculate minute lesions in soft tissue, and so multiple points can be needled in one treatment session, and the same procedure can be repeated many times until maximal healing is achieved. In addition, a needling procedure for preventing injuries can be repeated to maintain healthy homeostasis.

For example, when treating low-back pain, the lumbar muscles, gluteal muscles, hamstring muscles, calf muscles, hip flexor muscles, abdominal muscles, iliotibial band, pectoral muscles, and even neck muscles can be treated in the same session. The same procedure can be repeated in subsequent sessions until complete healing is achieved. The same needling procedure will also be effective with asymptomatic healthy persons for preventing low-back, hip, and neck problems.

Who will benefit from this book

Dry needling therapy is easy to learn and offers unique efficacy in treating soft tissue dysfunction. Increasing numbers of medical doctors, physical therapists, chiropractors, occupational therapists, physician assistants, and nurses have recognized the clinical value of dry needling therapy and are learning this modality and using it with their patients.

The ultimate purpose of dry needling is to integrate physiological systems to achieve homeostasis for better body fitness. This integration is achieved by normalizing tissue dysfunction caused by local or systemic pathology.

Many studies have shown that people who maintain an appropriate level of body fitness will have the additional benefit of prolonged life. Especially between the ages of 50 and 70, studies have shown mortality to be three times less in the most fit people than in the least fit.[12] Athletically fit people have more body reserves to call on when they do become sick. Proper exercise, good nutrition and regular de-stressing treatment can help body fitness for adults of all ages.

Based on a foundation of biomedical principles, dry needling can be practiced in many different ways according to any particular medical field. There is no reason that dry needling should be restricted to a particular style or technique. Every medical professional can develop their own style of dry needling once they understand the physiological mechanisms that underlie it.

Dry needling acupuncture is not the acupuncture of traditional Chinese medicine (TCM)

Dry needling has been developed on a foundation of the general principles of Western medical science. The understanding and practice of dry needling require that the practitioner has formal medical education, with comprehensive training which should include coursework in basic science as well as clinical courses like human anatomy, physiology, pathology, neurology, clinical diagnosis, etc. In addition, practitioners need clinical experience dealing with patients in terms of personal interaction, recording the medical history, and so on.

Traditional Chinese acupuncture developed about 3,000 years ago as an empirical clinical procedure. We have inherited much valuable experience from this ancient healing art, but this does not equal and cannot replace modern medical training, even though physiologically, traditional acupuncture is a type of dry needling therapy.

Confusion about traditional acupuncture can be avoided if we understand more of the history of its development. The distinguished scholar Professor Chen Fang-zheng, senior researcher of the Chinese Academy of Science and former director of the Institute of Chinese Culture at the Chinese University of Hong Kong, wrote in his recent book *Heritage and Betrayal: A Treatise on the Emergence of Modern Science in Western Civilization* (San Lian Shu Dian Press, Beijing, April 2009) that modern science could not evolve in Chinese culture as it did in the West because the ancient Chinese did not develop a method of logical enquiry into the objective world but focused only on practical aspects of their life. The same holds true in the development of traditional Chinese medicine.

Professor Chen Xiao-ye of the Academy of Chinese Medicine in Beijing also stated in a personal communication that TCM accumulated a great corpus of clinical experience, but did not develop consistent theories, so that today we have to formulate modern theories to explain its traditional methods. Professor Huang Long-xiang, Vice-President of the Acupuncture Institute at the Academy of Chinese Medicine in Beijing, came to the conclusion that the "meridian channel" theory of TCM has successfully accomplished its historical mission of preserving and developing acupuncture; now it has become the narrow neck of the bottle which is impeding further development of acupuncture medicine in the 21st century.[13]

For six decades, since the 1950s, the Chinese government has invested huge financial and human resources in studying acupuncture meridians. Researchers discovered and confirmed many "meridian *phenomena*" but no independent anatomical channels were found to match the meridian concept.

Such research, however, is not wasted, because it has clearly shown us that the concept of meridians was *invented* by the ancient doctors and that many "meridian phenomena" are of unknown physiology, but do have some relation to physical tissue, especially to our nervous system. Many laboratory scientists claim that they have discovered or confirmed the existence of meridian channels from research such as infrared imaging or similar procedures. If these researchers understood the neuroanatomy of the peripheral nervous system, the neurology and pathophysiology of the human body, and if they knew clinical needling mechanisms and had experience with real patients, they would interpret their results differently and reach different conclusions.

Why do many modern clinicians still cling to meridian theories if meridians are a human invention? There are social and empirical reasons. Practically, acupuncture based on meridian theory works. It is not uncommon in human intellectual history for mistaken theories to work quite well in terms of the empirical results. Also, in the tradition of Chinese medicine, theories and facts are not well differentiated and theories are often treated as facts.

The concept of meridians is a typical example of such confusion. Facts were often trimmed to fit the theories, which, in the words of Professor Huang Long-xiang, is like "cutting the foot to fit the shoe."[13]

Chinese medicine developed very slowly in the last 2,000 years because in both theory and practice it was subject to the dominance of traditional philosophy over human experience. Traditional Chinese medicine is no longer able to develop on its own as it is heavily dependent on a philosophical foundation that has become stagnant and fossilized. The theories of traditional acupuncture are no longer adequate for explaining the clinical mechanisms, benefits, and limits of dry needling.

We do not need to create new theories to explain how dry needling works. As with any modern medical procedure, the mechanisms, physiology, and clinical procedure of dry needling are based on universal scientific rules—the rules we discovered in mathematics, physics, chemistry, and biology.

Dry needling acupuncture has brought new concepts, a new system, a new interpretation and a new approach to learning and practicing healing therapy with needles. Both practitioners and patients will greatly benefit from this new approach.

Preface References:

1. Simons DG, Travell JG, Simons LS: *Travell & Simons' myofascial pain and dysfunction—the trigger point manual, Volume 1: Upper half of body*, Philadelphia, 1999, Lippincott Williams & Wilkins.
2. Gunn CC: *Gunn approach to the treatment of chronic pain: intramuscular stimulation for myofascial pain of radiculopathic origin*, ed 2, Livingstone, 1996, Churchill Edinburgh.
3. Melzack R, Stillwell DM, Fox EJ: Trigger points and acupuncture points for pain: correlations and implications, *Pain* 3:3–23, 1977.
4. Martin BI, Deyo RA, Mirza SK, et al: Expenditures and health status among adults with back and neck problems, *JAMA* 299(6):656–664, 2008.
5. Yuan J, Purepong N, Kerr DP, et al: Effectiveness of acupuncture for low back pain: a systemic review. *Spine* 33(23):E887–900, 2008.
6. Cherkin DC, Sherman KJ, Avins AL, et al: A randomized trial comparing acupuncture, simulated acupuncture and usual care for chronic low back pain, *Arch Intern Med* 169(9):858–866, 2009.
7. Heiderscheit B, Sherry M: What effect do core strength and stability have on injury prevention and recovery? In MacAuley D, Best T, editors: *Evidence-based sports medicine*, ed 2, Malden, Mass, 2007 Blackwell Publishing.
8. Fishbain DA, Goldberg M, Steele R, et al: DSM-III diagnosis of patients with myofascial pain syndrome (fibrositis), *Arch Phys Med Rehabil* 70:433–438, 1989.
9. Kraus H: Muscle deficiency. In Rachlin ES, Rachlin IS, editors: *Myofascial pain and fibromyalgia*, ed 2, St Louis, 2002, Mosby.
10. Bonica JJ: Management of myofascial pain syndromes in general practice, *JAMA* 732–738, June 1957.
11. Kraus H, editor: *Diagnosis and treatment of muscle pain*, Chicago, 1988, Quintessence.
12. Guyton AC, Hall JE: *Textbook of medical physiology*, ed 11, Philadelphia, 2006, Saunders, Chap 84.
13. Huang LX: Preface. In Ma YT, Ma M, Cho ZH, *Biomedical acupuncture for pain management, an integrative approach*, Edinburgh, 2005, Churchill Livingstone.

Acknowledgments

Our grateful acknowledgement is made to all our friends, students, and patients for their support and comments.

My heartfelt thanks go to my wife, Mila Ma, for her unwavering support and assistance.

This book owes an enormous obligation to the skills of our friend, Kellie White, the "dream come true" senior editor of Elsevier Publishing and her outstandingly professional team, and to Kelly Milford and Jennifer Boudreau for their patience, meticulous attention to details, and support through all stages of production.

Contents

Contents

Integrative Systemic Dry Needling: A New Modality for Athletes

All athletes experience injuries, as all people experience pain and disease in their lives. Some athletes are never completely able to recover from injuries that become chronic and make them more prone to new injuries. Some athletes come to believe that their performance is irreversibly impaired by injury while they are still in their prime, and some do have to face the reality that their athletic career is limited by chronic injuries. For many, however, this limitation is not inevitable. Some injuries can be successfully prevented, and it is possible to greatly improve recovery from both injury and surgery if the mechanisms of integrative systemic dry needling (ISDN) are understood by athletes themselves, their coaches, and their doctors.

Close examination of sports injuries indicates that most are related to soft tissue dysfunction. This is understandable, as soft tissue accounts for half of a human's body weight. Even for injuries that necessitate surgery, the final stage of recovery from both the injury and the surgery still depends on restoring the physiologic function of soft tissue.

ISDN is a unique medical procedure that is designed to restore and normalize soft tissue dysfunction. It is a new development in clinical technique that is different from both conventional dry needling and classic acupuncture, although it shares the same physiologic mechanisms as both methods. ISDN incorporates the analytic approach of conventional dry needling represented by Travell and Simons' trigger-point medicine[1] and Gunn's intramuscular stimulation[2] and synthesizes them into a unified pathophysiologic system. The treatment emphasizes both local problems and systemic dysfunction, because local injuries definitely affect the entire physiologic and biomechanical system. ISDN is thus a systemic and synthetic approach.

The basic techniques used in ISDN can be traced to the acupuncture that was developed in the ancient Chinese civilization, but its theoretical systems and clinical practice are based on modern medical science. Although ISDN is a division of modern integrative and experimental biomedicine, it maintains the benefits of classical acupuncture, including some of the traditional point system. However, ISDN does not depend on the theory or interpretation of classical acupuncture. The theoretical background and many of the clinical techniques of classical acupuncture are part of an ancient belief system based on empirical data that were appropriate to a particular culture. The unscientific origin behind classical acupuncture has impeded its further development, and ISDN has already metamorphosed from empirical practice into science-based 21st-century medicine.

Although it is a new integrative approach, ISDN is built upon the general principles of biomedical science that are familiar to and accepted by all health care professionals.

ISDN AND ATHLETES

ISDN can help all athletes, from so-called weekend warriors to dedicated professionals. It can enhance their physical performance, prevent common injuries, accelerate recovery from overtraining stress, promote rehabilitation after injury and surgeries, and prolong athletic careers by providing systemic maintenance.

ISDN achieves these goals not only because it reduces or cures the local injuries that commonly occur in sports but also because it emphasizes systemic balance and the restoration of physiologic homeostasis in both injured and healthy athletes. Optimal homeostasis ensures that the musculoskeletal system is balanced and thus produces effective mechanical movement; physiologic integration of the nervous, cardiovascular, endocrine, and immune systems; and a harmonious interaction between body and mind that can maximally support mechanical movement.

This is not a promise or a theoretical expectation but the result of my clinical experience, beginning in the 1960s. Especially since I began practicing in Colorado in 2000, I have come to better understand the physiologic mechanisms of dry needling as applied to athletes, systematically formulating my clinical procedure by working with both elite and weekend athletes and their coaches. Experience alone is not enough to justify such methods, but advances in evidence-based sports medicine have revealed much data that support my approach. This approach is successful because it effectively manages both chronic and acute stress in the athlete's musculoskeletal system. The term *effectively* is emphasized because athletes already have many techniques for minimizing chronic and acute stress, such as massage, physical therapy, warm-up stretching, and traditional acupuncture, and these techniques are effective, especially in young athletes whose physical adaptability is high. The majority of athletes, however, have passed their late 20s, and their musculoskeletal systems and other physiologic functions are changing. Chronic and acute stress slowly accumulate in the body, and physical deficiency gradually reveals itself. To restore physical capability, athletes need to restore homeostasis not only in local musculoskeletal structures such as a particular muscle group or joint, but also in the entire musculoskeletal system, and this must include balancing its physiologic and physical mechanics. Like all modalities in sports medicine, dry needling acupuncture or ISDN can be used by health care professionals to prevent and treat injuries, but in the context of sports, ISDN, as a nonspecific procedure, achieves these aims by reducing bodily stress and restoring and maintaining optimal homeostasis. With this homeostasis athletes can function better. They can better adjust to physical and psychologic challenges, and they can experience more rapid and more complete recovery from injuries.

The tenets of ISDN are to respect the human body and not interfere with it. It supports athletic activity in a natural way and never undermines the body with side effects.

ATHLETES EXPECT MORE THAN PAIN RELIEF

Working with athletes is a great pleasure for any health care professional. Because of their healthy bodies, positive emotion, strong willpower, good nutrition, and willingness to cooperate, they respond superbly to ISDN. With regular and well-designed maintenance procedures, patients can maintain optimal performance, and can even achieve better results than in previous years.

What is unique about working with athletes? Most seek medical attention at first for pain relief, which in most cases can be successfully accomplished because their well-trained bodies have maintained good self-healing potential. Whereas pain relief is enough for most nonathletic patients, athletes expect more than that. For them, pain relief is just a beginning. What they are seeking after suffering injury is to restore not only their original physical capability but also to acquire a level of good health that will minimize further injuries. I have seen elite athletes whose physical pain has ended as a result of conventional medical intervention, but so has their sports career. Many of these athletes may have had brighter and longer sports careers if they were properly treated, and even the injuries they suffered could have been prevented if proper procedures had been adopted sufficiently early. It is clear that if clinicians focus only on pain relief for athletes, they risk ignoring their patients' future performance and possibly prematurely ending their sports careers. ISDN aims to restore optimal homeostasis by reducing bodily stress so that the athlete's own biologic system can take care of pain relief.

CHRONIC AND ACUTE STRESS IMPEDE PHYSICAL PERFORMANCE IN SPORTS AND EXERCISE

The following description is an example of the kind of situation that can be successfully managed if the appropriate methods are used. Dara Torres (aged 42 in 2008), the American Olympian swimmer and mother of a 2-year-old daughter, is a historic figure in modern competitive sports. She missed the gold medal by 0.01 seconds, 24.07 to 24.06, in the 50-meter freestyle in the Olympic Games of 2008 in Beijing, losing to Germany's Britta Steffen—who was born 8 months before Torres won her first Olympic medal at Los Angeles in 1984. Australia's Cate Campbell, 16, took the bronze.

CNN reported on August 30, 2008, that Torres had had three surgical procedures on one shoulder since November 2007, and according to this report, Torres admitted that she was competing in the games with shoulder pain.

The historic achievement of Dara Torres is more than can be measured just by her medals. If she had been competing with less shoulder pain, however, she may not have lost that 0.01 second. If her musculoskeletal system had been carrying less acute and chronic stress from precompetition training, she would have been able to swim even faster. From the perspective of sport and exercise physiology, Torres could still expect to perform beyond her current physical limit if the acute and chronic stress in her musculoskeletal system could be reduced to the lowest level. Using the de-stressing effects of ISDN and other proper procedures, Torres and other athletes could continue to surpass their physical barriers and achieve new records.

Michael Phelps, at the age of 22, won eight gold medals in the 2008 Olympic Games. Enormous acute stress accumulated in his musculoskeletal system during those few days in Beijing, and this was in addition to the stress of his precompetition training. But his young body and the excellent condition of his musculoskeletal structure and of his cardiovascular, pulmonary, and metabolic systems were well able to meet the challenge. If this acute musculoskeletal stress could be effectively reduced right after each competition to quickly restore his body to its optimal physical condition, it is very likely that Phelps could improve his performance even more.

Since the 1920s, records show that the performance of runners has improved by about 10%. The triple jump record has increased by 30%, the long jump by 41%, and the high jump by 35%. The current records in pole vault are 80% higher than in

1896, but this increase is attributable chiefly to the introduction of the fiberglass pole. A significant factor in the setting of new performance records is the application of scientific methods in training, including nutrition and an understanding of the physics of forces involved in the motion of the human body. Chinese and Cuban athletes, for example, have shown great improvement since the 1980s for this reason.

Competition today is more intense than ever, and as records are being broken by ever-narrower margins, many people believe that athletes are nearing the absolute limits of human performance. Some try to meet this challenge by using artificial performance-enhancing substances. Steroids are used for at least two reasons: to build up muscle mass and to reduce muscle pain and inflammation. This behavior is now spreading to include other drugs that are specific to the demands of a particular sport, such as drugs that help to eliminate trembling in archery and shooting and drugs that promote rapid water loss so that weightlifters can reduce weight. Doping has become a serious concern of governments and sports officials, and today any exceptional performance is followed by testing for performance-enhancing drugs. Medal winners are tested and retested, their DNA is examined, and their blood may even be frozen for years to come.

LIMITATIONS OF HUMAN PERFORMANCE IN SPORTS AND EXERCISE

Do athletes have to use drugs to break past their physical limits? According to clinical evidence and research on the limits of human physical performance, the answer must be "no". Sports experts try to calculate the absolute limit of human performance by taking the highest value for each crucial physiologic factor such as maximal oxygen uptake, the greatest possible rate of burning energy, and the highest examples of physical stamina. A theoretical limit of human performance is then estimated by comparing these data with current performance records. Jamaican sprinter Usain Bolt lowered his own record in the 100-meter dash to 9.69 seconds in the Beijing Olympic Games, 0.03 seconds faster than the mark he set in May of the same year. Bolt knows that he could have achieved better; he visibly eased his pace when he saw that he already had secured the gold medal. According to research, the theoretical limit of the 100-meter dash could be as low as 9.2 seconds. The world record set by American athlete Jim Hines in 1968 was 9.95 seconds; thus, in four decades, the best performance improved by 0.26 seconds. Whether this research on performance limits can be considered reliable or not, it is beyond doubt that elite athletes will continue to break current records. This is because almost all athletes carry some level of both acute and chronic stress in their musculoskeletal systems as the effect of strenuous and often excessive long-term training. Younger athletes such as Michael Phelps can adjust and adapt to this stress, whereas older athletes are progressively less able to tolerate it and increasingly experience handicapped performance as a result of physical deficiency, soft tissue dysfunction, and chronic pain in their musculoskeletal system. ISDN can reduce this acute and chronic stress, and by improving and restoring the homeostasis of human movement, it can help athletes break through their current physical barriers to achieve better results, while prolonging their athletic careers for many years to come.

Many sports injuries are caused by repetitive overuse, which leads to soft tissue dysfunction and bone injuries such as stress fractures and bone spurs. The Chinese hurdler Liu Xiang was unable to compete in the Beijing Olympics because he injured his Achilles tendon right before the event. The world-famous Chinese basketball player, Yao Ming, suffered a stress fracture in his foot 8 months before the Beijing Games. The likelihood of such injuries can be greatly reduced if chronic and acute stress in the musculoskeletal systems are effectively managed.

ISDN AS AN EFFECTIVE TOOL IN CONVENTIONAL SPORTS MEDICINE

In addition to enhancing athletic performance and preventing injuries, ISDN can also be used to rehabilitate injured athletes. The most common injuries in sports are soft tissue dysfunction such as contusions, muscle strain, ligament sprain, swelling, inflammation, and deficient microcirculation. During recovery and rehabilitation, adhesion and the formation of scar tissue are major concerns. ISDN is an effective modality for managing most of these soft tissue dysfunctions. It has been shown to provide faster and more specific recovery than any other known method.

ISDN, if properly used, does not conflict with conventional sports medicine. In cases in which surgery cannot be avoided, ISDN does not replace conventional medical procedures such as physical therapy or surgery. Surgery may be followed by pain, swelling, deficient microcirculation, inflammation, soft tissue tension, adhesion of soft tissues, and restricted range of motion of joints. These conditions hinder the self-healing process that must take place after surgery. ISDN, combined with other rehabilitation modalities such as physical therapy, is a powerful method for accelerating this healing.

ISDN VERSUS CLASSICAL CHINESE ACUPUNCTURE AND TRIGGER-POINT MEDICINE

Acupuncture is one of the oldest techniques of sports medicine. From its beginnings more than 2500 years ago, traditional Chinese acupuncture was an indispensable part of Chinese martial arts. All the martial arts masters were also masters of acupuncture, and they used acupuncture to treat injuries incurred in the practice of martial arts. Contemporary ISDN is not the same as traditional acupuncture. The cornerstone of Chinese acupuncture, which has guided clinical acupuncturists for at least 2500 years with remarkable efficacy, is the so-called *meridian theory:* the theory that energy flows through pathways, or meridians, in the body. Careful research has shown that the notion of meridians is in fact invented, though it is derived from a combination of physiologic and anatomic features of the nervous, cardiovascular, endocrine, and immune systems. Although ISDN originated in traditional Chinese methods, it has developed from the ancient empirical approach to become a modern medical art rooted in evidence-based thinking and practice.

ISDN combines the essence of many different disciplines: anatomy, physiology, physics, kinesiology, physical therapy, neuroscience, trigger-point technique, and clinical experience, in addition to reflecting the results of both basic research and specialized research in the field of sports medicine. It is different from trigger-point therapy in that it encompasses a systemic approach for restoring homeostasis in local tissues and in the entire musculoskeletal system, whereas trigger-point techniques focus primarily on the local pathologic processes in soft tissue.

Traditional Chinese acupuncture was the major medical modality at the time of its ancient beginnings, and since then it has been gradually replaced in Chinese societies by herbal medicine, although it has persisted as a minor modality. Modern Chinese acupuncture is now quite different from what it was originally, just as modern needles are different from those that were used in the past. The human body and its diseases today are different from those of as little as 200 years ago: life expectancy is longer, and the spectrum of diseases is different. In the 1940s, the American medical doctor Janet Travell developed trigger-point medicine without any knowledge of Chinese acupuncture. She was intrigued to observe later that many of her discoveries about trigger points were already put into practice in Chinese acupuncture.

After practicing needling therapy since the 1970s, I now face new challenges with my athlete patients, both professionals and nonprofessionals. Nonathletes, for example, seek medical attention primarily for pain relief, but athletes, in addition to seeking pain relief, expect medical professionals to restore their physical function and performance capability. Since the early 2000s, this need has excited and motivated me to work with athletes and develop needling techniques for sports medicine. I extend my sincere gratitude to all the athletes and coaches with whom I have worked.

References

1. Simons DG, Travell JG: *Travell & Simon's myofascial pain and dysfunction: the trigger point manual*, ed 2, Baltimore, 1999, Lippincott Williams & Wilkins.
2. Chan Gunn C: *Gunn approach to the treatment of chronic pain: intramuscular stimulation for myofascial pain or radiculopathic origin*, ed 2, Edinburgh, 1996, Churchill Livingstone.

CHAPTER 2

Homeostasis and Stress in Sports and Exercise

Integrative systemic dry needling (ISDN), also known as *dry needling acupuncture*, is a nonspecific therapy for restoring and maintaining homeostasis by reducing physical stress. When exercise is performed under conditions of optimal homeostasis, it leads to health and the best possible sports performance. When exercise is performed under stress, it results in the deterioration of bodily function, which leads to illness and disability. Millions of people of all ages actively participate in physical exercise or some kind of sports, from simple running or cycling to more technical or skill-intensive activities.

People get involved in sports for many reasons, but all who do so are seeking to benefit from them. Proper exercise promotes health, which is desired by everyone, and a healthy body produces the best performance in sport. Properly performed sporting activities reduce physiologic and psychologic stress and promote homeostasis: that is, the optimal function of the biologic systems. Badly performed sporting activities increase bodily stress and may promote the premature decline of biologic systems. For both professional and nonprofessional athletes, understanding how to manage stress for the benefit of overall health is of basic importance, especially for those who want to achieve better sports performance.

This chapter focuses on the concepts of stress and homeostasis. In conventional biomedical practice, homeostasis is seen as a physiologic process studied more in physiology laboratories than by clinicians.

Athletes differ from nonathletic patients in that most athletes generally maintain a better level of homeostasis than other people. Sports injuries among athletes are usually musculoskeletal, whereas nonathletes may have more complex pathologic problems. Therefore treatment differs between the two groups. In dealing with athletes, an understanding of the homeostasis of biologic systems is essential.

HOMEOSTASIS IN SPORTS AND EXERCISE

Walter Cannon (1871–1945), the first professor of physiology at Harvard University, investigated the specific mechanisms whereby the human body responds to changes in the external environment while maintaining optimal function. He began with an idea of the French physiologist Claude Bernard (1813–1878): that people exist in an internalized fluid environment and have evolved mechanisms to ensure the optimal physiologic activity of cells and organs by keeping this environment constant. Cannon used the term *homeostasis* for this process of maintaining internal stability in a changing external environment. The human body, as a biologic system, is organized to respond psychologically and physically to constantly changing external conditions. It can tolerate only a narrow range of environmental conditions. Within the limits of its physiology, the body activates self-regulation mechanisms to maintain homeostasis, including self-repair mechanisms when damage occurs and compensatory mechanisms when self-repair cannot be achieved. Compensatory mechanisms ensure the continuation of body function for survival at the expense of homeostasis. These mechanisms provide a biologic response to the changing environment for the survival of the system. Sufficiently severe environmental conditions result in partial destruction of the orderly working of the body or in death, the complete cessation of systems-level function.

Homeostasis is critical to athletic performance. Homeostasis in sport and exercise—which is different from homeostasis in daily life—is called *sport homeostasis*. It implies the balanced mechanical function of the musculoskeletal system in addition to the traditional homeostatic condition of other physiologic systems, such as the cardiovascular or endocrine system. Human beings can experience optimal movement only when the musculoskeletal system maintains balance in both its mechanical and physiologic aspects. With optimal biomechanical homeostasis, body movement is at its best because all the muscles and joints are in harmonious coordination without the expense of compensatory mechanisms. For example, sports medicine research has demonstrated that lower back pain causes weakness of the core muscle, which results in slower movement of the hips and lower limbs. Athletes with lower back pain run more slowly and consume more energy with every motion. When the musculoskeletal system is functioning with this kind of reduced efficiency, athletes have reduced reaction time; they fatigue easily and are more vulnerable to injury; psychologic depression may be present and precompetition anxiety may be worse; and postexercise recovery may be delayed.

Therefore it should be understood that homeostasis of musculoskeletal mechanics is a part of physiologic homeostasis, which includes cardiovascular, respiratory, and metabolic physiology, and all these aspects are regulated by the same part of the brain: the hypothalamus.

STRESS IN SPORTS AND EXERCISE

Psychologists have conceptualized stress in three ways:

1. Stress is viewed as a stimulus if the person perceives events or circumstances as threatening or harmful (*stressors*).
2. Stress is a response to environmental challenges, if the person examines the physical and psychologic stress that stressors produce.
3. Stress is a process that involves continuous interactions and adjustments between the person and the environment.

On the basis of these concepts, *stress* can be defined as the condition that results when person-environment transactions lead to a perceived discrepancy between the demands of the situation and the resources of the person's biologic, psychologic, and social system.[1]

This definition may suggest that stress in sports and exercise should be understood as a condition that is challenging, threatening, or even harmful to the body. With perfect body condition, finishing a marathon is rewarding. With tight hamstring muscles, the same marathon is stressful. The tight muscles may be the consequence of excessive repetitive use, or overtraining, and now they also become stressors. If an athlete with tight hamstring muscles believes that a coming marathon will be a tough challenge, he or she may be comparing it with a previous easily accomplished marathon, understanding that his or her current training was handicapped or not completed because of tight hamstring muscles. If the athlete continues to feel the tight muscles, his or her thinking may evolve into anxiety and fear, which lead to psychologic stress, which in turn can cause homeostatic imbalance of the musculoskeletal, cardiovascular, respiratory, and digestive systems. Together, these imbalances manifest as precompetition anxiety. The physical demands on the working muscles send signals to the brain, a bottom-up pattern of stress activation. The athlete's thinking, which includes the memory of past experience, creates tension in the body, a top-down pattern of stress activation. These are examples of interaction between psychologic and physical stresses.

Physical training involves repeating a set of exercises with increasing intensity over an extended period. Selye[2] noticed that exposure to a particular stressor can increase the body's ability to cope with that stressor in the future through a process of physiologic adaptation. The increase in ability and performance with training shows how the body adapts to the required effort. Selye also recognized that severe and extended exposure to any stressor could ultimately exceed the ability of the system to cope. Runners who habitually train more than 45 miles a week at moderate to high intensity are known to have chronically elevated cortisol levels and negative mood states.[3] Full recovery from overtraining stress may take months of abstinence from the particular exercise.

OVERTRAINING STRESS

When the body can no longer tolerate any additional training stress, it will activate self-protective mechanisms to produce a condition of overtraining, which sport physiologists refer to as *overtraining syndrome*. This condition is highly individual, subjective, and identifiable only after the athlete's performance and physiologic function have suffered. The first sign of overtraining syndrome is a decline in physical performance with continued training. The athlete feels fatigued, with a loss of muscular strength, coordination, and working capacity. Other primary signs and symptoms are related to the autonomic nervous, cardiovascular, endocrine, and digestive systems, as well as to psychologic conditions. These conditions and their treatment are discussed in later chapters.

HOMEOSTATIC REGULATION IN SPORTS AND EXERCISE

Homeostatic regulation of the musculoskeletal system, in addition to other physiologic homeostatic regulation, is an important positive process of bodily adjustment in athletes. For example, research in evidence-based sports medicine has demonstrated that weakness of core muscles hinders movement of the limbs.[4] Through an understanding of homeostasis, it is clear how the musculoskeletal system is regulated during and after sports and exercise. Homeostasis is regulated by five physiologic layers[5]:

1. Organs and their local reflexes: Organs can regulate their own functions with built-in reflexes that do not need any higher level of control to function effectively. For example, local stress, such as tight muscles, can be reduced by local stimulation, such as stretching, massage, and dry needling through the local reflex mechanisms.

2. Autonomic and endocrine messengers: The autonomic nervous system and the endocrine system form two channels of communication from the central nervous system (CNS) to individual organs. Poor microcirculation, or local ischemia, is a major physiologic deficiency in overused muscles. Stimulation by needling balances the autonomic system to improve microcirculation and promote recovery from ischemia. This process also involves neuroendocrine messengers and their receptors in capillaries.

3. Brainstem regulation: The brainstem regulates autonomic outputs to the organs through a complex network of reflex centers. For example, during exercise the working muscles and the respiratory system initiate the signals that ascend to the brainstem and higher brain centers, which produce pronounced cardiovascular and endocrine responses to the physical demand.

4. Hypothalamic integration: The hypothalamus regulates endocrine messengers to the body, the autonomic output from the brainstem, and the movement of the musculoskeletal system to maintain homeostasis in response to physiologic challenges.

5. Inputs from higher brain centers: Brain areas above the hypothalamus use information received from the external world to form memory, emotion, and awareness. These higher processes can then alter the activities of the hypothalamus and brainstem. Before or during a sports event, an athlete may compare the present situation with memories of earlier similar situations and may assess the current experience as challenging or stimulating; on the other hand, the athlete may feel that the stress is undesirable or unmanageable. This positive or negative emotional reaction will influence the output from the hypothalamus and brainstem and, subsequently, the operation of the musculoskeletal system (Fig. 2-1).

Figure 2-1 shows the hierarchical or layered regulation of homeostasis. As depicted at the bottom of the figure, the individual organs, such as muscles, have intrinsic reflexive control mechanisms that allow them to operate by themselves when external conditions are constant. This local regulation is performed by the local reflex loop, which comprises the organs, the ganglia of the autonomic nervous system, and the spinal cord. These simple reflexes are sufficient for responding to strictly local needs. When local reflexive regulation is insufficient to meet rapid changes in demand or when the separate organs need to coordinate their function, as in sports activities, two parallel systems of communication—the autonomic nervous system and the endocrine system—are activated. These two systems are regulated by the brainstem and the hypothalamus.

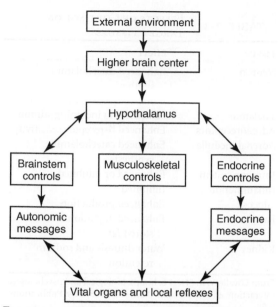

FIGURE 2-1 Schematic of homeostatic regulation over local organs. The local organs have self-regulating capacity. This self-regulation is determined by internal reflexes and actions of autonomic ganglia located in or near the organs. Local regulation is modulated in turn by descending influences from the autonomic nervous system, the brainstem, the hypothalamus, and higher centers in the central nervous system.

The hypothalamus coordinates the actions of the autonomic system and the endocrine system, and it has motor nuclei that store specific programs of survival-related behaviors. The autonomic nervous system and the endocrine system can initiate complex coordination among different organs and systems to meet changes in, or demands from, the external environment. When additional demands emerge as a result of the conscious processing of external information in the higher brain levels, as when the athlete starts to experience stressful thoughts during competition, the centers of the higher brain contribute to the shaping of inputs from the lower systems and outputs from the brain. For example, if pain or injury occurs during competition, the brain may modify the signals from the local organs, and the athlete will compare the current state with memories of previous experience to make decisions and develop coping strategies. These higher brain centers include the limbic system and the cerebral cortex.

This hierarchical regulation allows local processes to proceed on their own, leaving the human brain's finite resources for conscious processing free to manage new tasks. If more systemic coordination is needed to meet new challenges, as during intense competition, then maximal capacity of the cardiovascular system is required. In this case, endocrine and integrated autonomic regulation starts to work.

Each vital organ or organ system is capable of regulating its own function in response to slowly changing demands. If a muscle or a group of muscles is used repeatedly during a physical event, it will start to adjust. Muscles increase their metabolism, circulation, and mass in response to the physical demand. However, if the demand on the muscles exceeds what they are able to sustain, they will activate their self-protective mechanisms to resist any further stress: they become tight and inflamed, and the local reflex is inhibited. At this point, if the stressful demand is reduced or stopped, the muscles undergo a slow self-recovery process. Physical stress (e.g., tightness in soft tissue) or physiologic stress (e.g., inflammation and deficient microcirculation) suppresses self-recovery and inhibits both the reflex and feedback mechanisms that are necessary to restore homeostasis. Dry needling activates the reflex mechanisms to reduce both physical and physiologic stresses without disturbing or damaging the injured muscles, whereas stretching or massage may cause further injury.

The brainstem and hypothalamus receive information about the state of organs such as muscles, joints, and viscera, and they restore homeostatic physiology by sending back commands to the same organs by way of the autonomic nervous system and endocrine messages. Although they play different roles, all the autonomic, endocrine, and musculoskeletal systems are involved in the functioning of the motor system.

The skeletal motor system is a conscious and voluntary system. It has sensory nerves that give the brain information about the position and motion of the limbs. These nerves project to sensory areas of the cerebral cortex, and these cortical sensory projections allow people to be aware of the position and function of their muscles and joints.

The sensory and motor nerves are located directly in the cerebral cortex. The motor nerves run from the motor area of the cerebral cortex directly to individual muscle fiber bundles to command their movements, which enables people to be conscious of the position of their limbs and to have voluntary control of their movements. Each motor nerve fiber connects to a single muscle bundle to enable precise control of the target muscle.

The autonomic nervous system also has sensory and motor nerves. However, its sensory nerves ascend to the brainstem, not to the level of the cerebral cortex, and its motor nerves originate in the brainstem. As a result, humans have limited awareness of the state of their vital organs and, consequently, very little control over them. The autonomic nerve fibers reaching a target organ or tissue are highly branched, and the smooth muscle cells themselves are highly interconnected. This results in more widespread response on the part of the effectors.

The endocrine response to stress has two parallel pathways: the adrenocortical response, controlled by the hypothalamus and pituitary gland, and the adrenomedullary response, controlled by the sympathetic nervous system. During stress, the adrenal medulla secretes epinephrine and norepinephrine. This process is activated by sympathetic preganglionic fibers originating in nucleus of the solitary tract of the brainstem, influenced by messages from the paraventricular nucleus of the hypothalamus. Epinephrine, an endocrine messenger, acts on β-adrenoreceptors existing in many tissues and organs. It reinforces the activities of sympathetic nerves. Norepinephrine's role as a stress hormone is small.

The second major stress hormone is cortisol. Unlike epinephrine, cortisol plays a role in both normal physiologic activity and during periods of stress. Cortisol is needed for normal autonomic function and therefore for all forms of physiologic regulation at cellular level, as well as for metabolism. Some of the effects of cortisol on target tissues are listed in Table 2-1.

Without the tonic influence of cortisol, the action of the autonomic nervous system would be greatly diminished, and epinephrine would be less

TABLE 2-1	EFFECTS OF CORTISOL ON TARGET TISSUES
Tissue	**Effect**
Neuron	Enhanced catecholamine synthesis
Hippocampus	Enhanced memory function
Thalamus	Sensitivity to incoming stimuli
Adrenoreceptors	Enhanced β-receptor sensitivity
Adrenal medulla	Enhanced catecholamine synthesis
Immune system	Enhanced or inhibited
Inflammation	Inhibited
Glucose	Enhanced production
Fatty acid	Enhanced liberation from stored fat
Kidney	Water diuresis and sodium retention

From Lovallo WR: Stress & health: biological and psychological interaction, ed 2, Thousand Oaks, CA, 2005, Sage Publications, p 58.

effective at its target tissues. In addition to influencing normal tissue physiology, cortisol also participates in the stress response. During stress, cortisol potentiates the activity of the sympathetic nervous system to increase the release of stored glucose and fats. It performs the regulatory function of controlling stress so that an acute stress response will not threaten homeostasis. This important regulatory function is seen in experimental animals, which die as a result of poor regulation of the stress response if their adrenal glands are removed.

Cortisol and epinephrine reach all tissues via systemic circulation, and they work together to significantly alter the background environment in which all the tissues can function normally and to coordinate activity and responses across many tissues. Sports activity is an example of how coordinated activity of the musculoskeletal system is regulated by cortisol and epinephrine. Norepinephrine plays a less significant role in homeostatic regulation.

A third stress hormone is β-endorphin. In response to corticotropin-releasing factor (CRF) from the hypothalamus, the pituitary produces both β-endorphin and adrenocorticotropin hormone (ACTH). β-endorphin is an agonist of opiate receptors in the nervous system, producing analgesia and performing other physiologic roles such as balancing cardiovascular function. Supposedly β-endorphin functions as a physiologic and psychologic analgesic.

CENTRAL NERVOUS SYSTEM INTEGRATION OF THE STRESS RESPONSE IN SPORTS AND REHABILITATION

Mentality can influence emotions and cause psychologic stress and stress responses. Positive and negative emotions do not occur in isolation; they are part of particular patterns of brain activity, leading to distinct physiologic responses and behavioral reactions. These responses and reactions have a significant effect on the process of adjusting to stress during both sports activities and rehabilitation from injury.

Appraisal Model of Psychologic Stress

The appraisal model of psychologic stress[6] is illustrated in Figure 2-2. When people encounter an environmental stressor such as competition in sports, or illness or injury, they first test the situation for threat: Is the stressor a threat or a challenge, or is it irrelevant? This evaluation is based on beliefs, past experience, and commitment. Events are appraised as threatening if they violate beliefs, contradict experience, or reduce the ability to carry out a commitment. An ankle sprain is a minor inconvenience to a vacationer and may be ignored, but it can be a severe stressor to an Olympic athlete because of the athlete's commitment to the competition. To reduce or remove the threat, the athlete must adapt with new behavior and evaluate what resources are available to cope with it. An optimistic person interprets such an event as a challenge and will try his or her best to recover from the injury.

Such positive emotions, combined with problem-focused strategy, will occupy the athlete and produce a commitment to therapy and training. The athlete's life may be more stressful because of the need for therapeutic activity and behavioral adaptation, but he or she feels hopeful and in control of the situation. A pessimistic person

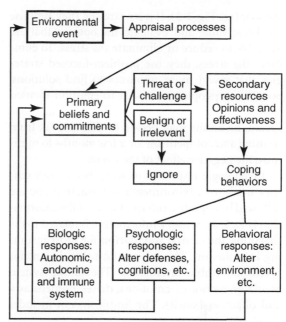

FIGURE 2-2 Appraisal model of psychologic stress. This model suggests that the primary appraisals of the threat value of an event and secondary appraisals of the effectiveness of available coping strategies have an effect on physiologic response to the event.

may see the stressor as a huge threat and may have no confidence in being able to manage the situation. Negative emotion makes life stressful, with uncertainty and anxiety. Both positive and negative responses to the event are stressful but generate different kinds of physiologic adjustment and different outcomes in reality. The athlete with positive emotion will benefit by reducing the stress and by feeling more energetic, whereas the one with negative emotion will feel more stressed and exhausted.

The example of the injured athlete shows that problem-focused strategies may be costly in terms of energy and time during the period of the stressful event, but they can lessen the intensity of the stress. Pessimistic strategies initially consume fewer resources but can be more costly in the long term because of a continuing drain of coping resources.

When people encounter any change in their environment, they compare it with memories of previous experiences to evaluate whether the change is a stressor (see Fig. 2-2). If it is a stressor, they appraise its threat value and evaluate the options that are available to reduce or eliminate the stress. To eliminate the stress, they use problem-focused strategies that invest more resources to find solutions. Sometimes people may resort to emotion-focused strategies. For example, if an athlete has an ankle sprain, he or she may decide to take a break from training and competition for a few months to minimize the negative effect of the event.

Psychologic responses to stress begin with sensory intake of environmental information and are followed by cognitive interpretation of the information (Fig. 2-3). Sensory information is relayed to the thalamus, the central way station for most incoming information. The information then is sent for prefrontal-limbic interaction. The limbic system regulates memories, emotions, drives, homeostasis, and olfaction (smell). The limbic system includes

diverse cortical and subcortical structures located mainly in the medial and ventral region of the cerebral hemispheres (Box 2-1 and Fig. 2-4).

The prefrontal-limbic interaction after information intake enables people to understand the nature, meaning, and importance of the event and to evaluate the available coping resources and the emotional characteristics of coping strategies. The thalamus also receives visceral signals and relays them to the amygdala. Furthermore, the prefrontal-limbic interaction provides the hypothalamus with the results of the appraisals and their associated emotion, which leads to changes in peripheral physiologic status. The hypothalamus combines input from the amygdala and the prefrontal cortex. The output of the hypothalamus and its engagement with the brainstem account for autonomic, endocrine, and musculoskeletal reactions to the challenge of stress.

The amygdala is responsible for forming memories of the emotional connotations of these events. The outputs of the hypothalamus activate physiologic responses to the appraised stress.

Two functional subsystems are incorporated in the brainstem pons and medulla (Fig. 2-5). The first is the central feedback loop subsystem, which serves to regulate the functional state of the entire central nervous system, causing it to switch focus to meet behavioral emergencies or to become quiescent when appropriate. This subsystem, consisting of

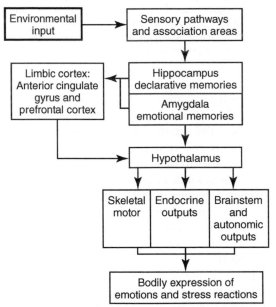

FIGURE 2-3 A simplified neurophysiologically based model of the primary process that activates autonomic, endocrine, and motor responses to psychologic stress. The hippocampus is essential for recognizing familiar events and facts (declarative memories). The amygdala is responsible for forming memories of these emotional connotations of these events. The outputs of the hypothalamus activate physiologic responses to the appraised stress.

BOX 2-1	SOME COMPONENTS OF THE LIMBIC SYSTEM

Limbic cortex
Parahippocampal gyrus
Cingulate gyrus
Medial orbitofrontal cortex
Temporal pole
Anterior insula
Hippocampal formation
Dental gyrus
Hippocampus
Amygdala
Hypothalamus
Thalamus
Basal ganglia

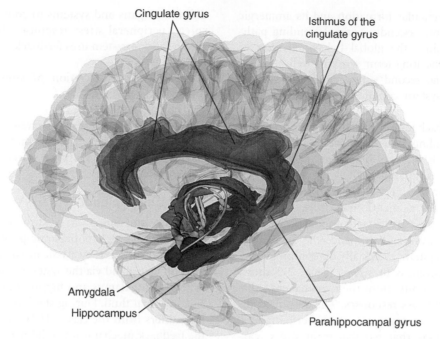

FIGURE 2-4 The limbic system forms a functional bridge between the cerebral cortex and the input and output structures of the nervous system. It is the basis of autonomic, endocrine, and behavioral responses to homeostatic challenges and events, with implications for survival and reproduction. It also helps that the memories of these events are stored and retrieved.

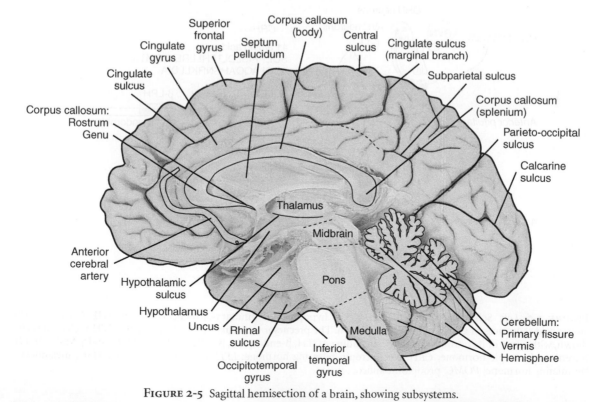

FIGURE 2-5 Sagittal hemisection of a brain, showing subsystems.

the pontine reticular formation and its aminergic nuclei and both ascending and descending pathways, determines the global behavioral state of the person: the long-term sense of well-being or dysphoria. The second subsystem, the brainstem response subsystem, contains the descending pathways that reach muscles and viscera. This subsystem also has feedback loops to and from the viscera and muscles, enabling reflex control over autonomic responses. This is a very important mechanism in dry needling stimulation.

Cortisol and epinephrine are the two primary stress hormones, as mentioned earlier. They act in concert with the peripheral components of acute response to stress and influence the entire central nervous system, eventually determining long-term responsiveness to stress. Figure 2-3 shows three sets of outputs from the hypothalamus that adjust bodily stress responses. The output to the endocrine system engages control over peripheral gland secretions that participate in stress reaction. Cortisol and epinephrine act in concert upon different organs and systems to coordinate widespread peripheral stress response. During stress, the endocrine system uses feedback to regulate the following:

- The short-term secretion of stress hormones themselves
- Gene expression in frontal-limbic areas that modulate long-term stress responsiveness
- The shaping of memories for emotionally significant events, which will then affect the appraisal process in the future[5]

Stress and the Endocrine System

In nonstressful conditions, cortisol secretion is regulated within the hypothalamic-pituitary-adrenocortical (HPAC) axis by classic negative feedback to the pituitary gland via the systemic circulation and to the hypothalamus and hippocampus by way of cerebrospinal fluid. During states of stress, regulation differs from the classic HPAC pattern in that the feedback mechanism is inhibited and the feedforward processes are enhanced (Fig. 2-6).

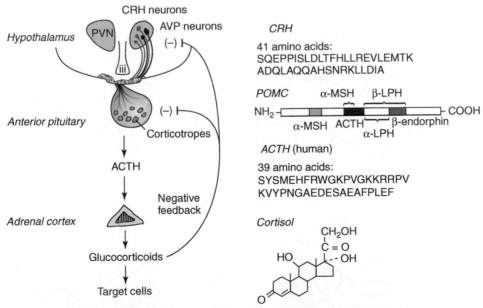

FIGURE 2-6 *Left,* Schematic representation of the hypothalamic-pituitary-adrenocortical axis (HPAC). *Right,* The amino acid sequences of CRH and ACTH are shown. The precursor molecular form from which ACTH is cleaved is also shown, with many of its hormone products, including ACTH, β-endorphin, β-LPH, γ-LPH, α-MSH, and γ-MSH. *ACTH,* Adrenocorticotropic hormone; *CRH,* corticotropin-releasing hormone; *LPH,* lipotropic hormone; *MSH,* melanocyte-stimulating hormone; *POMC:* proopiomelanocortin.

A central feedback subsystem, the corticotropin-releasing factor (CRF) system, contains specialized neurons that synthesize CRF and act together to integrate the CNS's response to stress. CRF, functioning also as a peptide transmitter, integrates sensory information from the cortex with emotional states and behaviors that are regulated by the amygdala and hippocampus to shape autonomic, hormonal, and behavioral responses to the stress. Some features of the central CRF system are summarized in Figure 2-7. The central CRF system binds the functions of the cortex, hypothalamus, and brainstem to integrate the outflow to the peripheral organs.

Cortisol acts upon two types of receptors: mineralocorticoid (type I) and glucocorticoid (type II). Type I receptors respond to low levels of cortisol, whereas type II receptors respond to high levels. During periods of stress, cortisol secretion increases and activates type II receptors. Insufficient cortisol secretion causes alterations in sensory thresholds and impairments in learning and memory ability. Excessive cortisol secretion is related to severe depression and to cognitive and mood disturbances. Repeatedly elevated or prolonged high levels of cortisol sensitize the amygdala and increase the CRF-gene expression. As a result, high levels of stress increase stress reactivity with far-reaching physiologic consequences. Gastrointestinal disorder is one of the consequences of amygdala sensitization, as is irritable bowel syndrome.[7]

Prolonged or repeated exposure to severe, life-threatening stress is followed, in some cases, by posttraumatic stress disorder (PTSD). Affected people may manifest psychologic distress, sleep disturbance, enhanced startle reactions, and alcohol or drug abuse. The research suggests that after prolonged and high levels of cortisol exposure at the amygdala, the central CRF system is sensitized and causes PTSD symptoms.[8] The central sensitization of the CRF system would have the effect of shifting the balance from a negative feedback process to a permanent feedforward process, which would result in a more reactive HPAC axis, accompanied by frontal-limbic alterations associated with anxiety. Patients with PTSD show reduced hippocampus volumes.[9] The hippocampus is the only area in the CNS that is known to spontaneously produce new nerve cells throughout life. High levels of cortisol exposure inhibit the growth of new cells and make existing cells more vulnerable to cell death.[10]

Another stress hormone, epinephrine, is regulated by the hypothalamic-sympathetic-adrenomedullary (HSAM) axis. During periods of stress, the hypothalamus and the brainstem send activating signals via sympathetic nerve fibers to the adrenal medulla, where the cells release stored epinephrine into circulation. The circulating epinephrine activates a stress response by increasing cardiac output and respiration rate, dilating peripheral blood vessels, releasing fuel from adipose tissue and the liver, and enhancing skeletal muscle contraction. The secretion of epinephrine and that of cortisol are

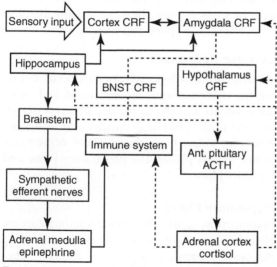

FIGURE 2-7 An oversimplified model of corticotropin-release factor (CRF) system. *Open lines* Part of the model indicates the classic feedback pathways of cortisol regulation in hypothalamus-pituitary-adrenocortical (HPAC) axis. CRF neurons found in different areas of the central nervous system and their communication with other parts of the central nervous system (CNS) manifest their extensive function during response to stress, regulating autonomic nervous system, endocrine system, and stress-related posture and locomotion. Cortisol acts on all cell types in the CNS and peripheral tissues, including the immune system. *ACTH,* Adrenocorticotropic hormone; *BNST,* bed nuclei of the stria terminalis.

linked together. The central CRF system activates both HPAC and HSAM pathways. Simultaneously, the pituitary secretion of ACTH results in cortisol secretion from the adrenal cortex via the HPAC axis and adrenal medullary secretion of epinephrine, which is activated by autonomic signals, via the HSAM axis. Both hormones work in concert to initiate and maintain stress responses and to establish memories of stress events. During stressful experiences, cortisol acts on the amygdala and hippocampus to consolidate the formation of declarative memories (the factual memory of events). These two stress hormones have different regulatory strategies. Cortisol is directed by negative feedback or positive feedforward processes between peripheral circulation and the brain neurons. Epinephrine, which does not pass the blood-brain barrier, is regulated by autonomic reflexes that are under the control of the hypothalamus, acted upon by cortisol.

Under the influence of long-term stress, the combination of sensitization of the amygdala and loss of hippocampus volume can permanently alter not only the cognitive process but also homeostasis, affecting energy balance and adaptive behavior, which results in health problems.

The brain organizes physiologic responses to meet homeostatic demands during stress. Homeostasis is regulated at different levels during stress responses. The cortex and limbic system exert the highest control over the entire system through cognitive processes to alter behavior with the goal of maintaining homeostasis. To reduce emotional agitation, coping behavior can be problem focused or emotion focused. The hypothalamus is responsible for the integration of most autonomic, endocrine, and motor system adaptations, according to commands from the cortex-limbic interaction. Departure from homeostasis can be regulated by reflex organization at the hypothalamic level. The brainstem receives signals from higher levels and also feeds back signals to higher and lower levels to coordinate the responses. At the lowest level, local organs use intrinsic reflex mechanisms to adjust local physiologic processes. If the stressors last too long, the entire system will adjust to the stress at the expense of homeostasis, resulting in both health problems and a decline in physical and psychologic performance.

Sports and Exercise as Physical and Psychologic Stress

Exercise is typical of the processes in which humans acquire the physical and physiologic ability to cope with physical stressors by repeated exposure to them. It is how people store physical ability and skill in conscious memory and transfer them into subconscious memory. For example, a person may initially practice a skill under the guidance of a coach. After the actions are repeated many times, an activity that was once difficult becomes a subconscious reflex through the wiring of the person's brain, which sends commands to his or her musculoskeletal motor system.

Two types of stress have been discussed: physiologic or physical stress and psychologic stress. Stress can start in the body and move to the mind, in a bottom-up way, or it may originate in the mind as ideas, anxiety, and fears. This pure psychologic stress is a top-down type. In daily life these two patterns of stress are not always distinguishable, and this is also true in sports and exercise.

Exercise Responses

Substantial physiologic adjustments occur during exercise in the nervous, cardiovascular, and endocrine systems in order to provide maximal oxygen and fuel to the exercising muscles and to remove metabolic toxins from them. These adjustments consist of two phases: the preparatory phase and the active phase.

Preparatory Phase

In competitive sports, thoughts about the future are often a source of psychologic stress. Such thinking can cause dramatic changes in physiologic functions before the start of any exercise that involves strenuous muscular activity and significant mental activity. The commands from the cortex activate hypothalamic and brainstem functions that regulate autonomic and endocrine outflow, as discussed previously.[11] Physiologists noticed that when trained runners were preparing to start a race, their resting heart rates doubled as the starter called out the starting commands.[12] The rise in heart rate was highest in sprinters starting a 60-yard dash (from 67 to 148 beats per minute).[13] The rise was less dramatic in those starting a 220-yard race (from 67 to 130) and even less in middle-distance runners starting an 880-yard run (from 62 to 122).

This preparatory phase obviously involves a top-down process. The anticipation of a planned, intentional activity causes the prefrontal cortex to activate the hypothalamus and the brainstem nuclei that are associated with sympathetic activation and suppression of parasympathetic activity; this results in increases in heart rate, cardiac output, sympathetic outflow to the blood vessels, and epinephrine secretion. The prefrontal cortical activity also regulates the motor cortex, the premotor cortex, and the supplementary motor cortex. All these centrally generated top-down outflows cause dilation of some muscle vascular beds, increase in muscle tone, and a rise in systolic pressure.

Active Phase

When the actual exercise starts, peripheral physiologic processes begin to exert more influence on the stress response. Feedback from the muscular activity to the brain centers, as well as local metabolic increase, further enhance the sympathetic outflow to the heart and blood vessels, which results in increased cardiac output and a redistribution of blood flow. This in turn provides the exercising muscles with significant increases of oxygen and nutrients. Meanwhile blood flow to uninvolved muscles, such as internal organs, decreases. A trained runner, with all these adjustments taking place, may maintain a level of effort equivalent to 85% of maximum for periods of 3 to 5 hours. Highly trained athletes may maintain sustained heart rates of 180 beats per minute, in comparison with their resting heart rates of 35 to 40.

The increase in sympathetic outflow causes more epinephrine secretion by the adrenal medulla. Epinephrine increases cardiac contractility and dilation of blood vessels in exercising muscles. In addition, epinephrine increases the liberation of free fatty acids from stored fat; the fatty acids circulate to the exercising muscles as fuel for increasing energy demand. The consumption of glucose by the exercising muscles results in a drop in blood glucose levels, which activates the hypothalamus and pituitary gland to increase the release of ACTH; this in turn leads to more secretion of cortisol by

the cortex of the adrenal gland, which liberates stored glucose in the liver and fat from adipose tissue. β-Endorphin is secreted by the pituitary gland along with ACTH. β-Endorphin is known as an *opiate analogue* and associated with analgesic physiologic processes. This analogue is thought to modulate discomfort during physical exercise.

Exercise Can Be a Positive or Negative Stressor

Sport and exercise are physically stressful to the body, and stress is usually regarded as undesirable. However, medical experts agree that well-managed exercise is beneficial for health and mood enhancement. People enjoy sports and exercise because they are different from negative events encountered at other times. People like this kind of activity because it produces a positive mood, and they experience benefits and satisfaction from it. In most cases, the body is capable of handling the substantial adjustments that are required by the demands of strenuous exercise.

The effect of a stressor depends on how it is interpreted; that is, whether the person perceives positive or negative consequences. A positive interpretation creates positive emotion, motivation, and mood, which result in positive adjustments of peripheral responses such as musculoskeletal locomotion. Negative thoughts about the situation lead to negative emotions and unwelcome consequences, such as an imbalance of the musculoskeletal system as a result of tight muscles. The emotional demands of competition, the desire to win, the fear of failure, and unrealistically high expectations can all be the source of psychologic stress.

With negative emotion, the musculoskeletal system is less balanced. If an event is interpreted as a negative stressor, more of the stress hormone cortisol is produced as a response. Higher levels and longer secretion of cortisol can change brain wiring, hamper physical performance, and harm health.

OVERTRAINING SYNDROME

During periods of intense training, athletes can experience unexplained levels of fatigue, as well as a decline in performance and physiologic function that cannot be restored by a few days of reduced training, total rest, or a carbohydrate-rich diet. These symptoms are collectively referred as *overtraining syndrome,* and it can last for weeks, months, or even years.[13] When athletes are subjected to excessive training, they may eventually exceed their ability to cope with or adapt to the training stress. If the intensity is increased from session to session beyond the body's ability to adapt, and if full recovery is not allowed, the training becomes a source of long-term physical and psychologic stress. For example, runners who train more than 45 miles a week at moderate to high intensity are known to have chronically elevated cortisol levels and negative mood states.[14]

Overtraining syndrome is subjective and highly individualized, which makes it difficult for athletes and their coaches to identify it as the cause of a decline in physical performance and bodily function.

The primary signs and symptoms of the overtraining syndrome are as follows:
- General fatigue that does not respond to normal procedures
- Loss of motivation and lack of mental concentration
- Feelings of depression, anxiety, irritability, excitability, and restlessness, and sleep disturbance
- Lack of appreciation for things that are normally enjoyable
- Change in appetite and weight loss
- Loss of muscle strength and coordination

It has been noted that both overtraining syndrome and clinical depression involve similar symptoms, brain structures, neurotransmitters, endocrine pathways, and immune responses, which suggests that they have similar origins.[15]

Some experts in sports medicine distinguish two kinds of overtraining symptoms: "intensity related" and "volume related." Athletes in different sports may exhibit signs of overtraining that are related to their specific training regimens. In the following section, we discuss overtraining syndrome as it relates to the nervous, endocrine, and immune systems.

RESPONSES OF THE AUTONOMIC NERVOUS SYSTEM TO OVERTRAINING

The symptoms of overtraining definitely illustrate an imbalance between the sympathetic and parasympathetic branches of the autonomic nervous system. People who engage in "intensity-related" activities, such as sprinters, may exhibit sympathetically dominant symptoms:
- Increased blood pressure and resting heart rates
- Elevated basal metabolic rate
- Emotional instability and sleep disturbance
- Loss of appetite

The symptoms can be parasympathetically related in people who engage in endurance activities:
- Decreased resting blood pressure and resting heart rate
- Early onset of fatigue
- Rapid recovery of heart rate after exercise

Sympathetically related symptoms occur more frequently than parasympathetically related ones. However, similar symptoms can also be experienced by athletes who have not trained excessively; thus care should be taken in making a clinical diagnosis.

HORMONAL RESPONSES TO OVERTRAINING

A physiologic imbalance of endocrine function has been recognized in athletes suffering from overtraining. Overtrained athletes often have higher-than-normal concentrations of urea in the blood, which is produced by increased protein catabolism. This is thought to be the mechanism responsible for loss of body weight in overtrained athletes. However, there are no conclusive data to confirm that higher levels of cortisol or epinephrine are related to long periods of overtraining. Serotonin is a major neurotransmitter that is believed to play an important role in overtraining syndrome. However, the concentration of serotonin in plasma does not match its concentration in the brain. Cytokines also play a significant role, inasmuch as the presence of circulating cytokines have been associated with trauma related to overtrained muscles, joints, and bones, as well as with infection.

Cytokines appear as part of the body's inflammatory response to injuries and infection. It is believed that excessive musculoskeletal stress, coupled with insufficient rest and recovery, causes local acute inflammation, which eventually evolves into systemic chronic inflammation. Systemic chronic inflammation activates circulating monocytes to synthesize large quantities of cytokines. Cytokine-induced symptoms of sickness are very much consistent with symptoms of overtraining.

IMMUNE FUNCTION AND OVERTRAINING

Research has shown that excessive training suppresses normal immune function, rendering athletes more susceptible to infection and disease.[16] Studies show that short periods of overload training temporarily impair the immune function, and prolonged overtraining amplifies this suppression of immunity, with low quantities of lymphocytes and antibodies. Intense training during illness decreases the ability of athletes to fight off infection and increases the risk of subsequent complications.[15]

SUMMARY

Sports and exercise are sources of physiologic and psychologic stress. The stressors can be the activities themselves or related conditions such as overtraining syndrome, postexercise pain or fatigue, or related injuries and rehabilitation.

This chapter introduced two concepts that are fundamental in acupuncture for sports and exercise and trauma rehabilitation: homeostasis and stress. All the following chapters focus on treating stress-related syndromes in sport and exercise and achieving trauma rehabilitation by reducing stress and restoring homeostasis.

The aim of ISDN is to reduce systemic stress in order to improve, balance, and restore optimal homeostasis by activating the local and systemic reflexes that involve the nervous, endocrine, cardiovascular, and musculoskeletal systems. During this de-stressing process, biologic survival mechanisms are stimulated at all levels, from molecular to organismic, to repair stress-related trauma and to approach homeostasis.

ISDN is capable of regulating stress-affected posture and locomotion to activate the integrative function of the central nervous and endocrine systems to restore homeostasis, and this de-stressing process in turn improves the balance and quality of posture and locomotion.

References

1. Sarafino EP: *Health psychology, biopsychosocial interactions,* ed 5, New York, 2006, John Wiley & Sons, p 84.
2. Selye H: *The stress of life,* New York, 1956, McGraw-Hill.
3. Luger A, Deuster PA, Kyle SB, et al: Acute hypothalamic-pituitary-adrenal response to the stress of treadmill exercise, *N Engl J Med* 316:1309–1315, 1987.
4. Heidersheit B, Sherry M: What effect do core strength and stability have on injury prevention and recovery? In MacAuley D, Best T, editors: *Evidence-based sports medicine,* Malden, Mass, 2007, Blackwell, pp 59–72.
5. Lovallo WR: *Stress & health: biological and psychological interaction,* ed 2, Thousand Oaks, Calif, 2005, Sage Publications, pp 41.
6. Lazarus RS, Folkman J: *Stress, appraisal and coping,* New York, 1984, Springer.
7. Greenwood-Van Meerveld B, Gibson M, Gunter W, et al: Stereotaxic delivery of corticosterone to the amygdala modulates colonic sensitivity in rats, *Brain Res* 893:135–142, 2001.
8. Bremner JD, Randall P, Scott TM, et al: MRI-based measurement of hippocampal volume in patients with combat-related post-traumatic stress disorder, *Am J Psychiatry* 152:973–981, 1995.
9. Gilbertson MW, Shenton ME, Ciszewski A, et al: Smaller hippocampal volume predicts pathologic vulnerability to psychological trauma, *Nat Neurosci* 5:1242–1247, 2002.
10. Sapolsky RM: Why stress is bad for your brain, *Science* 273:749–750, 1996.
11. Hobbs S: Central command during exercise: parallel activation of the cardiovascular and motor systems by descending command signals. In Smity OA, Galosy RA, Weiss SM, editors: *Circulation, neurobiology and behavior,* New York, 1982, Elsevier, pp 217–231.
12. McArdle WD, Foglia GF, Patti AV: Telemetered cardiac response to selected running events, *J Appl Physiol* 23:566–570, 1967.
13. Wilmore JH, Costill DL, Kenney WL: *Physiology of sport and exercise,* ed 4, Champaign, IL, 2008, Human Kinetics, p 301.
14. Lueger A, Deuster PA, Kyle SB, et al: Acute hypothalamic-pituitary-adrenal responses to the stress of treadmill exercise, *N Engl J Med* 316:1309–1315, 1987.
15. Armstrong LE, VanHeerst JI: The unknown mechanism of the overtraining syndrome, *Sports Med* 32:185–209, 2002.
16. Nieman DC: Immune response to heavy exertion, *J Appl Physiol* 82:1385–1394, 1997.

CHAPTER 3

Human Brain Plasticity, Sports, and Sports Injuries

This chapter is a brief review of some basic brain-body interactions and neural processes that occur during physical exercise and training. Understanding this interaction is essential for designing training programs, preventing potential sports injuries, and assisting rehabilitation by using integrative medical procedures. The aim of this review is to understand why dry needling is used and how it can benefit athletes by reducing physiologic stress during the different phases of their sports activities. Specific examples are treated in more detail in later chapters.

Brain research has revealed that every sustained activity—physical activities, as well as learning, thinking, and imagining—changes the brain and the mind. Thus each person's brain is different from those of all humans before him or her. Each time a new skill is learned or a new ability developed, the anatomy and function of the brain is modified on a substantial scale. Massive changes are associated with modern cultural specializations, such as sporting and artistic activities. The understanding of brain-body interaction is derived mostly from research on the brains of musicians, but the process of athletic training is very similar to that of musical training. Athletes, like musicians, have unique brains that differ from those of nonathletes, because sports are a highly specialized exercise of both brain systems and physiologic systems. How the brain is understood ultimately affects how human nature and human movement is understood as well. Sports are a typical two-way mind-body interaction. The processes of sports are motivated by mental processes. Training and exercise involve repetitive learning and memory storage. Sports performance is regulated by the brain systems both consciously and subconsciously. If injury occurs, the body will send feedback to the brain, which changes the behavior of the athlete for the purpose of both adaptation and survival. An understanding how the brain systems

regulate sports performance helps improve sports training, enhances physical performance, prevents potential injury, and accelerates rehabilitation from injury or surgery.

All the topics in this chapter deal with neuroscience and systemic physiology. Common important concepts can be found in relevant textbooks. This chapter focuses on knowledge that is clinically related to the integrative systemic dry needling (ISDN) therapy, and readers who are interested in basic concepts of neurophysiology may refer to Doidge.[1]

THE BRAIN AND PHYSICAL TRAINING

Modern sports are unique human activities. They involve strenuous, repetitive physical and psychologic training assisted by modern equipment. Professional athletes (and some amateurs) are always preparing for competition. In many cases, modern sports training is pushing human systems to their physiologic limits. Thus, because of the intimate brain-body interaction, understanding the brain in sports is of utmost importance. It is a two-way process in that the behavior of the athlete modifies the brain and the brain modifies behavior.

There is also interaction between genetic makeup and behavior. Most people assume that genes shape the person: behavior and brain anatomy. Nobel laureate Eric Kandel's work[2] shows that when people learn new skills, their minds also affect which genes in their neurons are transcribed. Thus it is possible to shape genes to some degree through sports and exercise, which in turn shape the brain's microscopic anatomy.

The nerve cells that make up the brain are signaling devices that operate according to built-in circuits, although the circuits themselves are plastic. Their signaling capabilities underlie all aspects of mental and physical life, from the generation of thought and sensory perception to the control and execution of movement. All physical activities in sports and exercise modify the brain systems, first consciously and then unconsciously. Athletes first learn coordinated motor skills through conscious mental processes and physical repetition. The learned skills are stored in the form of short-term memory. Short-term memory is created by a functional, nonstructural modification in the ability of neurons to signal each other. For example, the neurons representing a group of muscles signal each other, after proper training, with clearer, faster, and stronger communication. Further training transforms this short-term memory into long-term unconscious memory in the synaptic connections of different brain systems. Long-term memory involves an actual structural or anatomic change in the number of signaling sites. Repetitive training causes the ability to perform a particular motor skill to be embedded in the neural circuits that produce that specific behavior. This acquired skill becomes a subconscious reflex without any conscious recollection when athletes use it. Performance of complex motor tasks, such as pitching a baseball, requires higher-order planning before the memory systems

and primary motor cortex can be activated. Motor planning appears to involve many different areas of the cortex. Motor control involves a delicate balance between multiple parallel neural pathways and the recurrent feedback loops of the nervous system. Understanding the signaling properties of neurons, therefore, is essential for understanding the biologic basis of sports behavior.

Three basic principles of brain activity are crucial in sports and exercises: (1) experience changes the brain; (2) neurons that fire together wire together; and (3) neurons out of sync fail to link. First, athletes have different brains because of the exercise they have done or their general experience in sports. This principle also warns that coordination between the brains and the musculoskeletal system can be disturbed by the wrong kinds of experience, such as improper exercise or musculoskeletal imbalance or injury. The brain responds to body exercise, as do muscles. The second principle indicates that the athletes have different brains because of special connections between the neurons of their brains. The body has an ordered "map" in the brain (Fig. 3-1 and Fig. 3-2). For a particular sport, coordination between certain groups of muscles and powerful

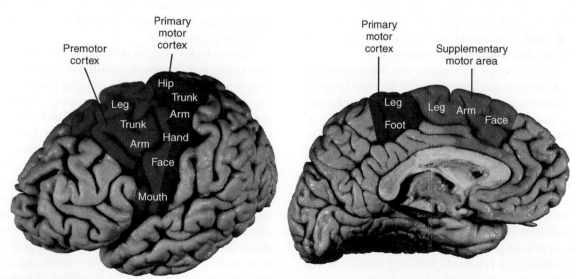

FIGURE 3-1 Organization of the primary motor cortex (M1). The different parts of the body are represented in a somatotopic manner disproportionately because of the fine control required in speech and fine manipulation of objects with the fingers.

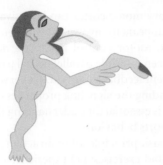

FIGURE 3-2 How the human body appears in the brain: the mouth and tongue and the tip of fingers require a greatly enlarged representation in the thalamus and cortex. Repetitive training in sports will change this map.

output from these muscles are needed. Repetitive training builds up and solidifies the neuronal connection between the parts of the brain map representing these muscles. These neuronal connections are wired together and fire together during exercise. The third principle is a reminder that wrong kinds of physical experience will erase the brain connection built by good experience. The wrong kinds of experience may include improper training or training with fatigued or injured muscles. If one part of the connection fires more slowly than others, as in the case of musculoskeletal fatigue from overtraining or injuries, the coordinated movement is disturbed or even destroyed. Athletes should perform only with coordinated and well-balanced physical systems and without pain or injuries.

Human beings have about 100 billion neurons. Each neuron can have as many as 1300 synapses (connections) with other neurons. The human cortex alone has 30 billion neurons and is capable of making 1 million billion synaptic connections. The number of all possible neural circuits is astronomical: 10 to the power of 1 million. These staggering numbers explain the complexity of the human brain, the most complicated known structure in the universe. Through these potentially massive microstructural modifications of the synaptic connections, the brain is capable of performing so many different mental functions and behaviors. Different systems of the brain connect with each other in larger aggregates, and their functions tend to become integrated, yielding new functions. Physical performance depends on such higher-order integration within the brain systems and between the brain and the body.

Physical exercise and sports involve the following processes. People consciously learn new motor skills by repetition and unlearning of old habits. After a certain number of repetitions, the new motor skills activate and strengthen related neuronal connections in the brain, so the skills are stored as short-term memory. Further training of these skills creates or modifies the neuronal connection in different parts of the brain. Once the brain map and circuit of the new skills are built, the skills become a long-term memory stored in different brain systems. This circuit formation is the result of repetitive training, and it is activated first in conscious stages and eventually in subconscious stages. When a motor skill is performed, it must first be planned; the planning occurs by activation, both conscious and subconscious, of brain circuits. This planning happens rapidly in the premotor cortex, which then sends commands to the neuromusculoskeletal system, which in turn executes the command according to the brain's directions by activating muscles and joints. During the action, the brain systems monitor motor and sensory feedback from the body and refine the execution of the action. Once it is finished, other brain circuits will be activated to start a new action. An example is gait: activity shifts from one group of muscles to another, as electromyography shows.

This is a highly coordinated mind-body interaction and is mostly subconsciously reflexive rather than consciously reflective. As training progresses, the muscles and joints become more coordinated so that they execute the planned order more smoothly, moving exactly according to the directed amount, no more and no less. The execution is precise, fast, clear, efficient, and powerful. This, in turn, solidifies the brain's circuit. In the presence of injury or a preinjury condition such as musculoskeletal fatigue, the execution is no longer so precisely coordinated nor so fast, clear, efficient, or powerful. In these circumstances, peripheral systems such as muscles and joints cannot execute the commands from the brain according to stored memory, and the subconscious reflexive coordination between the brain and the body is disturbed.

For example, if an athlete has lower back pain, the movement of his or her limbs is much slower and the range of motion of joints is limited because of fatigue or injury in the core muscles. If the condition persists, the feedback to the brain may unlearn or erase the previously stored memory to adjust to the fatigued or injured systems. This may lead to a handicapped performance and require more training to relearn the previous coordination and restore subconscious memory.

How do these physical activities affect the brain? So far, the data collected are from research on musicians. Studies of musicians who play stringed instruments have shown that the more they practice, the larger are the brain maps for their active left hands. The neurons and maps that respond to the type of sound produced by strings increase in number. In trumpeters, the neurons and maps that respond to "brassy" sounds multiply. Brain imaging shows that several areas of musicians' brains—the motor cortex and the cerebellum, among others—differ from those of nonmusicians. Imaging also shows that musicians who begin playing before the age of 7 years have larger brain areas connecting the two hemispheres. In people who meditate and meditation teachers, the insula—the part of the cortex that is activated by paying close attention—is thicker. Because of the plastic nature of the brain, not everyone uses the same areas of the brain for the same activities. As a result of this plasticity, the range of human activities is vast.

Research has revealed that exercise stimulates the production and release of brain-derived nerve growth factor (BDNF), a neuronal growth factor that redesigns the brain and plays a crucial role in influencing the brain's plasticity.[2] Even natural movement of the limbs, repeated consistently, stimulates the growth of new neurons. Exercise stimulates the sensory and motor cortices and maintains the brain's balance system. In addition, a healthy heart, healthy blood vessels, and a good diet invigorate the brain.

After the right kind of training, the neurons in the brain are better arranged for particular activities. When people are motivated to learn, the brain responds plastically. As brain maps get bigger, the individual neurons become more efficient in two

stages. Research data clearly demonstrate that as a monkey is trained to use its fingers, its brain map for the fingertip grows and takes up more space. After awhile, the individual neurons within the map become more efficient, and eventually fewer neurons are necessary to perform the task. As neurons are trained and become more efficient, they can process faster. This means that the speed at which people think is itself plastic. Speed of thought is essential in competitive sports and provides great benefits even in daily life. Research on animals also reveals that as an animal is trained at a skill, not only do its neurons fire faster but also their signals become clearer. Faster neurons are more likely to fire in sync with each other and become better team players. These neurons wire together more and form groups that produce clearer and more powerful signals, and powerful signals, in turn, have greater influence on the brain's physiology and structure.

Another important mind-body interaction is related to close attention, which is essential for long-term plastic change. In fact, lasting changes occur only when close attention is paid. Research has demonstrated that when people perform tasks automatically, without particular attention, the repetition will change brain maps, but the changes will not last. The ability to work on several tasks simultaneously does not build long-term memory. Attempting to learn new things with divided attention does not contribute to long-term change in brain maps.[3]

Physical training consists of learning new skills and unlearning old habits. Improving and refining sports skills involves the mental and physical processes of learning and unlearning, and the two processes involve different chemistry in the brain. When people learn a new skill and turn it into long-term memory, neurons in the brain fire together and wire together to form new connections, and a chemical process called *long-term potentiation* strengths the connections between the neurons. When the brain unlearns associations, old neuronal wiring is disconnected; this requires a different chemical process, *long-term depression*. Unlearning and weakening connections between neurons is just as plastic a process, and just as important, as learning and strengthening them. If people were capable of only building connections, the neuronal networks would become saturated. Unlearning skills or erasing existing memories is necessary to make room in the networks for new ones.

Nothing speeds brain atrophy more than being immobilized in an unchanging environment. The monotony undermines the dopamine and attentional systems that are crucial to maintaining brain plasticity.

IMAGINATION AND BEHAVIOR

Neuroscientific research reveals that physical ability can be influenced and even trained by mental imagination. The data clearly indicate that mental practice is an effective way to prepare for learning a physical skill with minimal physical practice. This knowledge could be very useful for athletes and their coaches.

Doidge[1] described the following experiments in his book *The Brain That Changes Itself*:

> "Everything your 'immaterial' mind imagines leaves material traces in the brain and in the body. Each thought alters the physical state of your brain connection. Each time you imagine moving your fingers across the keys to play the piano, you alter the tendrils in your living brain." (p. 213)

> "An interesting experiment with learning a simple routine on the piano shows how training the imagination improves physical performance. Two groups of people who had no experience of playing the piano were given a simple sequence of notes to learn. One group, the 'mental practice' group, sat in front of an electric piano keyboard, two hours a day, for five days, and *imagined* both playing the sequence and hearing it played. A second "physical practice" group actually played the music two hours a day for five days.… The level of improvement at five days in the mental practice group, however substantial, was not as great as in those who did physical practice. But when the mental practice group finished its mental training and was given a single two-hour physical practice session, its overall performance improved to the level of the physical practice group's performance at five days … We all do mental practice when we memorize answers for a test, or rehearse any kind of performance or presentation. But because few of us do it systematically, we underestimate its effectiveness. Some athletes and musicians use it to prepare for performances." (p. 202)

> "From a neuroscientific point of view, imagining an act and doing it are not as different as they sound … Brain scans show that many of the same parts of the brain are activated in imagination as are in action, and that is why visualizing can improve performance.

> In an experiment that is as hard to believe as it is simple, Drs. Guang Yue and Kelly Cole showed that imagining that one is using one's muscles actually strengthens them. The study looked at two groups, one that did physical exercise and one that imagined doing exercise. Both groups exercised a finger muscle, Monday through Friday, for four weeks. The physical group did fifteen maximal contractions, with a twenty-second rest between each. The mental group merely imagined doing fifteen maximal contractions, with a twenty-second rest between each, and at the same time imagining a voice shouting at them, 'harder! harder!'… At the end of the study the subjects who had done physical exercise increased their muscular strength by 30%. Those who only imagined doing the exercise, for the same period, increased their muscle strength by 22%. The explanation lies in the motor neurons of the brain that 'program' movements. During these imaginary contractions, the neurons responsible for stringing together sequences of instructions for movements are activated and strengthened, resulting in increased strength when the muscles are contracted." (p. 204)

This research suggests that imagining an act engages the same motor and sensory programs that are involved in actually performing it.

SUMMARY

Sports require high-level motor skills that require long-term training, and this process changes the brain. Sports injuries also change the brain's plasticity and impair the neuron wiring between different groups of muscles that have been built up by long-term training. When clinicians understand the interaction among brain plasticity, training, and injury, they will appreciate how important it is to prevent sports injury and, when prevention is impossible, to achieve complete recovery. With this understanding, the clinical importance of dry needling therapy presented in the next chapters can be better appreciated by clinicians, athletes and their coaches.

References

1. Doidge N: *The brain that changes itself,* New York, 2007, Penguin Books.
2. Squire LR, Berg D, Bloom FE, et al: *Fundamental neuroscience,* ed 3, New York, 2008, Academic Press, pp 491–516.
3. Kandel ER: *In search of memory the emergence of a new science of mind,* New York, 2006, W.W. Norton & Company.

CHAPTER 4

Musculoskeletal Systems and Human Movement

Human movement is a complex process involving an infinite variety of positional changes, which are controlled by a wide range of internal systems and external factors. A sequence of movement can be influenced by anatomic mechanics, physiologic conditions, psychologic factors, and sociologic and environmental interaction. This chapter focuses on the anatomic, biomechanical, and physiologic aspects of movement.

Most movements, including specific movements used in sports, have been previously learned and, after months or years of practice, have become reflexive and fluent. The neural processes that store, adapt, and are used in these learned movements are complex and integrate all the systems of the body to produce them. When people learn a new movement, action initially arises from a conscious decision, and active thought processes are needed to perform it. At the early stage of acquiring a new skill, considerable concentration is needed, and the movement may be clumsy. With practice, the motion is converted into a learned sequence of movements that will be stored in the different parts of the brain and can be reproduced with fluency and very little conscious thought.

The purpose of this chapter is to understand the mechanical character of movement; this understanding is essential in the use of dry needling acupuncture therapy to achieve the best integration of human movement (described in subsequent chapters).

SKELETAL SYSTEM

The design of the skeletal system is closely related to its function. The skeleton constitutes approximately 20% of total body weight. It consists of bones, cartilage, ligaments, and joints of the body; bones are the largest component. Joints, or articulations, are the intersections between bones, and ligaments connect bones at the articulations so as to strengthen the joints. The skeletal system is usually conceptualized as two parts: the axial and appendicular skeletons. The misalignment of a bone or a joint causes mechanical imbalance of the system, which increases the effects of stress. Thus an integrative understanding of the functional anatomy of the skeletal system is crucial in preventing and treating sports-related injuries. The major bones and muscles of the body are described in Chapter 12.

The skeletal system determines shape and body size. Although the general size and shape of the bones are inherited, structural adaptations can be caused by external forces (e.g., weight bearing) and influenced by the internal forces exerted by tendons, ligaments, and muscles. In the developing skeleton, the influence of weight bearing and muscular forces have a more substantial effect on the formation of the size and shape of the bones than the same forces have on a mature skeleton. The skeletal system performs many mechanical and biologic functions: leverage, support, protection, energy processing, storage, and blood cell formation. Some of these functions, such as leverage, support, and stress absorption, are critically important for human movement.

Levers and Torque

The skeletal system provides the levers and axes of rotation about which the muscular system generates movement. A lever is a simple machine that magnifies the force or speed of movement, or both. The levers are primarily the long bones of the body, and the axes are the joints where the bones meet. Human skeletal levers can be one of three types (Fig. 4-1). Human levers serve many different functions, including movement, manipulation of objects, and weight bearing. If a joint is misaligned, the lever structure is altered, and mechanical stress to the joint caused by external and internal

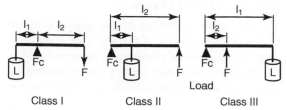

Class I   Class II   Class III

FIGURE 4-1 The three classes of lever. The lever arms are of lengths l_1 and l_2. Equilibrium is achieved if $l_1 \times L = l_2 \times F$. Mechanical advantage $(M_a) = L/F = L_1/L_2$. M_{a1} (class I lever) can be greater or less than 1; $M_{a2} > 1$, whereas $M_{a3} < 1$. *F*, Applied force; *Fc*, fulcrum; *L*, load.

forces increases, all of which result in injury to the joint or soft tissue. From the perspective of physics, human levers are constructed with mechanical disadvantage. This means that the muscles have to produce 50 pounds (22.7 kg) of force to hold a 5-pound (2.3-kg) object. However, this mechanical disadvantage is compensated by the gain in speed of the lever movement.

When a force is applied to a lever, the lever rotates about the fulcrum. *Torque* is an expression for how a force changes the angular motion of a lever, which signifies the angular velocity. To calculate the torque *M*, the magnitude of the force *F* is multiplied by the distance *l* between the force and the rotating point. In Figure 4-1, the torque is calculated as

$$M = F \times l$$

Equilibrium is achieved when the torque on the left equals that on the right:

$$M_L = M_R$$

Or:

$$L \times l_1 = F \times l_2$$

Human skeletal levers and torques are discussed in the following section.

Force and Stress on the Skeletal System

External and internal forces are always acting on the body, and it is important to understand their effects and how these forces can facilitate movement or, conversely, cause damage to the skeletal system.

The skeletal framework is a series of long and short bones connected at joints. Each joint has a specific design that allows for movement in certain directions. Movement at joints is produced by either internal or external forces. Internal forces are generated by muscle contraction, whereas the most important external force is probably gravity, inasmuch as it is always present and must always be taken into account when the factors responsible for movement are considered. Other external forces exist, such as the mechanical force produced by body contact in sports or physical impact during accidents. During movement, both internal and external forces need to be controlled precisely.

All people are aware of using gravity to facilitate movement. When people move in the direction of gravity, the prime factor in producing movement is gravity itself, and muscles are used to control or enhance the effect of gravity so that the required movement takes place. All downward movements, such as sitting down, stepping down, and bending down, are produced primarily by gravity; the muscles are used only to initiate the activity and control the speed of movement.

Some external forces are capable of causing injury during movement. Each time a person takes a step and the heel strikes the floor, a "ground reaction force" is transmitted through the whole body. As the speed of walking increases, so do the ground reaction forces, which leads to greater forces through the lower limb and an increased likelihood of injury. The human body has evolved mechanisms to attenuate the effects of ground reaction forces so that it is not damaged by their repeated occurrence. When the heel strikes the ground, the relatively soft heel pad on the sole of the foot absorbs some of the initial force. The knee flexes as the limb takes the load of the body, and this knee flexion movement, up to approximately 40 degrees, also has a shock absorption effect. Through small movements at the hip and spine, residual forces are further absorbed, which ensures that the effect of these forces is minimal by the time they reach the skull and brain. The healthy muscles are major cushions to absorb the physical forces from all directions to protect the tendons, ligaments, and bones. If the muscles are fatigued or injured, they cannot function as cushions and bone fracture may occur, such as stress fracture in the tibia in running and other sport activities.

Physical forces are transmitted in straight lines. Every time they meet an interface between tissues, some are absorbed by the soft tissues and bones, and others are deflected by anatomic design. No single, straight structure runs the length of the body, and thus force has no direct route to travel. All the long bones in the body are curved, as is the vertebral column. As externally applied forces are transmitted through the bones, the curvature of the bones absorbs or deflects the forces. By the time the forces have reached the cervical spine and the skull, much of the effect has been removed, and the impact on the skull and the vertebral column is kept to a minimum.

The curved bones transfer energy. When a force is applied longitudinally to a curved structure such as the femur, the bone deforms and the curvature increases, absorbing some of the forces rather than transmitting them to more vulnerable structures such as the cervical spine and skull. The absorbed forces form elastic (potential) energy, which is released as kinetic energy when the bone returns to its resting shape. This energy transfer is useful in many human movements. For example, a higher jump can be achieved if compressive forces are applied to the long bones of the lower limbs immediately before takeoff.

Nevertheless, there are limits to how far the skeletal framework can sustain internal and external stress. It is not uncommon that a sudden powerful muscle contraction or a repeated external force can cause bone fracture. One of the purposes of dry needling acupuncture therapy is to lower the stress in muscles so that they can absorb more force during sporting activity and thereby prevent or reduce stress-related injuries to the musculoskeletal system.

GENERAL REVIEW OF THE MECHANICS OF MAJOR HUMAN JOINTS

Knowledge of the mechanical torques operating at major joints helps clinicians understand how stress is distributed in joints and muscles and thereby how to restore musculoskeletal balance and treat soft tissue dysfunction.

Joints of Class I Levers

The mechanical advantage of this type of joint can be less or more than 1. If the joints are positioned properly, mechanical advantage is better; otherwise, the muscles must deal with a lower mechanical advantage, more physical work, and higher energy consumption. These factors cause muscle fatigue to build up more rapidly, with more physical stress in the joints and a higher likelihood of injury such as disc herniation or bone fracture.

Elbow

The elbow joint functions as both a class I and a class III lever, according to how it is used. It is a class I lever when the external force F acts on one side and the internal force F_m acts on the other (Fig. 4-2). The arm will be still if $F_m \times l_m = F \times l$, where l_m is

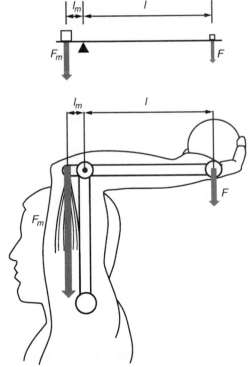

FIGURE 4-2 The elbow joint functions as both a class I and a class III lever, according to the function. The joint serves as a class I lever when the external force F acts on one side and the internal (muscle) force F_m acts on the other. The arm is held still if $F_m \times l_m = F \times l$, where l_m is the length of the lever arm generating internal force and l is the length of the lever arm being acted upon by the external force.

the length of the lever arm generating internal force and *l* is the length of the lever arm being acted upon by the external force.

The ball will accelerate if F_m increases, or $F_m \times l_m > F \times l$.

Neck

The center of gravity of the head lies anterior to the atlanto-occipital joint (Fig. 4-3). In normal adult cervical posture, the momentum arm of the extensor muscles ($l_{extensor}$) = 4 cm, and the momentum arm of the head's weight (l_{weight}) = 2 cm. Thus the extensor muscles use approximately half the weight of the head to support normal head posture. If the head is positioned forward, $l_{extensor}$ may reduce and l_{weight} will increase. In this head-forward posture, the extensor muscles have to use much more force to balance the head.

Lower Back

As Figure 4-4 shows, the traction force of the back muscles counterbalance the weight of the trunk. If the momentum arm of the body weight is three times longer than the momentum arm of the lower back muscles, these muscles have to use a force of three times the body weight to achieve this balance. In the act of bending forward, the lower back muscles must sustain a physical stress equal to several times body weight to maintain the posture.

Joints of Class III Levers

Both the muscle force and the weight or load are on the same side for these joints, but they pull in different directions (see Fig. 4-1). The mechanical advantage of these joints is always less than 1. That means that merely to maintain balance, the force supplied by the muscles has to be many times greater than the combined weight of the body parts and the load.

During abduction, the shoulder joint functions as a typical class III lever (Fig. 4-5). The elbow joint can serve as a class I lever for extension and as a class III lever for flexion.

Reaction Forces Inside the Joints

The bones of the skeleton are essentially levers and each joint serves as a fulcrum (see Fig. 4-1).

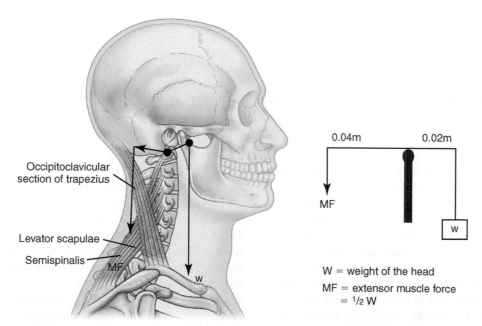

FIGURE 4-3 The cervical joint serves as a class I lever. The center of gravity of the head lies anterior to the atlanto-occipital joint. In normal adult cervical posture, the momentum arm of the extensor muscles ($l_{extensor}$) = 4 cm, and the momentum arm of the head's weight (l_{weight}) = 2 cm. Thus the extensor muscles use approximately half the weight of the head to support the normal head posture.

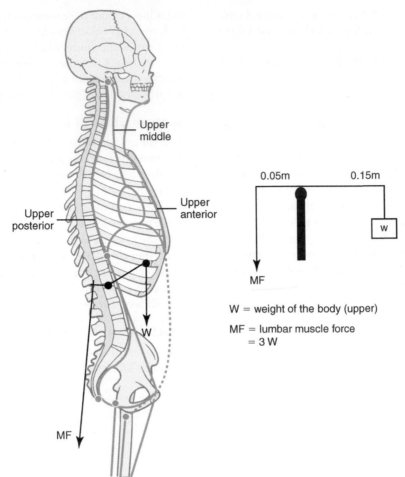

Upper
middle

0.05m   0.15m

Upper
posterior

Upper
anterior

W

MF

W = weight of the body (upper)

MF = lumbar muscle force
   = 3 W

W

MF

FIGURE 4-4 The traction force of the back muscles counterbalances the weight of the trunk.

Most of the skeletal muscles of the human body operate in first- or third-class lever systems with mechanical advantages less than 1 as the tendons of the muscles that operate the joints usually are inserted close to the joints. As Figure 4-1 shows, the fulcrum of the lever system sustains the physical force equal to the sum of muscle force and loading force. For example, in Figure 4-4, if the upper body weighs W = 50 kg (110 lb), the lower back muscles have to exert F = 150 kg (330 lb) to support the standing in normal posture, and the reaction force *Rj* to support the normal posture in the lumbar

joint Rj = 50 kg + 150 kg = 200 kg (440 lb). If low back pain occurs, the lower back muscles have to use much more force to support the posture, and the reaction force inside the lumbar joint is much higher. It is not surprising that an overloaded joint is more likely to be subsequently subject to wear and tear, resulting in osteoarthritis or other joint and muscle injuries. Therefore frequent de-stress treatment with dry needling technique introduced in this book is of great importance to maintain optimal physical performance and a career in sports.

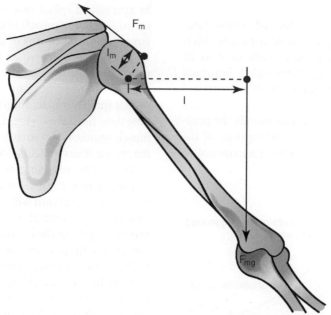

FIGURE 4-5 During abduction, the shoulder joint function as a typical class III lever.

Support of Body Weight

The skeleton can maintain a posture that supports body function while accommodating large external forces, as in sports such as weight lifting or jumping. The bones of the lower vertebrae, the pelvic bones, and the bones of the lower extremities are larger than their counterparts in the upper body (upper vertebrae, bones of the shoulder, and bones of the upper extremities), in proportion to the amount of body weight that they bear. The muscles that move these bigger bones are correspondingly bigger and stronger than their upper body counterparts.

Upper Limb

The upper limb consists of the shoulder girdle, the humerus, the radius, the ulna, and the bones of the wrist and hand. The design and structure of the upper limbs enable people to grasp and manipulate objects and to perform many other actions.

Muscle

Muscles are the major powerhouse of motion in both daily life and sports. Techniques in molecular biology were among the first methods to be used for understanding the mechanisms of muscle contraction. The physiologic and pathologic mechanisms of muscle are a focus of both sports science and pain medicine. Many textbooks deal with these topics, but this book focuses on the physiologic mechanisms that are related to sports performance, injury prevention, and rehabilitation after injury.

Protective Reflexes Through Sensory Feedback in the Musculoskeletal System

Any movement of the musculoskeletal system involves both acceleration and deceleration phases. If acceleration is not precisely controlled, or if deceleration is delayed or not strong enough, the resulting overacceleration of the body part can cause rupture of the muscles, tendons, and even bones. Two types of peripheral nerve cells are involved in this coordination to protect a muscle against unnecessary injury: muscle spindles and tendon spindles. Muscle spindles prevent overstretching of the muscle fibers, and tendon spindles prevent overcontraction. Tendinitis, a common injury in athletes, is usually the result of ignoring warnings from these two spindles.

Muscle Spindles

The muscle spindles are located throughout the muscle between regular skeletal muscle fibers (Fig. 4-6). A muscle spindle consists of 4 to 20 small, specialized muscle fibers called *intrafusal fibers* (inside the spindles), and certain sensory and motor nerve endings are associated with these fibers. A sheath of connective tissues surrounds the muscle spindle and attaches to the endomysium of the extrafusal fibers. The intrafusal fibers are controlled

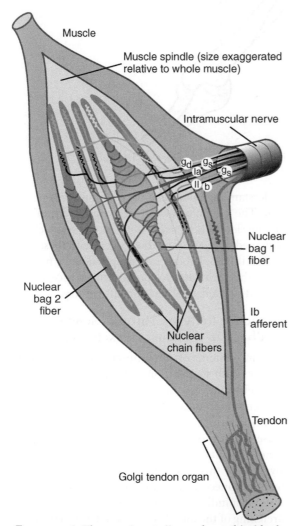

Muscle

Muscle spindle (size exaggerated relative to whole muscle)

Intramuscular nerve

Nuclear bag 1 fiber

Nuclear bag 2 fiber

Ib afferent

Nuclear chain fibers

Tendon

Golgi tendon organ

FIGURE 4-6 The muscle spindles are located inside the muscle between regular skeletal muscle fibers throughout the muscle. *gd*: γ-d motor neuron fiber, *gs*: γ-s motor neuron fiber, *b*: β-type sensory neuron fiber, *Ia*: primary sensory ending, *II*: secondary sensory ending.

by specialized spinal motor neurons: the γ-motor neurons. Regular muscle fibers are controlled by the larger α-motor neurons of the spinal cord.

The central region of an intrafusal fiber contains no or only a few actin and myosin filaments; therefore, it cannot contract but can only stretch. Because the muscle spindle is attached to the extrafusal fibers, any time those fibers are stretched, the central region of the muscle spindle is also stretched. In other words, when the muscle fibers stretch, so do the muscle spindles.

Sensory nerve endings wrapped around this central region of the muscle spindle transmit information to the spinal cord when this region is stretched, informing the central nervous system about the muscle length. In the spinal cord a sensory neurons synapses with an α-motor neuron, which triggers reflexive muscle contraction in the extrafusal fibers to resist further stretching. γ-motor neurons excite the intrafusal fibers, prestretching them slightly. Although the central region of the intrafusal fibers cannot contract, the ends can. The γ-motor neurons cause a slight contraction of the ends of these fibers, which stretches the central region slightly. This prestretch makes the muscle spindle highly sensitive to even small degrees of stretch.

If the muscle stretches enough that there is a risk of rupture, the spindle responds by sending a signal to the muscle to contract. This keeps the muscle from being injured. In response to that stretch, the sensory neurons send action potentials to the spinal cord, which then activates the α-motor neurons of the motor unit in the same muscles to increase the force of contraction to overcome stretching.

After the information is sent to the spinal cord from the sensory neurons associated with muscle spindles, the same signals continue to travel up to higher parts of the central nervous system, supplying the brain with continuous feedback about the exact length of the muscle and the rate at which that length is changing. This information is essential for maintaining muscle tone and posture and for executing movements. The muscle spindle functions as a servo mechanism to provide continuous correction to motion. The brain is simultaneously aware of errors in the intended movement, and so it sends descending commands to correct the muscle contraction at the spinal cord level.

If the muscles are fatigued or injured, as with overtraining, the muscles become shortened to resist physical stretching, the coordination between intrafusal and extrafusal fibers disintegrates, and central commands cannot be executed. If the fatigued or injured muscles are forced to work, worse injury results.

Tendon Spindles

Unlike muscle spindles, the tendon spindles give an inhibiting signal, which prevents the muscle from contracting. Tendon spindles are encapsulated sensory receptors and located just proximal to where the tendon fibers attach to the muscle fibers (see Fig. 4-6). Usually, 5 to 25 muscle fibers are connected to each tendon spindle. Whereas muscle spindles monitor the length of muscle fibers, tendon spindles are sensitive to tension in the muscle-tendon complex and serve as a strain gauge, a way of sensing changes in tension. The tendon spindles are so sensitive that they can respond to the contraction of even a single muscle fiber. These inhibitory sensory receptors perform a protective function by reducing the potential for injury. When stimulated, tendon spindles inhibit the contracting (agonist) muscles and excite the antagonist muscles.

Coordination between agonist and antagonist muscles is crucial in maintaining normal mechanical balance in the joint, as well as in protecting the muscles from overstretching.

When muscles are fatigued or overtrained, they become shorter and less flexible, with soreness or sensation of pain. If these symptoms are ignored and the muscles are forced to work, the stiff muscles will transfer the stress to the tendon, resulting in tendinitis. This indicates that in the treatment of tendinitis, both muscles and tendons should be treated simultaneously.

Figure 4-6 illustrates a situation in which reflexes protect the muscles and tendon from injury. If a person moves one arm backwards quickly toward its outermost position to do a powerful throwing action, and if the arm moves backwards too far or with too much speed, there is a risk of muscle or tendon rupture. Normally, the muscle spindles send a warning signal and the muscle contracts; the arm will then stops and turns back before it reaches

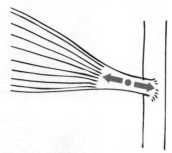

FIGURE 4-7 The direction of the forces sustained in the tendon causes tendinitis because the forces conflict.

the critical position. If the muscles are fatigued or injured, this movement will not be controlled precisely, and it is possible to tear or rupture the muscles or tendons.

When a muscle contracts, the tension in the tendons increases. Figure 4-7 depicts the direction of the forces sustained in the tendon. This shows how both conflicting forces contribute to tendinitis.

Other Protective Sensory Organs

Additional sensory organs around the joints and in the joint capsules transmit information used to adjust movements and protect the body from injury. Figure 4-8 shows three different sensory organs, each of them responsible for sending specific sensory information: Pacinian corpuscles are sensitive to pressure, Ruffini corpuscles are sensitive to position and speed, and the free nerve endings are sensitive to pain. These sensory organs are distributed in capsules, in perimysium around muscle, and in periosteum around bones. A kick on the tibia can cause severe and immediate pain, but if there is no damage, the pain will disappear in as little as 10 seconds. If an injury such as contusion occurs, the pain-producing substances will be synthesized, and the pain will persist.

MUSCULOSKELETAL RESPONSES TO STRESS

The curves in Figure 4-9 show stress reactions in muscle, tendon, and bone. Muscle is elastic, and in reaction to a relatively small stress, it extends

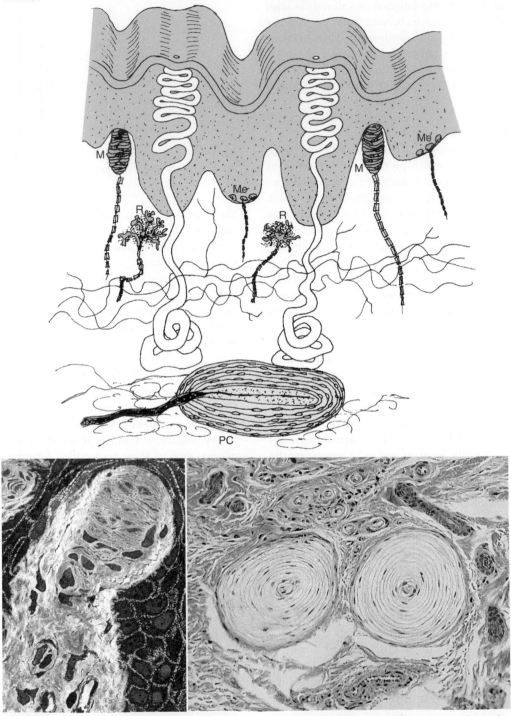

FIGURE 4-8 Each of the three different sensory organs is responsible for sending specific sensory information to the brain. Pacinian corpuscles are sensitive to pressure, Ruffini corpuscles are sensitive to position and speed, and free nerve endings are sensitive to pain.

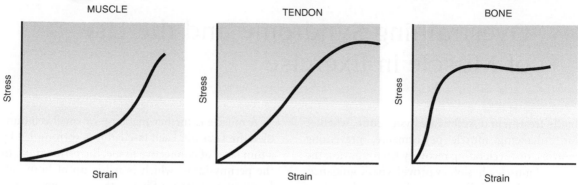

FIGURE 4-9 Stress reactions in muscle, tendon, and bone.

dramatically. The tendons are less elastic and more resistant to stress. The bones make small adjustments in response to pulling and pushing. However, with heavy loads, both bones and tendons can be stretched to some extent before breakage or rupture occurs. Muscle, on the contrary, becomes progressively stiffer as the load increases, before it ruptures. Clinical experience has demonstrated that at heavy loads, a muscle will rupture before a tendon ruptures or a bone breaks. A ruptured muscle often heals faster than a ruptured tendon or a broken bone; therefore, from this perspective, muscle injury is the least dangerous of these three types of injury.

SUMMARY

The mechanical properties of the human musculoskeletal system are reviewed briefly to show how this system reacts to mechanical stress and how injuries happen. This understanding is necessary for clinicians and offers a rationale for treating soft tissue dysfunctions in sports injuries. Of more importance is that this knowledge helps clinicians treat parts of the musculoskeletal system that are subject to fatigue and potential injury in any particular sport so as to prevent real injury later.

Readers are encouraged to learn more about the biomechanics of athletic motion in order to prevent injuries, to treat injuries properly, and to help patients to recover better and faster.

Additional Readings

1. Wirhed R: *Athletic ability and the anatomy of motion,* St Louis, 2006, Elsevier.
2. Greene DP, Roberts SL: *Kinesiology: movement in the context of activity,* ed 2, St Louis, 2005, Elsevier.

CHAPTER 5

Overtraining Syndrome and the Use of Muscle in Exercise

In the treatment of soft tissue dysfunction, whether for enhancing muscle performance, preventing injuries, or accelerating recovery from injuries, the study of muscle physiology provides basic guidance. Although detailed discussion of muscle physiology is beyond the scope of this book, this chapter briefly reviews some of the concepts that are relevant to clinical practice.

When people exercise, all types of muscles in the body—skeletal, cardiac, and smooth muscles—are activated and coordinated for the same purpose: to perform a successful movement. Skeletal muscles are under conscious control by the mind. Most skeletal muscles—for example, deltoids, pectorals, and biceps—attach to and move the skeleton. The human body contains more than 600 skeletal muscles. The thumb alone is controlled by nine muscles. Although the physical structures of smooth, cardiac, and skeletal muscles differ somewhat, their control mechanisms and principles of action are similar.

SKELETAL MUSCLE

Skeletal muscle is surrounded by a layer of connective tissue, which is called the *fascia,* or epimysium, of the muscle; it consists mainly of collagen fibers. The fascia is built up in the same way as the outer layer of a joint capsule. It provides a surface against which the surrounding muscles can glide, and it gives muscles their form. Thus a muscle and its fascia are anatomically and physiologically bound together. When a muscle is fatigued, inflamed, or injured, the muscle is shortened and resists any stretching, and the same happens to the fascia. In fact, damage to the fascia creates additional problems. An inflamed fascia may adhere to other fascia, which makes muscle movement difficult or impossible. Scar tissue forms, and the lack of mobility can become permanent. This is one of the major sources of chronic soft tissue dysfunction and pain.

A muscle is further made up of small cell bundles, the *fasciculi.* Each fasciculus is surrounded by a thin layer of connective tissue, the *perimysium.* In the perimysium—which is made up of both collagenous and elastic fibers—the nerve and blood vessels branch off before finally reaching the actual muscle fibers. Each fasciculus consists of a number of muscle fibers, or muscle cells. Each muscle fiber is surrounded by a very thin layer of connective tissue, which is called *endomysium* (Fig. 5-1).

The structure and function of muscle fibers is described thoroughly in textbooks on physiology. The rest of this section is a brief review.

A muscle fiber is composed of small structures called *muscle fibrils* or *myofibrils.* The fibrils lie in parallel and give the muscle cell a striated appearance. Fibrils are made up of smaller regularly aligned components called *myofilaments,* which are chains of protein molecules. The striated appearance is attributable to the presence of two types of myofilament: actin and myosin. When the muscle contracts, the actin filaments move longitudinally between the myosin filaments. As a consequence, the myofibrils shorten and thicken.

The connective tissue surrounding the muscle, the epimysium, extends and is continuous with the muscle's tendon. The muscles of the body have very different shapes (Fig. 5-2). When a muscle contracts, it produces a force, F, that affects the origin and insertion of the muscle equally but in opposite directions. A muscle and its fascia become shortened when a muscle is fatigued, inflamed, or injured, which may create a static force on tissues of both origin and insertion. If the shortened muscle is forced to stretch, the muscle creates warning pain and conveys the stretching stress to the tendons of both origin and insertion. The consequence is tendinitis, which is a symptom of tendons, muscles, and related soft tissues, including nerves, blood vessels, and fascia. This condition can become more

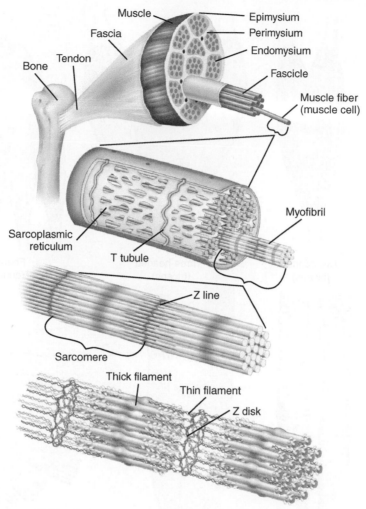

FIGURE 5-1 Anatomical configuration of the skeletal muscle.

serious in athletes when medication is used to block or suppress the warning pain signals.

The structure of the muscle exactly serves its function. For example, strap-shaped muscle is found in places where it is necessary to execute large ranges of movement quickly. Pinnate-shaped muscle can be found where movements over a small range but of great strength are required. To assess the effect of a muscle, the clinician must also know where it is attached in relation to the joint. The alignment of force of a muscle is dependent on its physiologic cross-section. The ability of a muscle to create a force to do work depends on two factors: its physiologic cross-section and its position in relation to the joint. This knowledge is very important in the treatment of muscular symptoms related to movement.

TYPES OF MUSCLE CONTRACTION

Muscle does two types of work: dynamic and static. In dynamic work, the origin and insertion of a muscle are affected by changes in muscle length. If the muscular force causes the origin and insertion to move toward each other, or if the muscle is shortened and contracted, the dynamic work is *concentric.* If the muscle force is exerted while the

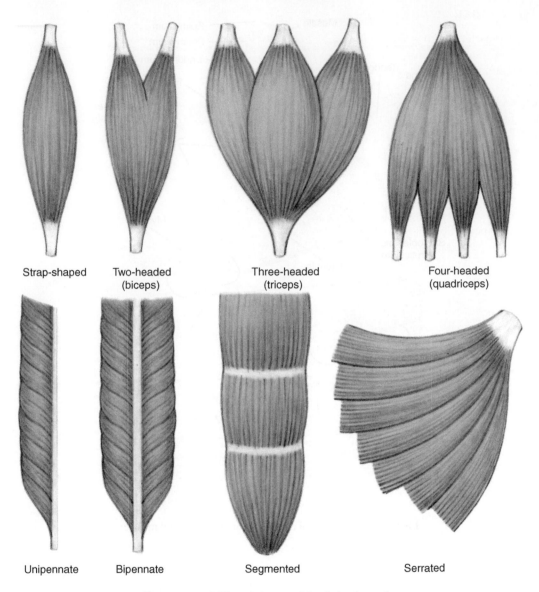

Strap-shaped   Two-headed (biceps)   Three-headed (triceps)   Four-headed (quadriceps)

Unipennate   Bipennate   Segmented   Serrated

FIGURE 5-2 Different shapes of the skeletal muscles.

origin and insertion are receding from each other, the muscle is working *eccentrically;* that is, it tries to shorten but is actually lengthened by external forces when it tries to halt a movement in a joint. In static (isometric) work, a muscle contracts without any movement taking place in the joint. The muscle can achieve its maximal speed or movement when working in the best possible conditions. Muscular performance is greatly reduced in the presence of any pathologic condition, including those that the person may not consciously realize, such as symptoms of overtraining.

Whenever muscles contract, whether the contraction is concentric, eccentric, or isometric, the force generated must be graded to meet the needs of the activity. The amount of force produced depends on the number and type of motor units activated, the frequency of stimulation of each motor unit, the size of the muscle, the muscle fiber length, and the muscle's speed of contraction.

MUSCLE FIBER TYPES

A single muscle has to perform different functions, some more dynamic, which require speed and strength, and some more static, which require endurance. A single skeletal muscle contains different fibers for different speeds of contraction and different amounts of strength: slow-twitch (type I) fibers and fast-twitch (type II) fibers. Slow-twitch fibers take approximately 110 milliseconds to reach peak tension when stimulated. Fast-twitch fibers can reach peak tension in about 50 milliseconds.

Although only one form of type I fiber has been identified, type II fibers can be further classified into two major forms: fast-twitch type a (type IIa) and fast-twitch type x (type IIx). A third subtype of fast-twitch fibers has also been identified as type IIc.

The difference between types IIa, IIx, and IIc is not fully understood. Type I fibers are more frequently recruited than type IIa and type IIx fibers, and type IIc are the least often used. Most muscles are composed of approximately 50% type I fibers and 25% type IIa fibers. The remaining 25% are mostly type IIx; type IIc fibers make up only 1% to 3%. Current knowledge about type IIc fibers is very limited. The exact percentage of each of these fiber types varies greatly between muscles and also between individuals, especially among athletes in different sports. Table 5-1 is based on the current knowledge of these fibers.

As mentioned earlier, the percentages of type I and type II fibers are not the same in all the muscles of the body. The arm and leg muscles usually have similar compositions of fiber types. People with a predominance of type I fibers in their leg muscles probably have a high percentage of type I fibers in their arm muscles as well. A similar relationship exists for type II fibers. The soleus muscle is the exception: It is composed of a very high percentage of type I fibers in everyone.

Different sporting or other activities require different muscular functions, which make use of different ratios of type I and type II fibers.

Type I Fibers

Type I fibers are very efficient at producing adenosine triphosphate (ATP) from the oxidation of carbohydrate and fat. As long as oxidation occurs, type I fibers continue producing ATP, which allows the fibers to remain active. Thus the ability to maintain muscular activity for a prolonged period (muscular endurance) depends on type I fibers, which have high aerobic endurance. They are recruited most often during low-intensity events, such as marathon running, and during daily activities, such as walking, for which the muscle-force requirements are low.

Type II Fibers

Type II muscle fibers have relatively poor aerobic endurance in comparison with type I fibers. In type II fibers, ATP is formed through anaerobic, not oxidative, pathways when oxygen supply is insufficient. Type IIa motor units generate considerably more force than do type I motor units, but they also fatigue more easily. Thus type IIa fibers appear to be the primary fiber type used during shorter, high-intensity endurance events, such as the mile run or the 400-m swim.

Type IIx fibers are not easily activated by the nervous system. Thus they are used rather infrequently in low-intensity activity but are predominant in highly explosive activity, such as the 100-m dash or the 50-m swim. Current knowledge of type IIx fibers is quite limited.

TABLE 5-1	CHARACTERISTICS OF FIBER TYPES OF SKELETAL MUSCLES		
Fiber Types	**Type I (Slow Twitch)**	**Type IIa (Fast Twitch a)**	**Type IIx (Fast Twitch x)**
Contractile speed	Slow	Fast	Fast
Fatigue resistance	High	Moderate	Low
Oxidative capacity	High	Moderately high	Low
Glycolytic capacity	Low	High	Highest
Motor unit strength	Low	High	High

The composition of a person's muscle fibers appears to be determined early in life, possibly within the first few years. Genes determine which α-motor neurons innervate individual muscle fibers. After innervation is established, the signals from α-motor neurons determine the differentiation of muscle types. Physical environment also affects the differentiation. There is some evidence that endurance training and strength training, as well as muscular inactivity, may cause a shift in the myosin isoforms. Training may induce a small change, perhaps less than 10%, in the amount of type I and type II fibers. Both endurance and resistance training have been shown to reduce the percentage of type IIx fibers and increase the proportion of type IIa fibers.

Researchers have further shown that aging alters the genetic expression of muscle fibers. Older people tend to lose type II motor units, which increases the percentage of type I fibers.

Athletes who participate in low-intensity but high-endurance sports have a high percentage of type I fibers, whereas those of high-intensity, short-term and explosive activities have more type II fibers. As anticipated, the leg muscles of distance runners, who rely on endurance, have a predominance of type I fibers (Table 5-2).[1]

Despite all these data, it is difficult to conclusively determine whether type I and type II fibers can be transformed into each other by prolonged intensive training. Each type of muscle fiber is controlled by a particular type of motor neuron. This innervation of a particular muscle fiber by a motor neuron may not change. It is possible that after a very long period of power training, muscle fibers that require a full oxygen supply may adapt to work with a smaller oxygen supply. It is presumed that type II muscle fibers can be trained to operate at a more consistent production of energy with improved blood flow and, therefore, better oxygen supply. As a result, less lactic acid is produced, and these type II fibers can work for a longer period of time before signs of exhaustion occur. It is, therefore, very important for athletes that they recover from, or at least mitigate, musculoskeletal stress or symptoms of overtraining as soon as possible after each event and before attempting the next one. This can be achieved with the help of needling techniques that are introduced in this book.

It has been observed that type I fibers change after prolonged work of relatively low intensity:

- The capillary net in the muscle around the type I fibers increases. This means that the ability to supply the operating fibers with oxygen and energy-providing substances also increases.

TABLE 5-2   PERCENTAGE OF MUSCLE FIBERS IN SELECTED MUSCLES OF MALE AND FEMALE ATHLETES

Athlete	Sex	Muscle	% Type I	% Type II
Sprint runner	Male	Gastrocnemius	24	76
	Female	Gastrocnemius	27	73
Distance runner	Male	Gastrocnemius	79	21
	Female	Gastrocnemius	69	31
Cyclist	Male	Vastus lateralis	57	43
	Female	Vastus lateralis	51	49
Swimmer	Male	Posterior deltoid	67	33
Weightlifter	Male	Gastrocnemius	44	56
	Male	Deltoid	53	47
Triathletes	Male	Posterior deltoid	60	40
	Male	Vastus lateralis	63	37
	Male	Gastrocnemius	59	41
Canoeists	Male	Posterior deltoid	71	29
Shot-putters	Male	Gastrocnemius	38	62
Nonathletes	Male	Vastus lateralis	47	53
	Female	Gastrocnemius	52	48

From Wilmore JH, Costill DL, Kenney WL: *Physiology of sports and exercise*, Champaign, IL, 2008, Human Kinetics, p 41.

- The number and size of mitochondria in the fibers increase. This means that the ability to produce energy increases at the required pace.
- The muscle endurance with submaximal loads increases. This means that a person can perform the same movement many more times.
- The size of the fibers changes very little or not at all. This means that there is no increase in strength.

Training with heavy loads affects mainly type II fibers. The main changes in type II muscles are as follows:

- The size (the cross-section area) of the fibers increases, and so more force can be produced. The increase of cross-sectional area results from the creation of more fibrils in the fiber. The number of fibers does not change. Genes for fibrils are activated.
- The fiber's ability to work with less oxygen increases, and so the fiber produces less lactic acid.

PHYSICAL PROPERTIES OF MUSCLE: TONE, TENSION, CONTRACTURE, THIXOTROPY, AND SPASM

Understanding the physical properties of muscle is of great importance for maintaining optimal muscle function and treating soft tissue dysfunction. Muscle tone depends on two things: (1) the basic viscoelastic properties of the soft tissues associated with the muscle and (2) the degree of activation of the contractile mechanisms of the muscle. Viscoelasticity is related to the biomechanical properties of connective tissues, whereas contractility depends either on physiologic contraction, which is controlled by motor neurons in the spinal cord, or on pathologic endogenous contraction, which is not. This endogenous contraction, defined as *contracture,* is often the pathologic cause of a reduction in the level and quality of muscle performance.

The concept of muscle tone means the elastic or viscoelastic stiffness, or both, in the absence of contractile activity (motor unit and contracture).[2] In some pathologic conditions, muscle tone may increase for any reason. This hypertonia includes a variety of conditions, such as spasticity, rigidity,

dystonia, and muscular contracture. The causes and mechanisms of different types of hypertonia may be quite different. Hypotonia, on the other hand, is the condition of loss of normal elastic stiffness of the muscle.

Muscle contractile activity may occur in three forms[2]:

1. Electrogenic contraction or stiffness, which is muscle tension resulting from electrogenic muscle contraction (determined on the basis of observable electromyographic activity) in normal muscles that are not completely relaxed. Under these conditions the α-motor neurons and the neuromuscular junctions are physiologically active.
2. Electrogenic spasm, which is specifically a pathologic involuntary electrogenic contraction.
3. Contracture, which arises endogenously within the muscle fibers independently of electromyographic activity. This concept is of critical importance in the treatment of soft tissue dysfunction in soft tissue pain management, both in sports and in ordinary activity.

Electromyographic recordings can identify electrogenic contraction arising from electrical activity of the motor nerves and muscle fibers, but it cannot identify endogenous contracture of skeletal muscle, because the latter does not depend on the propagation of action potentials in the muscle fiber. Contracture indicates the endogenous shortening of some muscle fibers in the absence of electromyography-initiated α-motor neurons of the spinal cord. The molecular mechanisms of this are explained by Mense and Simons.[2]

When muscle is suddenly mobilized, its stiffness can be reduced immediately without activating any electromyogenic process. This physiologic process is referred to as the *thixotropic property* of skeletal muscle. Human postural muscles do not show sustained electromyographic activity except for occasional minimal corrective bursts to maintain balance. This indicates that the tension in postural muscles that is necessary to maintain posture for long periods is produced by the mechanical properties of muscles and related soft tissues. This property also explains how muscle stiffness is reduced when needling therapy is applied to stiff muscles.

The sudden insertion of the needles may reduce the thixotropic viscosity of the muscles, so that static muscles can perform less restricted motion of the muscles and joints. This property may be related to changes in myoplasmic viscosity and connectin filaments.[3]

Muscle spasm is an involuntary contraction of a muscle or a segment within a muscle that can be caused by irritation of a nerve root, plexus, or peripheral nerve branch. Spasm caused by irritation of the nerve endings within a muscle may be limited to the muscle involved or may spread to other muscles because of reflex pain mechanisms.

Protective spasm may occur as a consequence of injury to an underlying structure, such as a ligament of bone. This type of spasm, which often occurs after a back injury, prevents movement and further irritation of the injured structure.

Segmental muscle spasm is the involuntary contraction of an uninjured segment of a muscle as a result of an injury to the muscle. The contraction of this segment creates tension for the injured part and strains the muscle. Pain associated with tension within the muscle may be limited to that muscle or be more widespread because of reflex or referred pain mechanisms.

Diseased viscera cause muscle spasm in particular locations. This reflex muscle spasm can be observed in patients with cardiac infarction, appendicitis, renal inflammation, and acute pancreatitis. Needling therapy is very effective in relaxing these spasms.

Contracture is the physiologic condition in which all or some of the fibers in a muscle are in a state of contractile activity unaccompanied by electrical activity.[4] Some contractures cause slight or moderate shortening of the muscle, which results in restriction of range of motion. Some cases of contracture are remedied by proper treatment, especially needling therapy. Stretching movements may damage the tissue structures if done improperly. A period of several weeks is usually needed for restoration of mobility in muscle that shows moderate tightness, but with needling treatments, this restoration can be achieved in a few days.

Individuals who spend most of the day in sedentary postures may develop adaptive shortening in the one-joint hip flexors (iliopsoas). Prolonged sitting with the knees partially extended places the foot in a position of plantar flexion and may result in adaptive shortening of the soleus. Wearing high-heeled shoes much of the time may also lead to the development of adaptive shortening of the soleus. Adaptive shortening of postural muscles can affect both balance and alignment. When adaptive shortening continues too long, it may become an irreversible histologic contracture.

Endogenous contracture is the commonest symptom that affects performance in sports, but it is ignored by clinicians in sports medicine. Needling is the most effective therapy for preventing and treating contracture. Detailed knowledge of the molecular mechanisms of contracture and its contribution to trigger-point formation is indispensable for clinicians, and readers are referred to a review and other new materials.[2]

Stiffness is another form of physiologic tension of skeletal muscle. A stiff muscle resists passive movement. Stiffness can be measured by examining the distance moved between origin and insertion during passive movement.

POSTURE AND MUSCLE IMBALANCE

Posture is the state of balance and coordination of musculoskeletal and visceral systems. Skeletal asymmetry is a major source of muscle strain inasmuch as compensatory muscular control is necessary to maintain a working posture and to keep the eyes level. For example, a length discrepancy between the lower limbs causes a chain reaction of muscular overloads of the entire musculoskeletal system. The tilted pelvis requires contraction of the quadratus lumborum muscle to curve the lumbar spine in order to bring the rest of the body over the pelvis. Consequently, the spine above is tilted to the other side. This tilt requires further compensation of neck muscles such as the sternocleidomastoid and upper trapezius. This sustained contraction and overload facilitates the development of trigger points inside the postural muscles, from gastrocnemius through soleus, adductors, iliotibial band, gluteus muscles, piriformis, iliopsoas, quadratus lumborum, muscles of the shoulder girdle, trapezius, and neck muscles.

Any of the muscles in this series can be the cause of a similar chain reaction if they are fatigued, rigid, shortened, or injured. This chain reaction degrades the coordination and function of the musculoskeletal system and creates musculoskeletal pain. It has been shown that trigger points in one muscle may reflexively inhibit the activity of a functionally related muscle in the same region.[5]

Postural pain has both muscular and ligamentous origins. The critical role of muscle overload and muscle strain in posturally induced musculoskeletal pain merits more clinical attention. A trigger-point structure develops within muscles that have been affected by acute episodic overload, by sustained contraction (as in asymmetric posture), by excessive repetition of the same movement, or by being left in a shortened position for a period of time. In addition to the pain caused by muscles, electromyographic data demonstrate that sustained tension on the joint capsule and ligaments can also cause pain.[6] Thus endogenous contracture, as well as a trigger-point structure, develops in joint capsules and ligaments. Knowledge of this physiologic process helps clinicians understand why athletes, and even nonathletic healthy people, need regular integrative systemic dry needling (ISDN) to restore and maintain normal physiology of the soft tissues.

FATIGUE IN MUSCLE AND THE CENTRAL NERVOUS SYSTEM DURING EXERCISE

Athletic fatigue is the inability to maintain the required power output for continuing muscular work at a given intensity. Fatigue has an extremely complex physiologic process. Current understanding of athletic fatigue involves the energy system of the muscles and central nervous system.

Fatigue may result from depletion of glycogen and phosphocreatine in muscles, which reduces ATP production. In short-duration exercise, such as sprinting, the fatigue is caused by increased concentration of H^+ from accumulated lactic acid, which impairs muscle contraction and ATP production. The central nervous system plays a role in most types of fatigue. Some fatigue results from a failure

of neural transmission at a neuromuscular junction, in which the transmission of nerve impulses to the muscle fiber membrane is prevented as a result of reduced synthesis of acetylcholine. The function of enzymes at a neuromuscular junction, such as cholinesterase, can fail because of low concentration or hypoactivity. Abnormal metabolism of intracellular calcium or potassium also can occur, inhibiting muscle relaxation. Perhaps the central nervous system limits exercise performance as a protective mechanism. Perceived fatigue usually precedes physiologic fatigue. Muscular and neural fatigue can be effectively reversed if a combination of procedures is used, including rest, nutrition therapy, and needling therapy for the fatigued muscles. If muscle fatigue is not properly treated, affected individuals have a higher risk of injury.

MUSCLE SORENESS: DELAYED-ONSET MUSCLE SORENESS (DOMS)

Muscle soreness is one of the many common symptoms that can be successfully treated by dry needling, even when the usual physical procedures such as massage, stretching exercises, or manipulation have had no effect. A sore muscle becomes inflamed, shortened, and weak, and this can lead to tendinitis, avulsion of muscular attachment, or abnormal bone growth. Early treatment by needling, especially right after exercise, is necessary and very effective for preventing the injury of muscle and soft tissues.

Muscle soreness results from exhaustive, high-intensity, or repetitive exercise. Mild muscle soreness is usually felt during and immediately after exercise; then a more intense soreness is felt a day or two later and may last for weeks (Fig. 5-3).

Acute muscle soreness during and immediately after exercise can result from accumulation of the end products of exercise, such as H^+, and also from tissue edema, which is caused by fluid shifting from blood plasma into the tissue when venous and lymphatic circulation become insufficient. Some acute soreness disappears within a few hours after exercise, and some can last for days or weeks if ignored or not properly treated.

Muscle soreness that is not felt until a day or two after heavy exercise is referred to as *delayed-onset muscle soreness* (DOMS). According to the

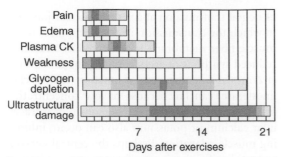

FIGURE 5-3 The delayed responses to exercise-induced muscle damage. These valuable data show that, under natural conditions, more than 3 weeks is necessary for complete histologic recovery from the ultrastructural damage (microtrauma or microtear).

author's clinical experience, the muscles that will later exhibit DOMS are already more sensitive to needling therapy than are those that will not. Thus needling therapy provides both early diagnosis and treatment of DOMS. The author has also observed that if the athlete receives ISDN treatment immediately or within 1 day after the exercise or competition, the DOMS symptoms are greatly reduced or even not felt by the athlete.

Knowledge of DOMS is limited, but almost all current research has demonstrated a connection between DOMS and eccentric muscle activity.[7] The levels of several specific muscle enzymes in blood, including myoglobin, increase from 2 to 10 times their normal levels after intensive exercise. This suggests that some structural damage may occur in muscle fibers after heavy training. Studies[8] support the idea that these changes might indicate some degree of muscle tissue breakdown. Examination of tissue from the leg muscles of marathon runners has revealed remarkable damage to the muscle fibers after intensive training and competition. Electron micrographs provide evidence of damage to the membrane of the muscle fibers and other cellular microstructural damage, such as Z-discs, after marathon running. Experts believe that this damage is responsible in part for localized muscle pain, tenderness, and swelling associated with DOMS.

DOMS also triggers an inflammatory reaction. The white blood cell count tends to increase after activities that induce muscle soreness; accordingly, some investigators believe that soreness results from inflammatory reactions in the muscle. In fact, substances released from injured muscle can act as attractants, initiating typical inflammatory processes. Monocytes in muscle are activated by the injury and provide chemical signals to circulating inflammatory cells. Neutrophils invade the injury site and release cytokines. Cytokines are immunoregulatory substances, which attract and activate additional inflammatory cells. Neutrophils possibly also release oxygen free radicals that can damage cell membranes. Macrophages invade the damaged muscle fibers and phagocytize debris. After the dead tissues are removed, muscle regeneration starts to replace the injured cells.

It is clear now that muscle soreness results from injury or damage to the muscle fiber and possibly the plasmalemma.[9] This damage sets up a chain of events at the cellular level to activate the repair process, involving energy sources, inflammatory reactions, and other molecular mechanisms. The precise cause of skeletal muscle damage and the mechanisms of repair, however, are not well understood.

Edema, or the accumulation of fluids in the muscular compartment, also can lead to DOMS. This edema is probably the result of muscle injury. An accumulation of interstitial or intracellular fluid increases the tissue fluid pressure within the muscle compartment, which irritates pain receptors within the muscle.

DOMS and related edema result in failure in the excitation-contraction coupling process and loss of contractile protein, which reduce the force-generating capacity of the affected muscles. Failure in excitation-contraction coupling appears to be the most important, particularly during the first 5 days after injury. Muscle glycogen resynthesis is also impaired when a muscle is damaged. Resynthesis is not affected for the first 6 to 12 hours after exercise, but it gradually stops completely as the muscle undergoes repair. This energy redistribution reduces the fuel-storage capacity of the injured muscle and makes it weak, such that muscle retraining may be needed. Maximal force-generating capacity gradually returns over days or weeks.

EXERCISE-ASSOCIATED MUSCLE CRAMPS

Athletes may experience cramp in skeletal muscles during the height of competition, immediately after competition, or at night during sleep. Investigators have not been able to pinpoint the cause of muscle cramping. Most exercise-induced or exercise-associated muscle cramps are unrelated to disease or medical disorder. Exercise-associated muscle cramps have been defined as painful, spasmodic, involuntary contractions of skeletal muscles that occur during or immediately after exercise.[10] Nocturnal muscle cramps may or may not be associated with exercise.

It was believed that muscle cramps were caused by disturbances in fluid and electrolyte balance, particularly sodium balance, in association with high rates of sweating, as is the case with heat cramps. This may be true for some exercise-associated muscle cramps, and more recent research suggests that these cramps result from sustained α-motor neuron activity, which is caused by aberrant control at the spinal level.[10] Muscle fatigue appears to cause this lack of control through an effect on both Golgi tendon spindles and muscle spindles. Muscle spindle activity increases and tendon organ activity decreases.

OVERREACHING

Overreaching is a systematic attempt to intentionally overstress the body, allowing the body to adapt to the training stimulus beyond the level of adaptation attained during a period of acute overload.[11] After this training strategy is adopted, there is a brief decrease in performance lasting for days or weeks, followed by improved physiologic function and physical performance. The difficulty with this kind of training is achieving its positive results while avoiding possible negative effects in the form of overtraining symptoms (described in the next section), recovery from which may take months or years.

Athletes who adopt overreaching training should consider a supporting program, especially regular dry needling therapy, to reduce the physiologic stress to the musculoskeletal system and other systems as well.

OVERTRAINING SYNDROME

Overtraining, in athletes, is an excessive stress that may produce systemic pathologic consequences, recovery from which requires months or years. Some athletes may develop overtraining syndrome during periods of intense overload training. They may experience a sudden unexplained decline in performance, physiologic dysfunction, or psychologic depression that extends over weeks, months, or even years. The precise causes for such breakdowns are not fully understood, and individual symptoms vary by the type of training. These symptoms cannot be remedied by the procedures normally used for nonpathologic fatigue. The nonpathologic fatigue that may follow one or more exhausting training sessions is usually relieved by a few days of reduced training, or rest, plus a carbohydrate-rich diet.

Symptoms related to overtraining syndrome are subjective and identifiable only after the individual's performance and physiologic function have deteriorated. This makes it very difficult to recognize that a deterioration in performance is caused by overtraining. The underlying causes of overtraining syndrome are often a complex combination of emotional and physiologic imbalances. Primary signs and symptoms[12] may include

- General fatigue
- Loss of muscular strength, coordination, and working capacity
- Change in appetite
- Weight loss
- Sleep disturbance
- Irritability, restlessness, excitability, or anxiousness
- Loss of motivation and vigor
- Lack of concentration
- Feelings of depression
- Lack of appreciation for things that normally are enjoyable

Hans Selye,[13] the founder of stress research, noted as long ago as 1956 that a person's tolerance of stress can break down as often from a sudden increase in anxiety as from an increase in physical distress. The emotional demands of competition, the desire to win, the fear of failure, unrealistically high goals, and the expectations of others can be sources of intolerable emotional stress, which can result in a loss of competitive desire and enthusiasm for training. Armstrong and VanHeest[12] made the important observation that overtraining syndrome and clinical depression share similar signs and symptoms, brain structures, neurotransmitters, endocrine pathways, and immune responses. This indicates alterations in the nervous, endocrine, and immune systems in the affected athletes. Physiologic symptoms accompanying the decline in performance often reflect changes in systems that are controlled by either the sympathetic or parasympathetic branches of autonomic nervous system.

Sympathetic symptoms from overtraining may include:

- Increased resting heart rate and blood pressure
- Elevated basal metabolic rate
- Loss of appetite
- Decreased body mass
- Sleep disturbance
- Emotional instability

Athletes who emphasize highly intensive resistance-training methods are more prone to sympathetic symptoms.

Endurance athletes are more likely to suffer from parasympathetic overtraining, and their performance decrements differ markedly from those associated with sympathetic overtraining. These parasympathetic overtraining symptoms may include the following:

- Early onset of fatigue
- Decreased resting heart rate and decreased resting blood pressure
- Rapid heart rate recovery after exercise

The symptoms of overtraining syndrome are particular to the different training regimens of different sports. Thus the concepts of "intensity-related" and "volume-related" overtraining are used to differentiate specific training stressors that produce unique signs and symptoms.[14]

Of the two conditions, sympathetic overtraining is the one whose symptoms are the most frequently observed. However, some people who are not overtrained develop symptoms associated with the autonomic nervous system. For this reason, the presence of these symptoms cannot always be assumed to be result of overtraining.

The endocrine system is definitely involved in the response to overtraining stressors. Athletes with overtraining may show altered blood concentrations of hormone during periods of overloading, which is suggestive of a reaction of endocrine function in response to excessive stress. When volume or intensity of training increases, the blood concentrations of thyroxine and testosterone usually decrease, and that of cortisol increases. The ratio of testosterone to cortisol is thought to regulate anabolic process in recovery; thus a change in this ratio is considered an important sign related to overtraining syndrome. Decreased testosterone coupled with increased cortisol result in more protein catabolism than anabolism in the cells. Furthermore, most overtraining studies have been conducted on aerobically trained endurance athletes. Hormonal modification during overtraining is complicated, and more research is needed for its interpretation for different individuals and types of training.[14] Many experts believe that no blood marker can conclusively define overtraining syndrome.

Armstrong and VanHeest[12] proposed that overtraining stressors activate the following two predominant hormonal axes involved in the body's response to stressors: the sympathetic-adrenal-medullary (SAM) axis, which involves the sympathetic branch of the autonomic nervous system, and the hypothalamic-pituitary-adrenocortical (HPA) axis.

This simplified outline is illustrated in Figure 5-4, which shows the interactions of the brain and immune system with these two axes. Thus it is highly likely that brain neurotransmitters play an important role in overtraining syndrome. Levels of serotonin, a major neurotransmitter, are elevated and therefore play a significant role in overtraining, but plasma concentrations of this important neurotransmitter do not accurately reflect those concentrations in the brain. In support of Armstrong and VanHeest's[12] model, a major role played by cytokines in overtraining syndrome has been proposed[15]: Trauma associated with overtraining in skeletal muscles, bones, and joints causes inflammation and elevates levels of circulating cytokines, which are responsible for the inflammatory response

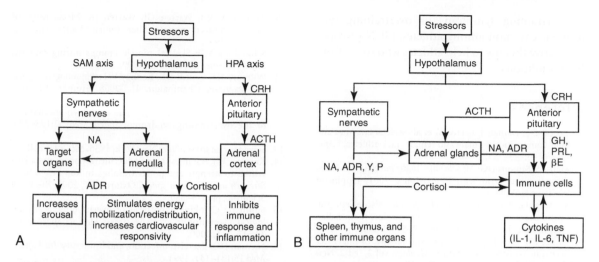

FIGURE 5-4 A, The hypothalamus mediates the stress of overtraining through two axes: the hypothalamic-pituitory-adrenocortical (HPA) axis and sympathetic-adrenal-medullary (SAM) axis. **B,** The brain-immune system interactions mediate the overtraining responses, and the cytokines play a potentially major role in the physiologic processes. *ACTH,* Adrenocorticotropin; *ADR,* adrenaline (epinephrine); *CRH,* corticotropin releasing hormone; *βE,* β-endorphin; *GH,* growth hormone; *IL-1,* interleukin-1; *IL-6,* interleukin-6; *NA,* noradrenaline (norepinephrine); *P,* substance P; *PRL,* prolactin; *TNF,* tumor necrosis factor; *Y,* neuropeptide Y.

to infection and injury. Excessive musculoskeletal stress from training, if accompanied by insufficient rest and recovery, sets up a cascade of events whereby a local acute inflammatory response evolves into chronic inflammation and eventually into systemic inflammation. Systemic inflammation activates circulating monocytes, which can then synthesize large quantities of cytokines. Cytokines act on the brain and body functions and induce symptoms consistent with those of the overtraining syndrome.

Overtraining, as a stress, certainly affects the normal function of the immune system. This system provides defense against invading bacteria, parasites, viruses, and tumor cells and also actively participates in tissue regeneration after injury. It depends on the actions of specialized cells, such as lymphocytes, granulocytes, and macrophages, as well as antibodies, for neutralizing foreign invaders, the pathogens that might cause illness.

Overtraining suppresses normal immune function, which increases susceptibility to infections and slows down both recovery from fatigue and the healing of injuries. This immune suppression is characterized by abnormally low concentration of both lymphocytes and antibodies. Invading organisms or endogenous conditions, such as bacterial flora and viruses inside the body, are more likely to cause illness when concentrations of active immune cells are low. Also, intense exercise during illness may decrease the ability to fight off infection and increase the risk of more serious complications.[16]

Overtraining syndrome is a systemic and complex issue that is difficult to diagnose and difficult to treat effectively with conventional procedures. With ISDN, therapy, this syndrome may be prevented and treated more effectively, especially in conjunction with other therapeutic procedures.

SUMMARY

Dry needling acupuncture is soft tissue therapy that normalizes the pathophysiology of soft tissues, leading to balance in the musculoskeletal system and the restoration of homeostasis. Thus it is critical for clinicians to understand the physiologic and pathologic processes of working muscles during athletic training and when those muscles are injured.

Overtraining symptoms or overtraining syndrome is common among athletes. ISDN provides an effective therapy to help athletes who suffer from these conditions.

References

1. Costill DL, Daniels J, Evens W, et al: Skeletal enzymes and fiber composition in male and female track athletes, *J Appl Physiol* 40:149–154, 1976.
2. Mense S, Simons DG: *Muscle pain: understanding its nature, diagnosis, and treatment*, Philadelphia, 2001, Lippincott Williams & Wilkins.
3. Mutungi G, Ranatunga KW: The viscous, viscoelastic and elastic characteristics of resting fast and slow mammalian (rat) muscle fibers, *J Physiol* 496:827–836, 1996.
4. Layzer RB: Muscle pain cramps, and fatigue. In Engel AG, Franzini-Armstrong C, editors: *Myology*, vol 2, ed 2, New York, 1994, McGraw-Hill, pp 1754–1768.
5. Headley BJ: Chronic pain management. In O'Sullivan SB, Schmitz TJ, editors: *Physical rehabilitation: assessment and treatment*, ed 3, Philadelphia, 1994, FA Davis, Chap 27.
6. Harms-Ringdahl K, Ekholm J: Intensity and character of pain and muscular activity levels elicited by maintained extreme flexion position of the lower-cervical–upper-thoracic spine, *Scand J Rehab Med* 18:117–126, 1986.
7. Schwane JA, Johnson SR, Vandenakker CB, et al: Delayed-onset muscular soreness and plasma CPK and LDH activities after downhill running, *Med Sci Sports Exerc* 15:51–56, 1983.
8. Wilmore JH, Costill DL, Kenney WL: *Physiology of sports and exercise*, Champaign, IL, 2008, Human Kinetics, p 41.
9. Armstrong RB, Warren GI, Warren JA: Mechanisms of exercise-induced muscle fiber injury, *Sports Med* 12:184–207, 1991.
10. Schwellnus MP: Skeletal muscle cramps during exercise, *Phys Sportsmed* 27:109–115, 1999.
11. Wilmore JH, Costill DL, Kenney WL: *Physiology of sports and exercise*, Champaign, IL, 2008, Human Kinetics, p 301.
12. Armstrong IE, VanHeest JL: The unknown mechanism of the overtraining syndrome, *Sports Med* 32:185–209, 2002.
13. Selye H: *The stress of life*, New York, 1956, McGraw-Hill.
14. Kraemer WJ, Ratamess NA: Endocrine responses and adaptations to strength and power training. In Komi PV, editor: *Strength and power in sports*, Oxford, UK, 2003, Blackwell Scientific, pp 379–380.
15. Smith IL: Cytokine hypothesis of overtraining: a physiological adaptation to excessive stress? *Med Sci Sports Exerc* 32:317–331, 2000.
16. Nieman DC: Exercise, infection, and immunity, *Int J Sports Med* 15:131–141, 1994.

Additional Readings

Wilmore JH, Costill DL, Kenney WL: *Physiology of sports and exercise*, ed 4, Champaign, Ill, 2008. Human Kinetics, Chap 13.

Chapter 13, "Training for Sport," is an excellent chapter that presents and discusses the optimal training model and overtraining syndrome with recent research data. This chapter will be an indispensable bridge between the understanding of overtraining pathophysiology and the clinical practice of treating overtraining symptoms with ISDN.

CHAPTER 6

Clinical Mechanisms of Integrative Systemic Dry Needling

In the practice of integrative systemic dry needling (ISDN), nothing is more important than understanding the biologic mechanisms of needling.

ISDN is a unique therapy because it entails the use of fine needles to inoculate minute intrusive "traumas," or lesions, into soft tissues to activate self-healing processes. When a needle is inserted into the human body, it breaks the skin—the first defense line of the immune system—and then inoculates lesions into all the soft tissues it encounters, including muscle fibers, nerve endings, blood vessels, fascias, tendons, ligaments, and even periosteum. Lesions remain when the needle is removed. The human biologic system activates all possible physiologic mechanisms to repair the lesions inoculated by needling.

The repair starts with an inflammatory reaction to destroy and eliminate the tissue that is lesioned and dead as a result of needling, and then genetic machinery is activated to synthesize new tissue to replace what is damaged. These processes require coordination of all physiologic systems, particularly the nervous, immune, endocrine, and cardiovascular systems, involving both central and peripheral mechanisms. These are built-in biologic survival mechanisms. No matter where the needles are inserted—in the face, neck, arm or leg—the local biologic mechanisms are the same (Fig. 6-1). Local symptoms, such as soft tissue pain in the shoulder, or nonlocal symptoms, such as headache, may respond to needling in the arms or in the legs. Because of this, ISDN therapy is nonspecific. Symptoms of different pathologic processes are improved or cured by the same "lesion" mechanism. However, different locations of the needling may result in somewhat different levels of therapeutic efficacy. For example, in the treatment of frozen shoulder, needling the painful shoulder area is more effective than needling the legs in most cases, although it has been observed clinically that needling the legs, the scalp, the ears,

or other part of the body can provide relief in the shoulder in some cases as a result of systemic reflex mechanisms.

These mechanisms used to be puzzling to medical practitioners and are still so today to those who compare ISDN therapy with pharmaceutical therapy. A sound physiologic basis has already been established by distinguished scientists and clinicians for why and how ISDN works. Pomeranz,[1] a prominent researcher in the field of acupuncture analgesia, said, "We know more about acupuncture analgesia than about many chemical drugs in routine use."

Nevertheless, knowledge of the complex biologic processes that underlie the apparently simple procedure of needling is still inadequate. To guide clinical practice, this chapter focuses on peripheral mechanisms. These mechanisms can be observed, predicted, and proved by any clinician who practices ISDN.

The fact that central mechanisms are not discussed in this book does not mean they are unimportant. On the contrary: They are critical in ISDN because the central regulations control and coordinate peripheral mechanisms. Needling signals are brought to the central nervous system (CNS) by sensory nerve fibers, first to the spinal cord and then to different spinal levels; to the brainstem, the thalamus, and the hypothalamus; and up to the cortex (Fig. 6-2).

Needling first stimulates the somatosensory system, when a needle punctures the skin and penetrates to the deep tissues and leaves lesions there. This system has many tasks ranging from the input for motor reflex to the higher orders of perception such as cognitive comprehension, perception of nociception and pain, and emotion.

Needling induces the coordination of all physiologic systems. Today with functional magnetic resonance imaging (fMRI) (Fig. 6-3), it is possible to

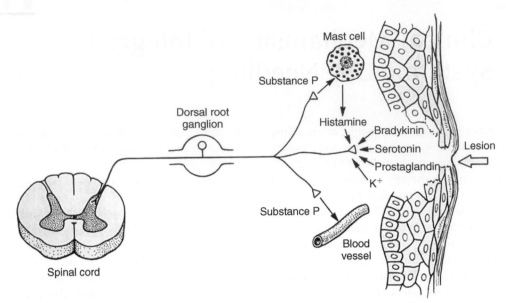

FIGURE 6-1 Lesion mechanisms of needling therapy. Needling introduces lesion into soft tissues, stimulates peptide-containing C fiber, and elicits axon reflex response. The damaged tissues release chemical signaling factors, as shown.

precisely locate the part of the brain that is activated by the needling. However, knowledge of how to interpret these images is still developing. A detailed discussion of central mechanisms is beyond the scope of this book, and for this reason, readers may refer to up-to-date research publications for more information.

In conclusion, ISDN is soft tissue therapy. In fact many different diseases, especially chronic diseases, either involve or are caused by soft tissue dysfunction. It is very important for clinical practice that the nature of soft tissue dysfunction be well understood.

WHY PATIENTS RESPOND DIFFERENTLY TO THE SAME ISDN TREATMENT

As mentioned previously, ISDN activates the built-in survival mechanism of the human body to achieve self-healing for many different pathologic conditions. Thus ISDN is effective for any symptoms that can be partially or completely healed through the biologic regulatory mechanisms of the body.

Humans inherit self-healing potential for biologic survival. However, this potential to self-heal is considerably affected by stress level, medical his-

tory, nutrition, and lifestyle, as well as by genetic endowment and age. Each person, therefore, has a different self-healing capacity, and this potential for self-healing is also changing dynamically. It deteriorates in people who abuse their health, and it improves in those who take good care of themselves. The efficacy of ISDN therapy, therefore, depends on two factors:

1. The level of self-healing potential of the body
2. The ability of the particular symptoms or diseases to heal

Patients' individual healing potentials are different, as are the status of their symptoms and the type of disease. This is why different patients respond differently to the same ISDN treatment. For two patients with the same medical diagnosis, patient A may enjoy miraculous results from ISDN therapy because of his healthy healing potential, and patient B may be disappointed after many sessions of treatment due to his weak and impaired healing potential.

Using an innovative, well-defined, and reliable evaluation procedure presented in this book, clinicians can categorize patients into four groups of responders to ISDN: excellent, good, average, and weak. Dung[2] discovered these important clinical

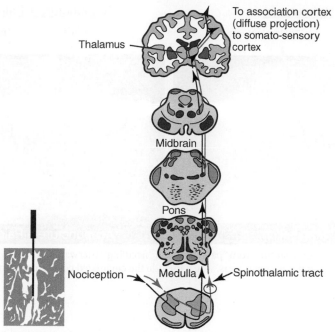

FIGURE 6-2 Needling stimulation brings physical and chemical signals all the way from the needling site to the cortex.

phenomena after research in which he examined more than 15,000 patients (personal communication).

Modern medical diagnosis can provide the necessary information about the nature of the symptoms and diseases, but individual self-healing potential is often ignored in medical practice.

NEEDLING IS SOFT TISSUE THERAPY

Clinicians have observed that needling therapy can be used with some efficacy in almost all known pathologic conditions, from soft tissue pain to Parkinson's disease, cancer, and even acquired immune deficiency syndrome (AIDS), with varying results. Needling therapy does not reverse many of these conditions but is able to improve some symptoms for some time. This merits specific clarification.

One of the most important concepts in ISDN medicine is that the nonspecific mechanisms of needling do not directly target any particular disease. Conventional medicine is designed to treat specific pathologic conditions with specific diagnoses and procedures. In almost all clinical cases, the benefit of ISDN therapy is the normalization of soft tissue function. The only exception is the occasional use of needling for anesthesia during surgery, which is not considered in this book.

Soft tissue encompasses muscles, connective tissues, and nervous tissues. In this book, the term is used to include muscles, ligaments, tendons, bursae, capsules, fasciae, peripheral nerves, blood and lymphatic vessels, and viscera with their associated soft tissue such as pleura or ligaments and nerves. The CNS is also considered soft tissue by some authorities. Soft tissue is distributed all over the body and accounts for 50% of body mass. It plays a role in all human activity, including mental activity (which is aided by blood vessels, for example). Therefore all pathologic conditions understandably involve soft tissue, and in many cases, the soft tissue is itself the pathologic focus of the symptoms or disease: for example, soft tissue pain in sport and daily activity.

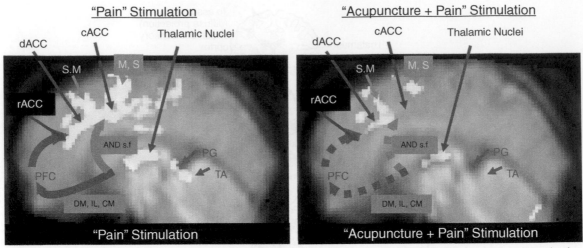

FIGURE 6-3 Cortical activation resulting from "pain" first and "needling" afterwards. A significant decrease in activation is seen in most of the pain signal processing areas, which include the cingulated cortex and the thalamus.

When needling is used for cases of drug abuse, it does not provide any pharmaceutical effect against the drug itself, but it reduces the tension in soft tissue that results from drug withdrawal.

The experience in Chinese acupuncture of more than two millennia of practice, as well as modern medical evidence, confirms that needling promotes normalization of dysfunctional soft tissue and restores homeostasis of biologic systems.

Soft tissue dysfunction manifests in the following symptoms:

- Inflammation
- Contracture of contractible soft tissues such as muscles, fascia, tendons, and ligaments
- Adhesion between different soft tissues
- The formation of scar tissue within the same tissue and between different tissues after chronic inflammation or injury
- Blood and lymphatic conditions such as deficient microcirculation and edema
- Trophic conditions of soft tissues
- Imbalance of musculoskeletal systems and inhibition of reflex

All human diseases involve soft tissue dysfunction to a certain extent. Many clinical symptoms are related to or produced by compensatory changes in soft tissue. The efficacy of medical intervention in treating many external injuries and internal dysfunction depends on how much the pathologic process of soft tissue—such as inflammation, contracture, adhesion, trophic deficiency, scarring, and blockage of local microcirculation—can be remedied. Chronic soft tissue dysfunction is a pathologic condition resulting from all these pathologic processes in soft tissue after acute or chronic injury. Compensatory adjustment may occur to enhance survival by sacrificing systemic homeostasis. For example, a person with a shorter lower limb continues to function by adjusting musculoskeletal balance. This compensatory adjustment favors immediate survival but can cause ongoing long-term homeostatic imbalance.

Thus soft tissue dysfunction and injury can happen at any time and in any environment as a result of external insults or internal imbalance, such as infection, physical invasions, overuse, cumulative injuries, diet abnormalities, internal pathologic conditions, improper or aggressive medical procedures, emotional stress, or changes in climate. This is why the incidence of soft tissue disease in human beings is so high.

After proper treatment of some acute dysfunctions of soft tissue, the tissue will heal and resume normal functioning. Some dysfunctions, however, may develop into chronic conditions. In some cases, dysfunctions or injuries of soft tissue start as chronic diseases. After injuries such as external physical tearing or internal tissue ulcer or inflammation, the result may be contracture, adhesion, scarring, and blockage of local circulation, tissue deformation, all of which lead to compensatory adjustment. The compensatory changes may become irreversible; therefore the dysfunctional soft tissue plays a major role in creating chronic symptoms and gradually sensitizing the CNS. Thus the term *chronic soft tissue syndrome* is used to describe a variety of chronic conditions.

TYPES OF SOFT TISSUE INJURY

Tissue destruction from physical deformation, tearing, breakage, necrosis, and blockage of circulation, which result in dysfunction and injury of soft tissue, can be classified as the following types:

1. Violent physical injuries: Crushing, beating, falling, compressing, and pushing and pulling are the common sources of contusions in body-contact sports.
2. Cumulative injuries: These are injuries caused by frequent or repeated actions of the same tissue.
3. Emotional stress: This can cause dilation or constriction of blood vessels and strong contraction or cramp in muscles, which results in damage to blood vessels. Emotional depression induces a slowing of humoral and blood circulation, which results in retention of fluid. This may lead to swelling or enlargement of tissues and organs, which may compress other tissues or organs, causing injury.
4. Unconscious injuries: These are the barely noticeable minor physical injuries of daily life.
5. Overloading fatigue: This type of injury includes overexertion (injury to limbs and muscles), overeating (injury to digestive organs), and overexercising (excessive physical training).
6. Injuries from chemical toxins: These include alcohol and drug abuse, smoking, overmedication, and exposure to pollutants.
7. Injuries caused by excess weight and obesity: These include cardiovascular injury and respiratory complications.
8. Postsurgical injuries: These include flesh wounds, internal bleeding, and nosocomial infection.
9. Disease-related injuries: An example of such a disease is rheumatoid arthritis, which causes inflammation, edema, and necrosis of soft tissues.
10. Environmentally related injuries: These injuries are caused by burns or temperature extremes.
11. Injuries caused by abnormal physiology: These injuries arise from imbalance between the sympathetic and parasympathetic nervous systems.

PATHOLOGIC PROCESS OF SOFT TISSUE DYSFUNCTION AND INJURY

Soft tissue dysfunctions—inflammation, contracture, adhesion, scarring, blockage of circulation, atrophy, and musculoskeletal imbalance—lead to further pathologic consequences.

Inflammation

Inflammation, or inflammatory response, is the physiologic process of local accumulation of fluid, plasma proteins, and white blood cells that is initiated as a result of physical injury, infection, or a local immune response. *Acute inflammation* refers to early and often transient episodes, whereas chronic inflammation occurs when the infection persists or when there is autoimmune disease. Inflammation is a built-in survival mechanism to protect the system from foreign invasion and to promote self-healing after tissue injury. Nevertheless, inflammation may get out of control, which results in pain or injury to tissues. Clinical evidence shows that ISDN needling brings inflammation down to the normal level at which it can assist in the process of healing. It should be noted that ISDN does not suppress inflammation but brings it to normal physiologic level.

Contracture and Cramp

Contracture is muscular contraction without CNS control, as defined in Chapter 5. After initial acute injuries, some soft tissues (muscles, tendons, ligaments, fasciae) become contracted and shortened as a protection against further injuries. Some contracture of soft tissue is described as *cramp* when it occurs in the context of exercise. Muscular contracture leads to contracture of related tissue such as fasciae, tendons, and ligaments.

Adhesion

Adhesion is scar-like tissue that forms between two surfaces inside the body as a pathologic consequence of soft tissue injuries. There are two types of soft tissue adhesion: one caused by external physical impact and the other by internal pathologic insult. Adhesions that develop in the limbs and spine cause more symptoms because of the greater amount of physical motion in those areas, and fewer symptoms are observed for adhesions in the face and abdomen.

Adhesion Caused by External Physical Impact

Violent force, cumulative stress, minor unnoticed impacts in everyday routine, overloading injuries, overweight conditions, and emotional abnormalities (stress or depression) cause injury of soft tissue such as broken capillaries and fibers. During recovery from these types of injury, soft tissues such as muscle, ligaments, blood vessels, nerves, and bones may adhere to each other.

Adhesion Caused by Internal Pathologic Insults

This type of adhesion can be caused by internal pathologic processes, invasive infections, environmental conditions, and postsurgical injuries.

Adhesion cannot be detected by instruments, and so it is often overlooked by medical professionals.

Scarring

External and internal scars are formed during the healing of soft tissue if the injury is severe enough or involves large areas. Internal scars are often pathologic factors for chronic soft tissue dysfunction.

Blockage of Circulation

Soft tissue injury may often include damage such as breakage of blood and lymph vessels, tearing of fibers, bleeding, and fluid retention. During the healing process, scarring and fibrillation can block

the normal circulation channels, which results in the retention of fluid in one area and reduced circulation in another. This condition can become the cause of chronic soft tissue dysfunction.

Atrophy

Atrophy results in abnormal anatomic structure. After inflammation and injuries, blood supply to the local tissues can be greatly reduced, causing trophic deficiency. With reduced exercise, the soft tissues such as muscles and tendons gradually deform.

Musculoskeletal Imbalance

Musculoskeletal imbalance can be the consequence of any or all the kinds of soft tissue dysfunction just mentioned. In the presence of these conditions, the biomechanical functioning of the musculoskeletal system and the joints becomes unbalanced, resulting in bad posture and a limited range of motion.

HISTOLOGIC FEATURES OF SOFT TISSUE INJURIES

Contracture

Contracture is a self-protective mechanism of soft tissue. It may be reversible or irreversible. When the shortening of the tissue is within the physiologic limits and is caused by overuse, overloading, misuse, or physical insults, it is reversible. Contracture from severe injuries, in which substantial amounts of tissue are destroyed, are irreversible. This may be the result of physical injury or surgery. During the self-healing process that follows surgical procedures, adhesion and scars are formed, and contractures resulting from these processes may be irreversible. For example, a leg may be permanently shortened after severe injury of the hamstring muscles or tendons.

Adhesion

During the self-healing that follows acute or chronic injuries, the regeneration of tissue can cause adhesion between neighboring tissues. This occurs between epimysia, endomysia, tendons and neighboring tissues, ligaments, and joint capsules. It may also be found between periosteum and nerve and neighboring tissues and between organs and related soft tissues. It is very important to prevent the formation of adhesions during the healing process.

Scarring and Fibrogenesis

After injury, self-healing proceeds in three stages: inflammation, cellular regeneration and differentiation, and tissue replacement. During this process, primordial cells and fibroblast cells are produced. They secrete fibrogen for the construction of tissue fibers. Usually the formation of connective fibers predominates over formation of muscle, capillary, and capsule tissues. Some of this scar tissue will be absorbed and some will persist, which may cause permanent dysfunction of the organs and soft tissue.

Circulatory Deficiency or Blockage

Contracture, adhesion, and scar tissue all disturb local microcirculation, both blood and lymph, which can cause ischemia, hypoxia, water retention, and accumulation of wastes. To improve microcirculation, it is equally important to relieve contracture and to reduce adhesion and the formation of scar tissue.

THREE STAGES OF SELF-HEALING OF SOFT TISSUE AFTER INJURY

After injury, soft tissues start the process of self-healing, which takes place in three stages:

1. Inflammation and immune reaction: The coagulation process and immune reaction release active biologic factors, such as platelet factors, and activated immune cells, such as white blood cells and macrophages, which digest the injured tissues.
2. Cellular regeneration and differentiation: Primordial cells regenerate and then differentiate into the same type of cells as the injured tissues.
3. Reconstruction of the injured tissues: Endothelial cells move to the injured parts to form the tissues and capillaries.

OSTEOFASCIAL COMPARTMENT SYNDROME

Soft tissue injuries increase the pressure in the space between the bone and fascia as a result of edema, contracture of soft tissues, and the consequential deficiency of circulation. Neighboring soft tissues such as nerves, blood vessels, and lymph vessels are adversely affected by the increased physical pressure. Edema, hypoxia, ischemia, tissue contracture, and necrosis may follow. Clinical data show that osteofascial compartment syndrome (OFCS) occurs when the compartmental pressure increases to 30 mm Hg. ISDN provides considerable relief in most cases of OFCS because of its efficacy in reducing edema.

PATHOLOGIC CONDITIONS OF HUMAN ORGANS INVOLVE CHRONIC SOFT TISSUE DYSFUNCTION

Chronic soft tissue syndrome is not limited to musculoskeletal tissue. Compensatory dysfunctions such as contracture, adhesion, scarring, and blockage of circulation also develop after visceral injuries. Listed here are some examples, but underlying these different types of visceral pathology is the same chronic soft tissue syndrome caused by inflammation, contracture, adhesion, scarring, and blockage of local microcirculation. The following information was collected by the author from research performed in China:

- Heart: Many cardiovascular diseases involve contracture or hypertrophy of cardiac muscle fibers, adhesion of fibers, scar tissue, and blockage of circulation.
- Lungs: Emphysema creates adhesion of alveoli and blockage of circulation.
- Stomach: Gastritis or gastric ulcer results in contracture and adhesion of muscle cells with the mucous membrane, accompanied by scars and blockage of circulation.
- Intestine: Chronic inflammation produces contracture and adhesion of soft tissues with scar formation and blockage of circulation.
- Urinary bladder: Chronic inflammation causes minor ulcers, which result in contracture and blockage of microcirculation.

BONE SPURS AND SOFT TISSUE DYSFUNCTION

Abnormal bone growth is often related to soft tissue dysfunction. Contracture, or shortened tissue, usually applies increased physical force to the bone. This results in an abnormal growth of bone material to adjust to the increased pulling force on the bone surface. In addition, shortening of the soft tissues, adhesions, scars, and blockage cause changes in the biochemical environment, and this type of biophysical and biochemical abnormality leads to abnormal growth of bone tissue.

ELECTRICAL ACUPUNCTURE

Electrical acupuncture stimulates specific peripheral nerves, which send strong impulses to the spinal cord and brain. With different stimulating frequencies, electrical acupuncture can induce different endorphins at different levels of the CNS. Endorphins have many physiologic functions, such as modulating pain mechanisms to relieve pain, relaxing cardiovascular systems, and improving immune activity by reducing physiologic stress. Electrical acupuncture stimulation, therefore, results in accelerated self-healing.

Endorphin mechanisms are nonspecific. Electrical acupuncture and needling stimulate the secretion of endorphins; however, chiropractic manipulation, massage, physical exercise, meditation, and taking a vacation can also have the same result to some degree. Nevertheless, electrical acupuncture provides special clinical mechanisms that greatly enhance the effects of ISDN. When a needle is inserted into damaged or unhealthy soft tissue, the needling process and the needling-induced lesions activate an anti-inflammatory response, relax the soft tissue contracture, and enable tissue regeneration. During insertion and removal of the needles, the tissue is only slightly stretched. Manipulating the needle can apply more of this tissue-stretching effect.[3]

If scar tissue from adhesion has already developed, more tissue stretching is needed to reduce it. The rhythmic contraction and vibration created by the electrical current facilitates the separation of tissue that is in the process of becoming adhered or has already adhered. This rhythmic contraction may also have the effect of loosening and breaking up scar tissue. In summary, the clinical value of electrical acupuncture stimulation is that it can reduce adhesion and prevent the formation of scar tissue, as well as improve blood and lymphatic circulation by subjecting the muscles to passive movement.

Electrical acupuncture should be applied cautiously. Because forceful movement is induced in the muscles, there is a potential for overcontraction, which can cause damage to muscle fibers. Such contraction, by applying excessive tension to the origin and insertion tendons, can lead to tendinitis or even breakage of the tendon fibers. The contracting muscles can cause physical impact between components of a joint, producing pain and damaging the joint structure. Strong muscle contraction even can break the bone. In view of these possibilities, electrical acupuncture should be used in a conservative manner with new patients: low intensity with minimal observable motion of muscle. It should start with frequencies of 2 to 10 Hz for short periods, such as 3 to 5 minutes. Once the patient feels comfortable with electrical acupuncture, the parameters can be modified.

NEEDLING SENSATION

Needling is a process of nociceptive stimulation with both mechanical and biochemical effects. Mechanical effects include physical pressure on and disturbance of the nociceptors of the sensory nerve endings. The biochemical effects are needle-induced neurogenic inflammation and the secretion of neuropeptides from nociceptive nerve endings and tissues, substance P, bradykinin, prostaglandins, serotonin, somatostatin, and calcitonin gene–related peptide (CGRP).

Sterile, disposable stainless-steel needles with plastic guide tubes are currently available, which technically facilitates needling. Once the needle touches or penetrates the superficial skin, the responses from the nociceptors of cutaneous sensory nerves are very diverse. The sensation could be nerve shock spreading proximally and distantly, sharp pain, tingling, and sometimes a stinging or burning sensation. Once the needle reaches deeper tissues, such as the fascia, muscles, blood vessels, and periosteum, the affected nerves are mostly muscular nerves and sensory nerves such as unmyelinated nerve endings (group IV, or C fibers) that innervate blood vessels and other soft tissues. Sharp pain is felt when blood vessels are penetrated, but otherwise the sensations may include dull ache, pressure, heaviness, distention, compression, soreness, tingling, numbness, and nerve shock. The sensation depends on the type of nerve fibers that the needle encounters and on the condition of the surrounding tissue, such as the presence of tissue perfusion and inflammatory mediators.[4]

Anything that has produced tissue damage or that threatens to do so in the immediate future can be defined as noxious, and the type of axon that responds selectively to the noxious quality of a stimulus is therefore, by definition, a nociceptor. Such axons are not pain receptors because nociception is not pain.

One important neurophysiologic occurrence during nociceptive needling is the antidromic activity of peripheral nerves. Needling as a nociceptive excitation stimulates the release of substance P from the unmyelinated nerve endings, which triggers a cascade of events that result in neurogenic inflammation, a sterile inflammation that is caused by antidromic neuronal activity in sensory nerve fibers through the release of endogenous substances with vascular and cellular actions. When nociceptive stimulation occurs, the action potential of sensory neurons travels in the periphery (not centrally) and releases those endogenous substances from the receptive endings. This indicates that a nociceptor not only is a passive sensor of noxious stimuli but also is capable of changing the chemical composition of its environment as part of its reaction to a tissue-threatening stimulus[5,6] (Fig. 6-4).

Stimulation of nociceptors activates the release of substances stored in the varicosities of the nerve ending.

Needling points on limbs may produce a brief sensation of electric shock, running up or down along the whole length of the limb. When the torso is needled, the sensation can be experienced as a local response. A few patients experience the unusual sensation of energy circulating from the needling site up to the head and down to the toes. This might happen because of the combination of cutaneous and muscular nerve conduction.

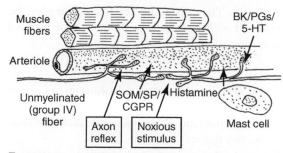

FIGURE 6-4 Antidromic neuronal activity during tissue-threatening stimulus. When noxious stimulation occurs, the sensory nociceptor senses the tissue injury and releases endogenous substances that change the chemical environment as part of the reaction. The action potentials propagate distantly (against afferent direction), a sensation often felt during needling therapy. The free nerve endings terminate on the wall of an arteriole. In the varicosities of the nerve ending, neuropeptides such as substance P (SP), somatostatin (SOM), and calcitonin gene–related peptides (CGRP) are stored. The mechanical stimulus also acts indirectly on the ending by releasing endogenous algesic substances from the blood such as bradykinin (BK), prostaglandins (PGs), or serotonin (5-HT). Substance P causes vasodilation, an increase in vascular permeability, and degranulation of mast cells, which release histamine as a vasodilator. (Adapted from Mense S, Simons DG: *Muscle pain*, Philadelphia, 2001, Lippincott Williams & Wilkins, Fig. 2.7.)

The diversity of the sensations can be explained by the types of nerve fibers stimulated by the needling (Table 6-1). Patients should be warned that some needling sensations such as aching or soreness may last for 1 or 2 days.

A needling-induced lesion stimulates the epidermis, dermis, and underlying connective tissues (elastic fibers, collagen, basal lamina, deeper fascia), muscular tissues (skeletal muscles and smooth muscles of blood vessels) and nervous tissues (nerve fibers of sensory neurons and postganglionic

TABLE 6-1	NEEDLING SENSATION AND THE RELATED NERVE FIBERS IN THE MUSCLES	
Types of Afferent Nerve Fibers	**Velocity (Milliseconds^{-1})**	**Types of Sensation**
Type I (Aα) (Muscle spindles and tendon spindles)	72–120	None or numbness
Type II (Aβ)	42–72	Numbness, pressure
Type III (Aδ)	12–36	Heaviness, distention, pressure, compression, aching
Type IV (unmyelinated, C)	0.5–1.2	Soreness, tingling, and burning pain

neurons). The cells injured by the needling will be replaced with fresh cells of the same type without scar formation.

The needling mechanisms are both local and systemic:

1. Local skin reaction and cutaneous microcurrent mechanism
2. Local interaction between needle shaft and connective tissues
3. Local relaxation of current muscle shortening and contracture, which improves local blood circulation through the autonomic reflex
4. Neural mechanism: nociceptive and motor neuronal activation, CNS-mediated neuroendocrine activity, segmental and nonsegmental pathways
5. Blood coagulation and lymphatic circulation
6. Local immune responses
7. DNA synthesis to replace the injured tissues and repair the lesions

LOCAL SKIN REACTION AND CUTANEOUS MICROCURRENT MECHANISM

Skin, with its neurovascular-immune function, serves as the first line of the body's defense system. When needling breaks the skin, it triggers a cascade of physiologic reactions to the intrusion. The needles encounter the following components of the skin:

1. Afferent somatic neuron fibers (cutaneous $A\delta$ and C fibers) and sympathetic nerve fibers (for controlling sweat glands and fine blood vessels)
2. Fine arterial and venous blood vessels (nutrition supply and temperature regulation)
3. Lymphatic tissue, mast cells (immune function)
4. Connective tissues (structural and functional support)

When a point changes from a latent phase to a passive phase, local neurogenic inflammation increases its sensitivity. Around this sensitive point, the electrical conductance of the skin increases and its resistance decreases, possibly because of fluid and ions that are present as a result of inflammation. Inserting a needle into this point will provoke an acute local inflammatory defensive response from all the aforementioned skin components. The first visible sign is the flare response, which is the

formation of redness (dilation of capillaries) around the needle. This vasodilatation of the autonomic nervous system is mediated by substance P, secreted by cutaneous nociceptive sensory nerves. Then an immune reaction is triggered by mast cells, which produce histamine, platelet-activating factor, and leukotrienes. At the same time, the needle-induced lesion promotes interaction between the blood coagulation system and the immune complement system.

The body surface always has a layer of electric charge because the human body is bathed in the electromagnetic field of the earth. Normally, dry skin has a direct current (DC) resistance of 200,000 to 2,000,000 ohms. At sensitive points this resistance is reduced to 50,000 ohms.[7] However, Melzack and Katz[8] found no difference in conductance between traditional ISDN points and nearby control points in patients with chronic pain. This phenomenon can be explained by the dynamic nature of the sensitive tissues. It is understandable that the area of sensitized tissue is larger in patients with chronic pain, whereas the same location in healthy persons is less or not at all sensitized. In a healthy person, the DC resistance of sensitive points is the same as for other areas. There is 20 to 90 mV of resting potential across the intact human skin, negative on the outer surface and positive on the inside.[9] Most sensitive points show a measurement of 5 mV higher than for nonacupoint areas.[7]

The insertion of a metal needle makes a short-circuit in the skin "battery," thus generating a microcurrent, called the *current of injury,* moving from inside to outside. The tiny lesion created by the needle causes a negative potential at the needling site and produces 10 mA of current of injury, which benefits tissue growth and regeneration.[10] These microcurrents induced by the needling are not sufficient to initiate nerve pulses to the spinal cord, and so the microcurrents do not create a tolerance to needling in the same way that tolerance develops for drugs such as morphine. This means that repetitive needling will not have a diminishing therapeutic effect. In case of electrical ISDN stimulation for more than 3 hours, however, the analgesic effect does gradually decline. Han[11] suggested that perhaps long-lasting electrical stimulation increases the release of cholecystokinin octapeptide (CCK-8), which is an endogenous antiopioid substances.[12] This effect is the body's attempt to maintain the natural balance. Without this balancing mechanism, the positive electrical stimulation and its results would create negative side effects and ultimately destroy the organism.

NEEDLE MANIPULATION: MECHANICAL SIGNAL TRANSDUCTION THROUGH CONNECTIVE TISSUE

Needle manipulation is an important technique in classic acupuncture, but not in ISDN. The ancient Chinese doctors believed that needling could not be effective without needle manipulation. Modern clinical evidence indicates that this is not the case and that therapeutic efficacy can be achieved without any manipulation as long as lesions are created. Nonetheless, needle manipulation can add value to ISDN treatment in many cases if the physiologic and mechanical mechanisms of it are understood.

A research team at the University of Vermont College of Medicine has proved that manipulation promotes tissue healing by producing biomechanical, vasomotor, and neuromodulatory effects on interstitial connective tissue.[3]

When a needle is inserted into the body tissue, there is an initial coupling between the metal shaft of the needle and elastic and collagen fibers. This affinity is caused by both surface tension and an attraction between the metal of the needle and the electrical charge of the connective tissue. Once this coupling has occurred, frictional force takes over. Then the rotation of the needle increases the tension of the fibers by winding them around the needle, which pulls and realigns the connective fiber network.[12]

The experienced practitioner detects the needle's resistance to rotation (needle grasp), and the patient feels some sensation. This "needle grasp" process affects the extracellular matrix, the fibroblasts attached to collagen fibers, and possibly capillary endothelial cells.

As a response to this physical deformation, the cells initiate a cascade of cellular and molecular events, including intracellular cytoskeletal reorganization, cell contraction and migration, autocrine release of growth factors, and the activation of intracellular signaling pathways and nuclear binding proteins that promote the transcription of specific genes. The aforementioned effects lead to synthesis and local release of growth factors, cytokines, vasoactive substances, degradative enzymes, and structural matrix elements. Release of these substances changes the extracellular surroundings of the needled tissue and results in the promotion of healing at this location. These results may also affect more distant connective tissue, thus spreading the healing process with long-term effects. This is how mechanical signals produced by simple manipulation of a needle can generate a cascade of downstream physiologic healing effects.

According to clinical evidence, this type of mechanical signal transduction, which results from correct needle manipulation (rotation or as a piston), may desensitize sensory receptors and restore a normal pain threshold. It is very common, especially with acute injuries, that pain, sensitivity, and swelling subside during or shortly after needling.

The mystery of needle manipulation was clarified by Langevin and colleagues,[3,12] and a proper understanding of it is indispensable for clinicians. It is important to understand that although the success of ISDN treatment does not require needle manipulation, clinical practice is enhanced if the practitioner knows how this technique helps reduce tissue stress and promote self-healing.

LOCAL RELIEF OF MUSCLE SHORTENING AND CONTRACTURE

Needling provides local relief of concurrent muscle shortening and contracture. Local muscle pain stimulates the muscle to generate sensitive points, persistent involuntary contracture, and shortening of the muscle fibers, which results in muscle tension and stiffness. There are four common sources of local muscle pain: (1) mechanical, chemical, or physical injury (e.g., burning); (2) repetitive strain, overstretching, or contraction beyond the muscle's natural limits for a long time; (3) diseased viscera that project pain to the body surface, partially through the mechanism of segmental neuronal reflex; and (4) referred pain associated with a diseased joint and its accessory structures.

Local muscle pain involves afferent sensory fibers (nociceptors), muscle fibers, and blood vessels. The nerve endings of sensory fibers contain neuropeptides, substance P, CGRP, and somatostatin. Under pathologic conditions, neuropeptides may be released from the sensory nerve endings and influence basic tissue functions such as neuronal excitability, local microcirculation, and metabolism. When tissue-threatening (noxious) stimulation occurs (mechanical, physical, or chemical), neuropeptides are released from the sensory nerve endings, and this triggers a cascade of events that lead to neurogenic inflammation. Substance P and CGRP cause vasodilation and increase the permeability of the microvasculature. Histamine is liberated from mast cells when they are exposed to substance P. All these substances diffuse to neighboring tissue, which results in an expansion of the inflammation.

Once this neurogenic inflammation spreads, fluids and proteins shift from the blood vessels into surrounding interstitial spaces. This process releases vasoneuroactive substances: bradykinin from protein (kallidin) in the blood plasma and serotonin (5-hydroxytryptamine [5-HT]) from platelets. Leukotrienes and prostaglandins are released from the tissue cells surrounding the injured site. All these substances increase the sensitivity of affected nerve endings. Thus the noxious stimuli result in sensitiveness (sensitized nociceptors) and then spontaneous pain (nociceptor excitation) in the localized region of muscle.

When nociceptors are sensitized, their firing threshold decreases. After this kind of physiologic alteration, any slight stimulus, such as light pressure, may cause the nerve ending to fire impulses to the CNS. This same amount of pressure would not elicit any response from normal, unsensitized nerve endings. If the sensitization continues to increase, it may further lower the firing threshold of the nociceptors, and they may spontaneously send impulses to the CNS, which causes a sensation of pain.

Repetitive strain and overuse are common types of muscle activity that cause local pain. If muscles are used in a movement repeatedly without adequate recovery time between repeats, or if they are held under load in a relatively fixed position for prolonged periods, as with unbalanced exercise, then discomfort, soreness, or pain develops, with a peak of discomfort during the first day or two. Pain makes muscles sensitive to palpation; it restricts their range of motion and sometimes causes slight swelling. In this type of injury, some disorganization of the striation of muscle fibers has been observed, and a lack of myofibrillar regeneration could persist as long as 10 days.[13] Changes in blood chemistry profiles have been noticed, including increases in plasma levels of interleukin-1, acid-reactive substances, lactic dehydrogenase, serum creatine, phosphokinase, aspartate aminotransferase, and serum glutamic oxaloacetic transaminase. Most of those enzymes are involved in muscle metabolism.

The literature of Chinese traditional acupuncture indicates that diseased viscera project pain to predictable points or areas on the body surface. This is a manifestation of the segmental mechanism of the viscerosomatic neuronal reflex. For example, an inflamed kidney may cause sensitivity or painful spasm in the lumbar area, resulting in lower back pain with sensitive points palpable from T10 to L5 on the back muscle (erector spinae). For some patients, additional sensitive points may appear in the neck region. This segmental mechanism plays a very important role in treatment of pain symptoms and is discussed in detail later in the chapter. Needling these sensitive points that are associated with diseased organs relieves the pain and other symptoms such as cramping, inflammation, and ulcers.

Joint disease and dysfunction can cause muscle pain. Because of the segmental reflex, the activity of sensory nerves influences the activity of efferent nerves from motor neurons of the same muscle. However, the muscle is also affected by the sensory nerves of neighboring muscles and joints. He and associates[14] described how stimulation of knee joint nociceptors excites afferent motor neurons of both flexor and extensor muscles. It is possible that sensory input from a joint will lead to a contraction in neighboring muscles. The contracted muscles may, in turn, put stress on the joint and its accessory structures such as capsules, ligaments, and discs. All these structures will produce pain under these circumstances because they are richly innervated by sensory nerves.

All types of different muscle pathophysiologic processes converge to a similar consequence in the muscles that maintain posture: The muscles become tense, stiff, and shortened, and sensitive points and enlarged contraction knots are formed within the muscles. Some of the contraction knots, if not released immediately, become persistent muscle contracture, which results in a chronic condition.

Sensitized spots are also found in other soft tissue that is richly innervated by sensory nerves such as tendons, ligaments, superficial and deep fascia, and, possibly, periosteum. Modern clinicians call these sensitive spots and contracture trigger points *dermopoints, motopoints* (neuromuscular attachment points), *nodes,* and so forth. All of them show some aspects of the acu-reflex points of traditional Chinese acupuncture. Physiologically, these points can be called *reflex points.*

Sensitive points vary in their histologic composition and pathophysiologic phases. Some consist mostly of sensitized nerve fibers, whereas others, in addition to the sensitized nerve receptors, contain knots of contracted muscle. Internal factors such as diseased organs and arthritis lead to the creation of sensitive points all over the body. Their locations are actually highly predictable, partly because of the segmental mechanism or special features of the sensory nerve fibers. In acute injury, sensitized points are formed according to the type of injury and the body anatomy involved. For example, a mild ankle sprain (inversion injury) causes elongation of ligaments on the lateral side of the ankle, whereas a severe ankle injury may tear the ligaments between the fibula and tibia, as well as the lateral ligaments. With a good knowledge of anatomy, clinicians can find the most effective sensitive points for treatment.

Any muscle, tendon, or fascia that harbors sensitive or painful points may resist stretching and may become tense, stiff, shortened, and painful. Most sensitive points used for pain treatments are on muscle, but points on tendons, ligaments, and fasciae are of the same importance and should not be ignored clinically.

Before pathologic contracture is discussed, it is important to review membrane depolarization and the five stages of healthy muscle contraction.

Depolarization can be simply described as follows: When a cell is not agitated (Fig. 6-5), the outside of the cell membrane is electrically positive and the inside is negative. When electric impulses or bioactive molecules stimulate a cell, positive Na^+ ions flow into the membrane so that the outside

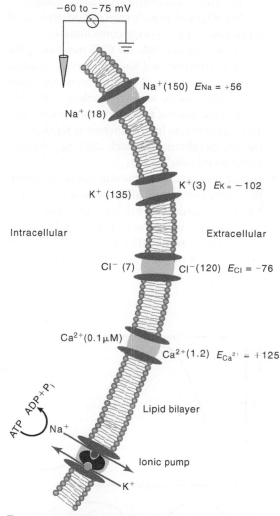

FIGURE 6-5 Differential distribution of ions inside and outside of plasma membrane of neurons and neuronal processes. Ionic channels for Na^+, K^+, Cl^-, and Ca^{2+} are shown. Concentration of the ions (in parentheses) are given in millimoles except that for intracellular Ca^{2+}. *ADP,* Adenosine diphosphate; *ATP,* adenosine triphosphate; E_{Ca2+}, extracellular calcium; E_{Cl}, extracellular chloride; E_K, extracellular potassium; E_{Na}, extracellular sodium; P_i, inorganic phosphate.

becomes less positive, which means that electricity flows into the cell. Then positive K⁺ ions flow out to restore the polarity of the outside. Finally, Na⁺ ions are pumped out and K⁺ ions are pumped in, by molecular channels, so that the concentrations of Na⁺ outside and K⁺ inside are restored. This represents one cycle of depolarization (Figs. 6-6 and 6-7). The depolarization consumes metabolic energy.

All five stages of muscle contraction are related to depolarization and energy consumption:

1. Electrical impulses from the CNS travel along the motor neuron fiber and reach the nerve terminal to depolarize the terminal membrane, which causes the terminal (nerve ending) to release acetylcholine into the space of the neuromuscular junction.
2. The acetylcholine in the junction space depolarizes the membrane of muscle cell (the postjunctional membrane).
3. In the muscle cell, a membranous organelle, the sarcoplasmic reticulum, attaches to the cell membrane and stores calcium. The depolarization of the cell membrane causes depolarization of the sarcoplasmic reticulum, which results in the release of calcium into the cell plasma.

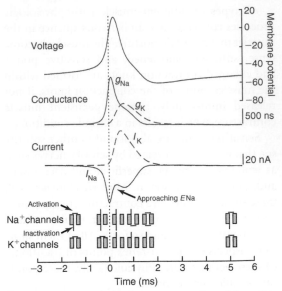

FIGURE 6-6 Depolarization, or generation of the action potential, is associated with an increase in membrane Na⁺ conductance and K⁺ current. Activation of Na⁺ channels allows Na⁺ to enter the cell, depolarizing membrane potential. E_{Na}, Extracellular sodium; g_{K}, conductance of potassium; g_{Na}, conductance of sodium; I_{K}, intracellular potassium; I_{Na}, intracellular sodium.

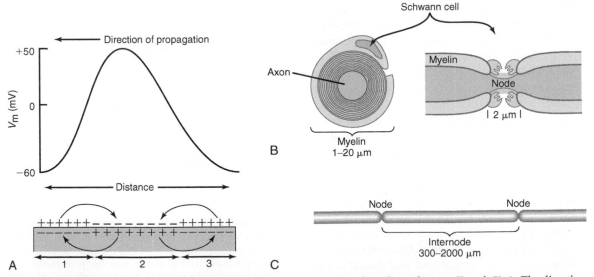

FIGURE 6-7 Propagation of the action potential in unmyelinated *(A)* and myelinated axons *(B and C)*. **A,** The direction of depolarization is from region 3 to region 1. Region 3 starts repolarization after depolarization. Region 2 is undergoing depolarization. V_{m}, membrane voltage. **B,** In vertebrate myelinated axons, the axon is exposed to the external medium at the nodes of Ranvier. **C,** Action potential is generated at the nodes of Ranvier, at which the Na⁺ channel is of high density. Conduction velocity is greatly increased in myelinated fibers.

4. The high concentration of cytoplasmic calcium stimulates two long linear molecules, actin and myosin, to move against each other so that the muscle cell becomes shortened.

5. After this contraction, calcium ions are pumped back into the sarcoplasmic reticulum through channels on the membrane of the sarcoplasmic reticulum. The concentration of cytoplasmic calcium thereby declines, which leads to a decoupling of actin and myosin. In this way, the muscle relaxes to its original length. If a person wants to maintain a posture, he or she voluntarily sends continuous impulses to the relevant muscles to keep coupling actin and myosin, and the muscles will maintain this contraction until the person stops sending these impulses.

These steps represent normal physiologic contraction.

The same steps are compared with the mechanism of pathologic contraction in Chapter 3, but it is reviewed briefly here because it is a very important mechanism in clinical ISDN practice. Simons[15] provided a very good explanation of this process with the name "energy crisis hypothesis." His hypothesis is modified as follows (Fig. 6-8):

1. When afferent sensory nerves are sensitized (the location feels sensitive) or excited (pain is felt at the location), efferent motor nerves are activated to release excess acetylcholine into the neuromuscular junction space.

2. Excess acetylcholine prolongs depolarization of the postjunctional membrane.

3. This results in longer depolarization of the membrane of the sarcoplasmic reticulum and leads to a longer period of high concentration of cytoplasmic calcium.

4. The high concentration of cytoplasmic calcium prolongs actin-myosin coupling. The sustained shortening of the muscle cell compresses local blood vessels. This compressed microcirculation (ischemia) obstructs the provision of energy and reduces oxygen supply.

5. The actin-myosin coupling continues because the concentration of cytoplasmic calcium remains high, and molecular pumps cannot return the calcium to the sarcoplasmic reticulum because the energy supply is low or absent.

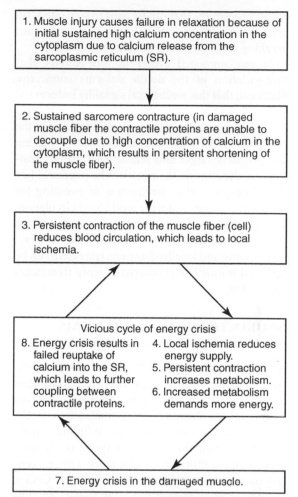

FIGURE 6-8 Energy crisis hypothesis (suggested by Dr. David G. Simons). Energy metabolism and the cellular process of muscle fiber contracture in a sensitive acu-reflex point. *SR,* Sarcoplasmic reticulum.

This is how ischemia, hypoxia, low energy supply, and muscle shortening continue to develop into a vicious circle unless interrupted by appropriate treatment. Muscle that is in contracture during such an energy crisis has a higher temperature than does normal muscle tissue. This pathologic contraction is endogenous, not initiated by voluntary impulse, and may persist indefinitely. According to clinical experience, any method of interrupting this energy crisis helps relax the muscle and reduce pain. Needling, electrical stimulation, physical stretching, proper exercise, and injection of appropriate drugs are all procedures that can be used to separate actin from myosin to relax the shortened muscle, thus breaking this energy-consuming vicious circle.

It was suggested earlier in this chapter that manipulation of the needle deforms connective fibers and that this mechanical signaling induces tissue healing. According to clinical evidence, manipulation also helps to stretch muscle and break the energy crisis at some acu-reflex points. Needling can precisely target and release endogenous contracture deep inside the muscle. The processes just described prove the effectiveness of needling for muscle relaxation, restoring local blood circulation, and promotion of tissue healing without any side effects. If local sensitization or endogenous contracture is acute and localized, muscle relaxation can be achieved immediately; otherwise, more treatments are needed.

NEUROCHEMICAL MECHANISMS OF ACUPUNCTURE ANALGESIA

Soft tissue pain often starts to subside immediately after needling therapy and even completely disappears within a few days. After needling, the peripheral mechanisms of normalizing soft tissue dysfunction are operating. Without central command from the brain and spinal cord, however, peripheral organs cannot work without central coordination; therefore the role of the CNS is important. Even though this book focuses on clinically observable and measurable physical parameters such as musculoskeletal balance, the basic background of the central mechanism of needling is indispensable for understanding peripheral mechanisms.

The neurochemical mechanisms of acupuncture analgesia have been investigated extensively in many Chinese, Japanese, South Korean, and North American universities. Han's[10] laboratory at Beijing Medical University and Pomeranz's[1,11] laboratory at the University of Toronto have contributed solid scientific data explaining the neurochemical processes of acupuncture analgesia.

The explanation of acupuncture analgesia is simplified for the purposes of this textbook. For example, after pain impulses reach the spinal cord,

at least six neural pathways transmit those impulses from spinal cord to cerebral cortex, and numerous neurochemicals are released at different sites to modulate pain signals, including three different endorphins (enkephalin, β-endorphin, and dynorphin), acetylcholine, cholecystokinin, serotonin, adrenocorticotrophic hormone (ACTH), somatostatin, substance P, vasoactive intestinal peptide, neurotensin, CGRP, gamma-aminobutyric acid (GABA), epinephrine and norepinephrine, and cytokines. More substances will probably be discovered in addition to this long list. However, a detailed description of interactions among neurochemicals is beyond the scope of this book.

The purpose of needling treatment is the integration of physiologic systems. This integration is achieved by normalizing any dysfunction that is caused by local or systemic pathologic condition.

The neurochemical mechanisms of needling provide analgesia (pain relief); promote homeostasis and tissue healing; improve the immune system, digestive system, cardiovascular system, and endocrine system; and promote psychologic adjustment for systemic integration. The integrated nature of these mechanisms explains why problems as different as asthma, tinnitus, irritable bowel, and gastric ulcers are all improved in the course of needling treatment for pain management. Needling therapy restores the body's control system and promotes self-healing through a systemic integration that is suppressed during disease or injury.

The systemic integration of physiologic and even anatomic functions of the human body by ISDN therapy is understood to result from activating the reflex circuits at different levels of the nervous system: the spinal cord segments, the brainstem, the hypothalamus and thalamus, the upper part of the limbic system, and the cortex.

GENERAL REVIEW OF THE NEEDLING REFLEX

Figure 6-9 illustrates the reflex circuits that are currently understood to be the mechanisms of needling. This illustration is not specific for pain management. Needling is nonspecific in nature, and this example illustrates the general physiologic

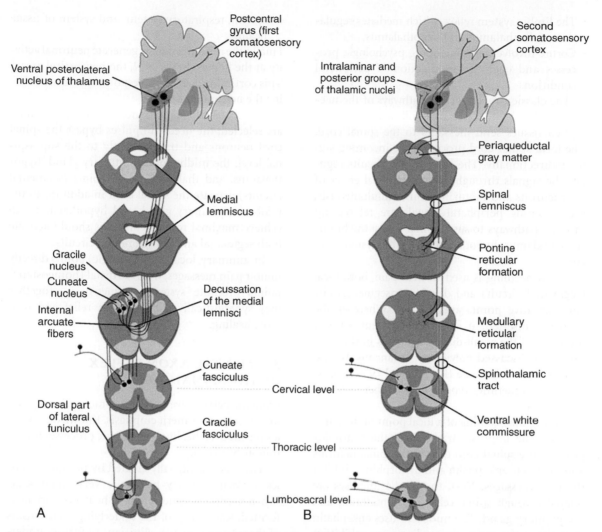

FIGURE 6-9 Anatomic depictions of ascending pathways that represent the needling reflex at different levels (see text). **A,** Nerve entry. Large-diameter afferent nerves enter the spinal cord and terminate in the first somatosensory area of the cerebral cortex through thalamocortical axons. **B,** Organization of the spinothalamic tract and remainder of the anterolateral system. The spinal cord itself terminates with primary axons. Second-order axons cross the middle line and ascend through the spinal cord and brainstem to terminate in the thalamus. Collateral extensions of these axons terminate in the reticular formation of the pons and medulla. This organization represents part of the needling pathways.

process of needling therapy. Needling-induced reflex responses occur at different levels of the nervous system:
- The segmental axon reflex, which consists of spinal interneuron and motor neuron reflexes, including interneuron inhibition and excitation responses and autonomic nerve reflexes

- The brainstem and pontine reticular formation reflexes, which mediate visceral physiology
- The midbrain periaqueductal gray reflex, which mediates the descending control of pain
- The thalamus and hypothalamus reflexes, which mediate homeostasis regulation of the system

- The limbic system reflex, which mediates regulation of the thalamus and hypothalamus
- Cortex involvement, including psychologic processes and cognitive modulation of peripheral conditions

The classic concept of the pathways of the needling reflex is illustrated as follows: Painful or injured tissues send messages to the spinal cord. The local spinal cord processes the incoming signal bidirectionally. The local spinal circuits regulate the signals through the biochemical effect of interneurons and motor neurons. Simultaneously, the incoming peripheral signals are relayed up through pathways to supraspinal levels: the brainstem, thalamus, hypothalamus, limbic system, and cortex.

When needling is used to treat pain, both local (segmental circuit) and distal (nonsegmental circuit) sensitive points are selected. Wherever the needle is inserted, it stimulates afferent sensory receptors of the small-diameter nerves in skin and muscle as discussed previously: cutaneous Aδ and C fibers, muscular type III (Aδ) and IV (C) muscle fibers, sometimes type II muscle fibers, and Aβ muscle fibers.

During the needling of a local point in the painful area, the impulses travel from the acu-reflex point to the spinal cord to activate spinal neurons and to secrete enkephalin and dynorphin to inhibit the pain messages. Next, the needle impulses are relayed through spinal cells to the midbrain and the pituitary gland. The midbrain uses enkephalin to activate the raphe-descending pain-inhibition system.

The pain-inhibition system secretes monoamines, serotonin, and norepinephrine to inhibit pain transmission in two ways:

1. Inhibition of ascending pain messages
2. Activation of spinal cord neurons to synergistically inhibit incoming pain message from painful tissues: The pituitary gland and hypothalamus, activated by the needling signals from the spinal cord, release β-endorphin into the blood and cerebrospinal fluid, which promotes physiologic analgesia and homeostasis of numerous systems, including the immune system, cardiovascular

system, respiratory system, and system of tissue healing.

Finally, the needling signals generate neuronal activity at the highest brain level, the neocortical area.[16] This cortical processing is responsible for modulating the perception of pain.

When distal points (nonsegmental circuits) are selected, the needle impulses bypass the spinal cord neurons and travel directly to the supraspinal level: the midbrain and pituitary gland, hypothalamus, and thalamus. Local points (segmental circuits) activate the spinal cord in addition to the midbrain, pituitary gland, and hypothalamus. To achieve maximal results, clinicians should activate both segmental and nonsegmental circuits.

In summary, local (symptomatic) points directly inhibit pain messages, whereas distal (homeostatic) points promote systemic homeostasis. Together they synergistically enhance pain relief and promote healing.

SEGMENTAL AXON REFLEX OF THE SPINAL CORD

From the perspective of clinical practice, local physiologic responses merit emphasis. Knowledge about lesion-induced healing physiologic processes is continuously growing.

The lesion artificially created by needling mimics accidental injury but on a very small scale. When needling-induced lesions heal, no scarring is formed. Knowledge of the underlying mechanisms of these lesions enables clinicians to further understand the local axon reflex induced by needling.

After a needle is inserted into tissue, the surrounding area becomes reddened. Accompanying this flare is edema or swelling, as the tissue fills with fluid. The region surrounding the lesion becomes sensitive because of chemical reactions caused by the injury. An individual C fiber terminates over a wide area of skin, and so a needling-induced lesion probably affects only a fraction of a fiber's many branches directly. Action potential generated at the directly involved branches also affect the other peripheral branches, as well as the main or parent axon that conducts the signal to the CNS. At all the peripheral terminals of a C fiber, substance P and CGRP are released toward two principal targets: the smooth muscles surrounding peripheral blood vessels and histamine-rich mast cells. This causes the arterial smooth muscles to relax, thus increasing the flow of blood into the neighborhood of the damaged tissue. Thus water and electrolytes flow out of capillaries into extracellular space; this process is referred to as *extravasation*. Histamine released from mast cells leads to a pronounced inflammatory response. All of this is important for promoting the infiltration of damaged tissue with cellular elements that will protect against infection and promote repair. The local chemical changes resulting from the lesion cause greater sensitivity of the surrounding tissue. The chemical changes sensitize the protein receptors inserted into nociceptive axons (Fig. 6-10). This primary hyperalgesia is a direct result of the axon reflex.

The response of nociceptors is affected by the histamine released by mast cells and by the edema that results from extravasation. Histamine selectively interacts with only a subclass of the most slowly conducting C fibers in which histamine receptors are inserted into the membranes of their axon terminals.[16] These histamine receptors and possibly other independent histamine receptors are related to itch, which may happen in some cases of injury.

Edema causes a general reduction in the pH of extracellular fluid from 7.4 to below 6.0. As outlined earlier, the protein receptors inserted into nociceptive axons are sensitive to the concentration of H^+. Thus activation of one branch of a C fiber leads to increased sensitivity of all its branches, and all neighboring nociceptors, to noxious stimulation.

Injured tissue releases two powerful pain-inducing chemicals: prostaglandin and bradykinin. They are lipids of the prostaglandin family and the nonpeptide bradykinin. Prostaglandins are derivatives of arachidonic acid, a membrane fatty acid that is itself a major component of the lipid bilayer of cell membranes. Damage to tissue and the resulting disruption of cell membranes cause the release of arachidonic acid into extracellular fluid, in which it is broken down by the enzyme cyclooxygenase (COX) to form prostaglandin.

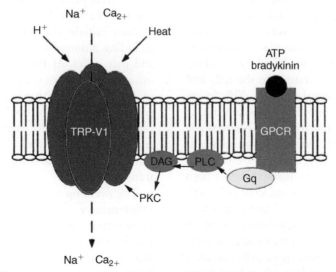

FIGURE 6-10 Polymodal nociceptor consists of a family of receptor channels referred to as *transient receptor potential* (TRP). The subfamily TRP-V1 channels respond to many different noxious stimuli, including heat and H^+ produced in response to tissue swelling. The noxious stimuli open a nonspecific cation channel that, through an influx of Na^+, depolarizes the nociceptor axon. Adenosine triphosphate (ATP) and bradykinin, the signals of tissue damage, bind to a G-protein coupled receptor (GPCR). Through a series of steps, the TPR-V1 is phosphorylated, which leads to a sensitization of the receptor. *DAG*, Diacylglycerol; *Gq*, a family of G proteins; *PKC*, protein kinase C; *PLC*, phospholipase C.

BLOOD COAGULATION SYSTEM AND IMMUNE COMPLEMENT SYSTEM

Activation or normalization of immune function is one of the most important physiologic processes of needling. Whether needling promotes activation or normalization of the immune system depends on the baseline performance of the system. Whether immune activity is suppressed, as it is in infection, or overactivated, as in cases of inflammation, needling gradually brings immune function to its normal level.

Needling is used effectively for acute inflammation of soft tissues caused by injury from accidents, sports, and all kinds of pathologic conditions (e.g., tonsillitis; inflammation of the parotid gland, lymphatic vessels, and nodes; appendicitis; pancreatitis; postoperational infections; bacterial dysentery; hepatitis B; nephritis; and other hypoimmune reactions). ISDN is also used for improving hyperimmune response in cases of chronic inflammation such as hyperthyroidism, Hashimoto thyroiditis, sinusitis, asthma, allergy, urticaria, gastritis, rheumatoid arthritis, diabetes, and low leukocyte count during chemotherapy. ISDN is a safe and beneficial adjunct therapy for all these conditions.

Research in some Chinese universities has yielded more knowledge of the molecular mechanisms of immune modulation as mediated by needling. Needling causes a minute trauma to the cells and very small, invisible internal bleeding. This lesion activates the immune response, thus promoting tissue healing and the restoration of homeostatic balance, which stimulates restorative control mechanisms and results in healing of the whole body.

Chemicals from connective tissue that have been needled, such as collagen fibers and mast cells, activate blood coagulation factor XII (Hageman factor). In addition to causing blood coagulation, factor XII activates other factors to attract immune cells to the site of needling. The needled tissue cells stimulate mast cells to produce peptides such as bradykinin and histamine, whose peripheral function includes vasodilatation and increased vascular permeability.

The enhanced vasodilatation of capillaries improves blood flow to the site, which enables immune cells to move from blood circulation to trigger the defensive immune reaction around the lesion. Chemicals are released to activate immune cells and excite nociceptive sensory fibers.

When the needle is removed, tissue repair processes are stimulated, the lesioned cells are digested, and protein synthesis is mobilized. The lesion-induced healing is directed by systemic neurohormonal mechanisms. The pituitary gland starts to increase the blood volume of adrenocorticotropic hormones (ACTH), which triggers the synthesis and secretion of physiologic corticosteroids and other hormones. This process protects the body from stress, including reduction of the inflammatory reaction. Descending neural control systems from the brain inhibit and desensitize the nociceptive nerves in both the spinal cord and the peripheral nervous system. These systems also balance the autonomic nervous system, which normalizes blood flow and energy metabolism. Finally, the body's homeostasis is improved or restored, and local tissue healing and pain relief are accelerated.

SUMMARY

ISDN therapy is a drugless and nonspecific inoculation into the body that causes minute lesions, which in turn initiate the mechanisms of self-healing, including autonomic homeostasis, tissue healing, and pain relief. At the needling site, a cutaneous microcurrent circuit is created to produce a current of injury (about 10 mA), which stimulates tissue growth. Mechanical stimulation from the needle, especially from needle manipulation, deforms the connective collagen and elastic fibers; this causes transduction of signals for tissue healing and gene transcription.

The needling and its lesion also induce a local inflammatory reaction against the intrusion. Endogenous (nonvoluntary) muscle contracture, which creates an energy crisis in the shortened muscle, can be relaxed by needling the corresponding acu-reflex points, to restore normal muscle physiology. This occurs through segmental and nonsegmental neural mechanisms. Needling signals from local (segmental) points are processed at both the spinal cord and supraspinal cord centers (midbrain, thalamus, pituitary gland, and cortex), whereas signals from distant (nonsegmental) points may be directly relayed to supraspinal cord centers. These mechanisms enhance one another to activate descending control systems, which include the secretion of chemicals and hormones into the blood and cerebrospinal fluid to restore homeostasis and facilitate the neural modulation of pain relief.

Responses to needling treatments vary because of physiologic differences among patients. In an average clinic population, about 28% of patients respond strongly, 64% respond adequately, and 8% respond weakly.[2]

Differentiation of patients and predictive prognosis are an important part of treatment procedure in ISDN therapy. An understanding of the needling mechanisms enables the development of a practical protocol for all pain symptoms. The neuromuscular acu-reflex point system introduced in this book simplifies the process of point selection and ensures more predictable and effective pain management.

In this chapter, the peripheral effects of needling stimulation have been discussed, and both peripheral and central mechanisms are summarized as follows.

It is clear that needling stimulation, with both peripheral and central effects, activates the physiologic processes of complex, innate survival mechanisms in order to restore and maintain homeostasis. The peripheral effects involve creation of needle-induced lesions, cutaneous microcurrents, mechanical signal transduction through connective tissues, local relief of muscle shortening and contracture, and other local reactions.

The central effects are a form of CNS response as a result of peripheral sensory stimulation. This response includes the neural-immune interaction, the humoral and autonomic nervous system pathways, and the efferent nerves present in other hypothalamic neural circuits. The peripheral and central effects of needling stimulation are physiologically inseparable.

Newly available molecular imaging tools such as high-resolution and high-sensitivity positron emission tomography (PET) and high-field fMRI enable clinicians to investigate in vivo the mechanisms of the human brain, especially higher brain (cortex) mechanisms, such as neurochemical and hemodynamic responses to needling stimulation.[17] The information gained from these tools will help clinicians better understand the mechanisms of needling and select more effective clinical procedures, although the interpretation of these data needs more development.

The central effects of neeldling stimulation activate the four determinants of homeostasis: (1) nervous system, (2) immune system, (3) endocrine system, and (4) cardiovascular system. They also depend on interactions between these systems and those controlled by neural pathways such as the autonomic nervous system.

Each acu-reflex point produces both a local and central systemic effect. Findings of fMRI corroborate clinical data in demonstrating that stimulation of any sensory nerve endings produces analgesic effects in the spinal cord and brain. Clinicians distinguish between the stimuli at different acu-reflex points according to whether more local effect or systemic effect is needed. If local effect is the priority (as in cases of localized inflammatory soft tissue pain), the treatment may focus on the local symptoms. If a systemic effect is desirable (as in cases of fibromyalgia or headache), the treatment should include both local and systemic treatment.

For example, elbow and paravertebral acu-reflex points between C4 and T1 are selected for treating elbow pain, whereas knee and paravertebral acu-reflex points between L2 and L5 are selected for treating knee pain. These combinations of symptomatic acu-reflex points (as in the elbow or the knee) with paravertebral acu-reflex points are based simply on the segmental innervation of the spinal nerves. However, the neck and shoulder should be treated together in some patients with knee pain because the knee pain may change the entire posture and cause imbalance of the spine.

References

1. Pomeranz B: Acupuncture analgesia—basic research. In Stux G, Hammerschlag R, editors: *Clinical ISDN: scientific basis*, Berlin, 2001, Springer, p 17.
2. Dung HC: Physiology in acupuncture. In *Anatomical acupuncture*, San Antonio, TX, 1997, Antarctic Press, Chap 7.

3. Langevin HM, Yandow JA: Relationship of acupuncture points and meridians to connective tissue planes, *Anat Rec* 269:257–265, 2002.

4. Levine JD, Fields HL, Basbaum AI: Peptides and the primary afferent nociceptor, *J Neurosci* 13:2273–2286, 1993.

5. Gamse R, Posch M, Saria A, et al: Several mediators appear to interact in neurogenic inflammation, *Acta Physiol Hung* 69:343–354, 1987.

6. Lembeck F, Holzer P: Substance P as neurogenic mediator of antidromic vasodilation and neurogenic plasma extravasation, *Naunyn Schmiedebergs Arch Pharmacol* 310:175–183, 1979.

7. Becker O, Reichmanis M, Marino AA, et al: Electrophysiological correlates of acupuncture points and meridians, *Psychoenerg Syst* 1:195–212, 1976.

8. Melzack R, Katz J: Auriculotherapy fails to relieve chronic pain, *JAMA* 251:1041–1043, 1984.

9. Jaffe L, Barker AT, Vanable AW Jr: The glabrous epidermis of cavies contains a powerful battery, *Am J Physiol* 242:R358–R366, 1982.

10. Pomeranz B: Effects of applied DC fields on sensory nerve sprouting and motor nerve regeneration in adult rats. In Nuccitelli R, editor: *Ionic currents in development*, New York, 1986, Liss, pp 251–258.

11. Han JS, Tang J, Huang BS: Acupuncture tolerance in rats: Antiopiate substrates implicated, *Chin Med J* 92:625–627, 1979.

12. Langevin HM, Churchill DL, Cipolia M: Mechanical signaling through connective tissue: a mechanism of the therapeutic effect of ISDN, *FASEB J* 15:2275–2282, 2001.

13. O'Reilly KP, Warhol MJ, Fielding RA, et al: Eccentric exercise-induced muscle damage impairs muscle glycogen repletion, *J Appl Physiol* 63:252–256, 1987.

14. He X, Proske U, Schaible H-G, et al: Acute inflammation of the knee joint in the cat alters responses of flexor motoneurons to leg movements, *J Neurophysiol* 59:326–340, 1988.

15. Simons DG: Referred phenomena of myofacial trigger points. In Vecchiet L, Albe-Fessard D, Lindblom U, editors: *Pain research and clinical management: new trends in referred pain and hyperalgesia*, vol 27, Amsterdam, 1993, Elsevier, Chap 28.

16. Cho Z-H, Na C-S, Wang EK, et al: Functional magnetic resonance imaging of the brain in the investigation of acupuncture. In Stux G, Hammerschlag R, editors: *Clinical acupuncture: scientific basis*, Berlin, 2001, Springer, pp 83–96.

17. Dubner R, Ruda MA: Activity dependent neuronal plasticity following tissue injury and inflammation, *Trends Neurosci* 15:96–103, 1992.

CHAPTER 7

Physiology of Acu-Reflex Points

A sensory axon reflex is the body's first response to needling, which elicits reflex responses at different levels from local spinal segment to cortex. To obtain specific results from nonspecific needling, selecting the best acu-reflex points for particular condition is the primary procedure.

Sensory axon reflex "points" are distributed all over the body (except for the nails, the hair, and part of the cornea; this is why pain is not felt when nails and hair are cut). Needling induces both mechanical and lesion-created stimuli in the body, which results in local and systemic reflex responses. Whenever health declines, some peripheral sensory nerves become sensitized. This sensitization can be caused by peripheral pathologic insults such as injury, or by visceral pathology, or by central sensitization such as pathologic changes in the anatomy and/or the functional and neurochemical profile of the central nervous system.

If this sensitization, especially when it is peripheral, is not neutralized, the sensitized reflex nerve will sensitize other peripheral nerves, possibly through both central sensitization and functional interconnectedness between different parts of the body. For example, when low back pain occurs at the L2-L5 level, it can be found that the superior cluneal, inferior gluteal, popliteal and sural nerves have already been sensitized. If the pain persists, the lateral and medial pectoral nerves also become sensitized. Why this happens in such an interconnected pattern is little understood, and what is currently known is just the tip of an iceberg. Nevertheless, the limited knowledge of this interconnectedness has already offered guidance in clinical practice: a systemic approach to restoring homeostasis. For instance, when pathologic conditions of the core system (e.g., low back pain) are treated, the interconnected peripheral nerves of the lower limbs will be treated at the same time. Or when knee pain is treated, the core systems, such as the lower back and even the neck, will not be ignored.

Thus a competent clinician should have both analytic and synthetic understanding of human anatomy, the pathologic condition that is currently being examined, and, particularly for sports medicine, the nature of human movement. This chapter provides the background for this understanding.

The ancient Chinese practitioners noticed this systemic functional interconnectedness between different parts of human body at least 3000 years ago, and they created "meridian theory" to explain it. With modern scientific knowledge of the human body and its pathology, clinicians are replacing empirical practice with evidence-based scientific practice. Modern Western medical professionals independently discovered similar techniques for treating soft tissue dysfunction and with a deeper analytic understanding, such as Janet Travell's trigger-point approach and C. Chan Gunn's intramuscular stimulation approach.

Needling therapy, presented as integrative systemic dry needling (ISDN) therapy in this book, is an integration of modern approaches to needling. It represents a synthesis of the theories and techniques of Janet Travell and C. Chan Gunn with other dry needling techniques and classical acupuncture. According to modern medical training, there is no conflict between these needling therapies, and each therapy has its advantages and limitations. This synthesis integrates the different clinical wisdoms and in this way enables clinicians to go beyond the limitations of each modality.

Each peripheral nerve, whether muscular or cutaneous, has a physiologic relationship with other distal peripheral nerves, as described previously. The sensitized tibial nerve on the leg, for example, can affect the greater occipital nerve from the posterior ramus of CII. Thus all the peripheral nerves form a physiologic network. This network is of great clinical importance, particularly in explaining the process and development pattern of chronic pathologic processes, especially chronic pain.

The origins of muscle pain can be categorized into five types: (1) trigger points, (2) muscle tension, (3) muscle spasms, (4) muscle deficiency (weakness), and (5) other soft tissue dysfunction, such as that of the fascia, tendon, or ligament. All these dysfunctions sensitize peripheral nerves, locally and even systemically.

The entire peripheral nerve network is a system that includes both modern trigger points and classic acu-reflex points. This system is the integrative neuromuscular acu-reflex point system (INMARPS). It is neuroanatomically defined and physiologically based. A basic understanding of the correspondence between the human nervous system (especially peripheral nerves) and these trigger points, or acu-reflex points, is crucial in the physiologic interpretation of the INMARPS. Many authors claim the discovery of "traditional meridians." However, in view of the relationship between the peripheral nervous system and acu-reflex points, this revelation actually concerns neither anatomic nor physiologic features of the human nervous system.

In this chapter, the physiology and anatomy of the INMARPS are described in detail. The purpose is to provide the anatomic and physiologic understanding of the acu-reflex point system that is necessary for clinical practice.

PATHOPHYSIOLOGIC FACTORS THAT CONVERT LATENT ACU-REFLEX POINTS TO PASSIVE POINTS

Muscle pain associated with passive acu-reflex points can be caused by a wide array of clinical conditions. Inflammatory diseases of muscle are the most common cause of muscle pain, and inherited myopathies are another possible source of muscle symptoms. In addition, nonpathophysiologic behavioral conditions such as stressful posture and repetitive overuse of muscles can cause myopathies.

Some possible conditions are briefly reviewed for consideration in dealing with clinical cases. This review demonstrates the complicated origins of muscle pain and how multidisciplinary approaches are required for many patients.

The causes of muscle pain and the appearance of passive acu-reflex points may be mechanical, pathologic (caused by chronic diseases), or iatrogenic (caused by drugs). Mechanical causes of muscle pain can be subdivided into ergonomic, structural, and postural pain syndromes. Ergonomic stress includes unfamiliar eccentric exercise, excessive exercise, and repetitive exercise syndromes. These are the primary causes of muscle pain for most athletes. Some of the most common mechanical stresses are discussed as follows.

Delayed-onset muscle soreness (DOMS) occurs after eccentric exercise and also after exercise of an ischemic muscle.[1] Exercise under these conditions causes injury to the muscle fiber and consequent muscle soreness. Natural healing may take 3 weeks to complete. Muscle fiber destruction after maximally eccentric contraction happens in a similar way as the changes that are seen in exercised ischemic muscle.[2-4] Untrained eccentric exercise also produces immediate damage to muscle and delayed muscle soreness in the days afterwards. Muscle soreness is the result of local muscle damage, inflammation, and nociceptor sensitization.[5] Repetitive exercise may entail repeated eccentric or lengthening contractions. Keyboard entry, for example, has been the cause of forearm pain and lateral epicondylalgia. The injury in lateral epicondylalgia occurs during the "down-stroke," or lengthening, phase of movement. When making a keyboard stroke, the finger is flexed while the wrist remains held in an extended position, in such a way that the extensor digitorum is lengthened while contracted.

Hypermobility syndromes also cause passive acu-reflex points and muscle pain. These syndromes produce multiple mechanical stresses. When ligaments are too slack to maintain joint stability, muscles are then recruited to keep up joint integrity; this results in structural stress. The mechanism of injury appears to be the muscular stress or overload that arises from the effort necessary to maintain integrity of the joint.

A head-forward posture is a common cause of pain in the neck, shoulder, facial joints, and back. It places stress on the extensor muscles of the neck and shoulder (longissimus cervicis, semispinalis capitis, semispinalis cervicis, splenius capitis, splenius cervicis, the suboccipital muscles at the base of the skull, and the trapezius and levator scapulae muscles). This posture is often associated with posterior displacement of the mandible and temporomandibular joint pain. Myalgic syndromes of the posterior cervical muscle and shoulder muscle are thus frequently associated with head pain and headache. Myalgic headache is often the result of postural or ergonomic stress on the shoulder and neck muscles.[6]

Pelvic torsion–related pain is associated with leg-muscle shortening or leg length pseudo-inequality and may possibly be related to lumbar and pelvic floor myopathy. In pelvic torsion, rotation of the pelvic iliac bone causes an ipsilateral high positioning of the posterior superior iliac spine and a low positioning of the anterosuperior iliac spine, which results in inequality of leg length. Scoliosis that results from pelvic torsion produces an asymmetry in shoulder height and mechanical stress on neck and shoulders, which can cause myalgic headache, neck pain, and shoulder pain.[7-11]

Sacroiliac joint dysfunction, or sacroiliac joint hypomobility, is another common problem in many athletes. It can cause pelvic and spine dysfunction that results in widespread axial muscle pain. Pain may be felt in the sacroiliac joint region of either the hypomobile side or the normal side and can be referred to the low back, the shoulders and neck, and the legs.

Somatic dysfunction, or muscle-joint dysfunction, is a limitation of range of motion caused by muscular restriction of joint motion. These restrictions can be painful and are often associated with palpable passive acu-reflex points.

Static overload occurs when mechanically stressful positions are held for prolonged periods of time. The active muscles gradually become fatigued. A fixed posture held for a long time causes pain in postural muscles. Another postural problem that is common in daily life is the eye-hand dominance habit: The head is rotated to bring the dominant eye closer to reading material that is on the contralateral hand-dominant side. Another example is back pain that is often related to the habit of carrying a child on one hip, often seen in mothers.

Nerve root compression produces acute or chronic myofascial pain, causing sensitized trigger points, muscle tension or spasms, and muscle deficiency. Passive acu-reflex points can develop acutely when an acute disc herniation occurs, and this can precede any neurologic disorder such as weakness, paresthesia, sensory loss, or inhibition of reflex. Such neurologic disorder always occurs within days of the onset of muscle pain. Needling can relieve the pain, but it may be for only days or hours. In such cases, the patient should be referred to a neurologist while the needling treatment continues.

Muscle imbalance is also a common cause of muscle pain. Usually an imbalance caused by muscle weakness will lead to mechanical asymmetries, as in the case of the leg-length-inequality syndrome and low back pain. In addition to medical treatment such as needling, physical correction using a heel lift or butt lift should be considered.

The causes of muscle pain just discussed are related to abnormal musculoskeletal mechanics. The second category of causes of muscle pain is related to medical illness, such as autoimmune disorders, infectious diseases, allergies, hormonal and nutritional deficiencies, viscerosomatic pain syndromes, and iatrogenic drug-induced muscle pain syndromes. The relationship of some of these conditions to muscle pain is more difficult to confirm. When such an illness is identified and treated, the muscle pain is reduced or resolved, but clinicians must be cautious about assuming a causal relationship.[12]

Autoimmune diseases, particularly connective tissue diseases, also create passive acu-reflex points. For any muscular pain of head, neck, or shoulder, the possibility of polymyalgia rheumatica must certainly be considered. Even though needling helps relieve the pain, consulting a physician for the appropriate test is necessary in these cases.

Infectious diseases produce passive acu-reflex points. Lyme disease is perhaps the most prevalent of the infectious diseases associated with myofascial pain. In some patients, intractable widespread muscle pain and chronic fatigue have been positively associated with Lyme disease (in which elevated immunoglobulin G titers and normal immunoglobulin M titers are indicative of past, not recent, exposure). Some affected patients develop joint pain. Post–Lyme disease syndrome is characterized by diffuse joint and muscle pain, fatigue, and subjective cognitive difficulty.[13] Other infectious or parasitic diseases also manifest as widespread pain and resemble Lyme disease.

Allergies may cause widespread muscle pain. Food allergy is an example. Needling therapy may offer the relief from both allergy and muscle pain.

Viscerosomatic pain syndromes occur when visceral disorders exist. Internal organs are associated with somatic segmental referred pain syndromes. Endometriosis, for example, is associated with abdominal myofascial pain. Interstitial cystitis and irritable bowel syndrome are associated with chronic pelvic pain syndromes. Liver disease can cause local abdominal and referred shoulder pain that manifest as a regional pain syndrome.

Nutritional deficiencies also cause muscle pain. Vitamin D deficiency is extremely common among patients with musculoskeletal pain.[14] Iron deficiency causes a metabolic stress that produces fatigue and muscle pain. Iron deficiency is also associated with restless leg syndrome; in this way, it can cause a secondary aggravation of the muscle pain.

Many drugs can induce muscle pain, and this type of pain is widespread and diffuse. The statin family of cholesterol-lowering drugs is an example.[15]

This brief review is not complete, but it is evident that muscle pain and the appearance of related passive acu-reflex points can be caused by many different pathologic conditions, and those mentioned are not an exhaustive list. Careful attention should always be paid, and different medical modalities should be considered in complex cases.

DYNAMIC PHYSIOLOGY OF ACU-REFLEX POINTS

Acu-reflex points have different anatomic characteristics in different parts of the human body. However, all acu-reflex points have one element in common: They become sensitized, or even painful, when there are pathologic conditions such as external injury or internal disease. Research data and clinical observation have improved the understanding of why acu-reflex points become sensitive.[16,17] Table 7-1 lists a number of pain-producing substances that appear in the sensitized spots. An examination of the biochemical environment of those sensitized spots reveals that the pain-producing substances are almost the

TABLE 7-1	PHYSIOLOGIC PARAMETERS OF SENSITIZED ACU-REFLEX POINTS
Measurement of Biochemical Substances	**Active TrPs* in Comparison with Latent TrPs and Normal Muscles**
Pressure pain threshold	↓ $P < 0.08$
pH	↓ $P < 0.03$
Substance P	↑ $P < 0.01$
Calcitonin gene–related peptide	↑ $P < 0.01$
Bradykinin	↑ $P < 0.01$
Serotonin	↑ $P < 0.01$
Norepinephrine	↑ $P < 0.01$
Tumor necrosis factor α	↑ $P < 0.001$
Interleukin-1β	↑ $P < 0.001$

* *TrPs*, Trigger points.
From Shah JP, Philips T, Danoff J, et al: Novel microanalytical technique distinguishes three clinically distinct groups: (1) subject without pain and without myofascial trigger points; (2) subject without pain with myofascial trigger points; (3) subject with pain and myofascial trigger points [Abstract], *Am J Phys Med Rehabil* 83:231, 2004.

same as the biochemical substances released from injured tissue as mentioned in the previous chapter. The biochemical similarity between sensitized acu-reflex points and injured tissue indicates a physiologic matching between these two conditions, and it is possible that the sensitization of acu-reflex points is caused by inflammatory mechanisms similar to those that cause tissue injury.

Because acu-reflex points are distributed all over the body, their anatomic configurations are varied and depend on their location. For example, some acu-reflex points are themselves motor points; therefore they are neuromuscular in nature. Some are associated with nerve trunks and blood vessels; therefore they may be considered neurovascular in nature. Some are located in the bone foramina with nerves and blood vessels, and some are associated with ligaments and tendons innervated by both sensory and motor nerve fibers. Because of such diverse configurations, they have been given many different names, such as *trigger points,*[2] *acu-reflex points, neuropoints,* and *dermopoints.* From the clinical perspective of needling therapy, all the points are termed *acu-reflex points,* because needling causes axon reflex responses at different levels of the nervous system. The prefix "acu-" indicates that many of the points are classic acupuncture points, although they are trigger points as well (*acus* means "needle" in Latin). In this way modern, biomedically based trigger-point medicine and the empirical wisdom of traditional acupuncture are combined into the INMARPS.

THREE DYNAMIC PHASES OF ACU-REFLEX POINTS

The sensitization of acu-reflex points is a dynamic physiologic process consisting of three phases: latent, passive, and active.

Latent acu-reflex points represent normal, non-sensitized tissues. Passive acu-reflex points have a lower mechanical threshold than does normal tissue and start to fire impulses to the spinal cord and the brain upon normal pressure. The same amount of pressure does not induce impulses on latent points. Active acu-reflex points have the lowest mechanical threshold and continuously fire impulses to the spinal cord and the brain even without pressure, and this continuous firing may finally sensitize the neurons in the spinal cord and brain. As the mechanical threshold decreases, the physical size of a sensitized acu-reflex point increases. The transition from latent to passive phase or from passive to active phase is a *continuous* process without any clear demarcation, and so there is no quantitative measurement for differentiating acu-reflex points of different phases. The pressure used to palpate the acu-reflex points is usually about 2 to 3 lb (0.9 to 1.4 kg). In the clinic, the author uses the thumb to press the points; the pressure is about 2 to 3 lb when the thumbnail turns color from pinkish to whitish. However, there is no standard pressure for examination of acu-reflex points. The pressure used in palpation may need to be adjusted, inasmuch as some patients are less tolerant of pressure because their acu-reflex points are sensitive or painful, even before any pressure is applied.

In healthy people, most acu-reflex points are latent. In the presence of pathophysiologic disturbances, such as muscle injury, chronic pain, or disease, nonsensitive (latent) acu-reflex points are gradually transformed into sensitive (passive) acu-reflex points. Almost everyone has a number of passive acu-reflex points but are not consciously aware of them until an experienced practitioner palpates these points with a proper amount of pressure, at which time those locations may feel sensitive or painful. The majority of acu-reflex points encountered in clinical practice are passive acu-reflex points.

As pathologic disturbance continues to develop in the body, the pain becomes more intense, and finally passive acu-reflex points become active. Active acu-reflex points feel painful without any palpation, and patients are able to pinpoint the precise location of these points or areas.

According to clinical cases, direct and indirect events stimulate or activate the transition of acu-reflex points from latent to passive phases and from passive to active phases. Acute injuries, overuse fatigue, repetitive motion, compression of nerves such as radiculopathy, and joint dysfunctions such as arthritis *directly* turn the acu-reflex points sensitive. Fever, cold, visceral diseases (e.g., those in the heart, lung, gallbladder, and stomach), and emotional distress *indirectly* sensitize the acu-reflex points.

PHYSICAL PROPERTIES OF ACU-REFLEX POINTS

The physical properties of acu-reflex points affect their physical representation in terms of quality (sensitivity) and quantity (size and amount).

The physical properties of acu-reflex points include three parameters: sensitivity, specificity, and sequence.[3] These properties indicate the severity or chronicity of pain symptoms and visceral pathologic processes, the status of central sensitivity, and the process of aging.

Sensitivity

Passive acu-reflex points may ache or feel sensitive, sore, or painful when palpated with proper pressure (about 2 to 3 lb [0.9 to 1.4 kg] at the fingertip, with variation as discussed previously). The amount or intensity of the sensation is termed *sensitivity*. Some patients describe their reaction to palpation as "a little bit sensitive," whereas others may cry out in intolerable pain. The latter patients clearly feel more pain from the same palpation, and their symptoms are either more severe or more chronic.

Such patients may need more treatment to achieve pain relief than do patients with less sensitive acu-reflex points. In other words, the degree of sensitivity of an acu-reflex point is proportional to the amount of pain: The more sensitive the acu-reflex points are, the more pain is felt by the patient, the more treatment will be needed, and the more likely it is that the symptoms will recur.

Specificity

Specificity refers to the size and precise location of a passive acu-reflex point. In the beginning of the passive phase, the area or surface size of a sensitive acu-reflex point is relatively small and difficult to locate, which is an indication of the early stage of transition from latent to passive phase. This condition is referred to as *high specificity*. When symptoms become more severe, the sensitivity of the acu-reflex point spreads to surrounding tissues; as a consequence, the surface size of the passive acu-reflex point grows, and the point becomes more easily palpable. This condition is referred to as *low specificity*. Some practitioners have found that careful palpation reveals large sensitive regions, from 16 to 200 cm^2 (about 1.5 to 5 inches in diameter) surrounding a sensitive point.[4]

It is more difficult to locate a smaller, less sensitive, or more specific acu-reflex point than a bigger, more sensitive, and less specific one. Therefore the smaller acu-reflex point is defined as being more specific. An acu-reflex point is more specific when it is limited to a small area and as less specific when it is larger and covers a broader area. Specificity is inversely proportional to sensitivity: Specificity decreases when sensitivity increases, and vice versa.

Sequence

Acu-reflex points appear in the human body according to two models: systemic or symptomatic.

All physically and physiologically healthy persons have fewer acu-reflex points than do persons who are not healthy. If an initially healthy person starts to develop chronic problems such as chronic diseases, degenerative problems related to age, poor diet, bad posture, or lack of exercise, then more passive points will appear symmetrically all over the body. This phenomenon—the formation of passive acu-reflex points appear all over the body in particular locations when homeostasis declines—is referred to as the systemic pattern or model of *acu-reflex point formation*. Of most importance is that in the systemic model, all passive acu-reflex points are formed in predictable locations and in a predictable sequence. The predictable sequence determines which acu-reflex point becomes sensitive first and which point is sensitized next. This predictability in all people, healthy or sick, provides a quantitative basis for evaluation of a patient's health and allows the development of a standardized treatment protocol for acupuncture therapy, whose purpose is to restore homeostasis. These predictable acu-reflex points are called *homeostatic acu-reflex points*, inasmuch as they are related to homeostatic decline. Once homeostasis is restored, homeostatic acu-reflex points are gradually desensitized and eventually disappear, although some may stay for the rest of the patient's life.

If a healthy person sustains an acute injury, as in vehicle accidents or sports, or is afflicted with an acute disease, such as a cold or muscle sprain, sensitive points appear around the injured area or in related skin or muscle segments. These local sensitive points are termed *symptomatic acu-reflex points*. An acute injury is an example of the symptomatic model of acu-reflex point formation. The local appearance of symptomatic acu-reflex points reflects the individual features of the specific acute injury or disease. Each patient may exhibit a particular sensitization pattern of symptomatic acu-reflex points.

In physically healthy bodies, homeostatic acu-reflex points transform from latent phase to passive phase according to a highly predictable pattern. For example, the H1 deep radial point (located on the deep radial nerve where the nerve enters the lateral side of the forearm to innervate the extensor muscles of the wrist and fingers) is always the first one to become sensitive, and this is true for everybody.

The number of sensitive homeostatic acu-reflex points in the body serves as a quantitative indicator of the patient's health. Usually, a healthy person has few sensitive homeostatic acu-reflex points. If a healthy person has acute pain, a few sessions of treatment relieve the pain. Less healthy people have more sensitive acu-reflex points and, therefore, need more sessions to achieve relief of even minor acute pain. Thus the number of sensitive homeostatic acu-reflex points in the body is the quantitative indicator of (1) health status, (2) self-healing capacity (healthy persons heal better and faster), and (3) the number of treatments needed to achieve symptom relief. This quantitative indicator provides clinicians with a reasonably objective method for evaluating patients and predicting the outcome of the treatment.

Suppose that two patients complain about similar symptoms of low back pain, but patient A has 20 passive homeostatic acu-reflex points, whereas patient B has more than 40. To achieve pain relief, patient A is likely to need two treatments, whereas patient B may need eight. Moreover, patient A is likely to enjoy long-term or permanent relief from pain after two treatments, whereas it is highly possible that patient B will experience a relapse of the symptoms a few months after the initial eight treatments. Because patient A is healthier than patient B, patient A will (1) experience faster therapeutic results with fewer needling treatments, (2) enjoy longer and complete pain relief, and (3) be less likely to experience a relapse of the same pain symptom.

ELECTROPHYSIOLOGY OF ACU-REFLEX POINTS

Muscles and nerves are excitable tissues generating electrical signals when stimulated. When undisturbed or at rest, they are electrically silent. Barlas and colleagues[1] investigated the electrical activity at trigger points, and they found two significant components: (1) intermittent high-amplitude spike potentials and (2) continuous, lower amplitude, noise-like recordings, which they called *spontaneous electrical activity.*

The author discovered similar electrical activity in response to peripheral pain in the neurons of the spinal cord and mid-brain (periaqueductal gray matter) in rats. In normal tissues, the neurons in the spinal cord and the periaqueductal gray matter are silent. When pain or inflammation is present in the muscles, the spikes and spontaneous electrical activity appear in both the spinal cord and the periaqueductal gray matter. As the pain intensity increases, the frequency of spikes increases and may reach more than 200 per second. Spike frequency in the nervous signaling system translates electrophysiologically into pain intensity.

NEEDLING RESTORES NORMAL ENERGY METABOLISM IN SOFT TISSUE DYSFUNCTION

Weinstein and Britchkov[13] demonstrated that muscular contraction knots are the histopathologic characteristics of trigger points. Gunn[18] also suggested a similar histologic structure of the shortened muscles with palpable sensitive or painful bands or points (Fig. 7-1).

Careful examination of pathologic activity in passive or active acu-reflex points and the muscles harboring them reveals that in addition to pronounced pain symptoms, at least two other abnormal phenomena are present:

- The surface temperature of most acu-reflex points is a little higher than that of normal tissues ($0.3°$ to $0.5°C$). This can be a sign of inflammation. Cooler temperatures in and around some acu-reflex points have also been reported, possibly attributable to vascular constriction in some cases.
- The affected muscles are tight and resist stretching.

In 1950, medical scientist Y. Nakatani, from Kyoto University in Japan, discovered that acu-reflex points on the skin have a high level of electrical conductivity. Moreover, the electrical conductivity of some acu-reflex points increased significantly during sickness. He found 370 such points, incorporated them into the classic meridian system, and called them *ryodoraku* points. *Ryodoraku* in both Japanese and Chinese languages means "meridian point with good electrical conductivity."

In 1977, Nakatani noticed that ryodoraku points were situated on areas containing sweat glands and inferred that the higher electrical conductivity of ryodoraku is caused by the high conductivity of the sweat glands. Modern *ryodoraku* theory focuses on interactions between the sympathetic nervous system and the somatic nervous system.[6]

In healthy skeletal muscle fibers (cells), calcium is stored in the sarcoplasmic reticulum. When a

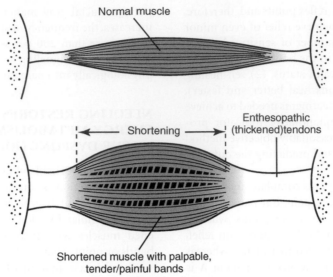

FIGURE 7-1 Muscle contracture caused by radiculopathy or other muscle injuries.

motor nerve fiber sends impulses to the muscles, the impulses initiate an action potential in the membrane of the muscle fiber. This action potential spreads into the sarcoplasmic reticulum (whose membrane is continuous with the muscle membrane), which results in release of calcium into the cytoplasm. The high concentration of cytoplasmic calcium triggers the coupling between two linear proteins (actin and myosin). After coupling, these two linear proteins slide against each other, which leads to shortening of the muscle fiber. This coupling and sliding between the two protein molecules consumes a large amount of energy. If there are no further impulses from the motor fiber after the initial shortening, the sarcoplasmic reticulum takes back the calcium into storage, and the concentration of cytoplasmic calcium drops accordingly. The low level of cytoplasmic calcium causes a decoupling of the contractile proteins (actin and myosin), which relaxes the muscle fiber.

If a muscle fiber is damaged, the sarcoplasmic reticulum is unable to take back the cytoplasmic calcium into storage. The two contractile protein molecules cannot decouple because of the high concentration of cytoplasmic calcium. This results

in persistent contraction of the muscle fiber, even without any further impulse from the motor nerve. If this energy-consuming process (the energy crisis) continues, sensitive muscle bands or acu-reflex points are formed. The sensitive bands, or trigger points, become a permanent contracture if the energy crisis persists for long enough.

Because acupuncture needling creates a tiny lesion, with bleeding, in the tissue, the contracting muscle immediately relaxes, and blood circulation improves. Thus acupuncture needling breaks the vicious circle of energy crises in trigger points inside the muscle.

The needle-created lesion disturbs the surrounding tissue and generates an electrical current of as much as 500 mA/cm,[8] which is called the *lesion current*. In addition, small local bleeding caused by the lesion stimulates secretion of numerous growth factors such as platelet-derived growth factors and neurotrophic factors.[9]

The electrical current and the bleeding promote healing and regeneration of damaged tissues and induce DNA synthesis of new proteins and collagens that repair damaged cellular organelles and restore normal function. A lesion may last for at least 2 days before the body heals it, which means that the stimulation it causes may also last as long. During the healing period the cells with lesions are digested and replaced by fresh tissue cells of the same type. This explains why acupuncture needling can achieve long-lasting results. After the needles are removed the needle-induced lesions keep working for at least a few days.

Acu-reflex points are mainly composed of sensitized sensory nerve receptors. This sensitized condition is a dynamic process: Acu-reflex points appear and grow when health deteriorates, and they may disappear as health is restored. Normal physiologic homeostasis reduces the sensitivity of acu-reflex points, whereas acute injuries or chronic diseases sensitizes them.

Acute injuries and acute diseases create local sensitive points. These are called *symptomatic acu-reflex points,* and they appear in different locations in individual patients, depending on each patient's injury or disease.

Some latent or active acu-reflex points appear as a result of the vicious circle of the metabolic energy crisis. Such acu-reflex points maintain a temperature higher than that of surrounding tissues because of sustained muscle contraction. The muscle contraction is itself an energy-demanding process, but when it is sustained, an environment of low energy and low oxygen (hypoxia) is created as a result of reduced blood circulation. Needling is able to relax the muscle, which breaks the vicious circle and restores normal blood circulation (Fig. 7-2).[19]

TEN BASIC ANATOMIC FEATURES OF ACU-REFLEX POINTS

Nerves are the major component of all acu-reflex points, but each point has a particular neural configuration. For example, different acu-reflex points may consist of cutaneous nerves, muscular nerves, α-motor nerves, and γ-motor nerves; some contain both afferent and efferent fibers; and some contain nerves and blood vessels. These different neural configurations result in different physiologic mechanisms of sensitization. Dr. H. C. Dung, professor of anatomy at the University of Texas Health

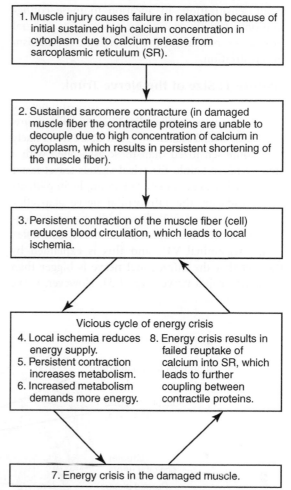

FIGURE 7-2 Energy metabolism and cellular process of muscle fiber contracture in a sensitive acu-reflex point. The energy crisis hypothesis is suggested by Dr. David G. Simons. *SR,* Sarcoplasmic reticulum.

Science Center at San Antonio, summarized the 10 basic anatomic features of acu-reflex points derived from his laboratory research and clinical experience.[20] The order listed as follows is physiologic. For example, an acu-reflex point with a large nerve trunk sensitizes faster than one with a shallow nerve; an acu-reflex point in deep fascia will sensitize more slowly than one with a shallow nerve. The anatomic configuration contributes to the predictable sequence and location of acu-reflex point sensitization. In addition to these configurations, functional anatomy, such as postural mechanics, may affect the physiologic mechanism of sensitization.

Feature 1: Size of the Nerve Trunk

Acu-reflex points are always associated with nerves, either cutaneous or muscular. The acu-reflex points associated with a bigger nerve trunk are more likely to become sensitized than these associated with a smaller nerve trunk. Electrical signals travel faster along thicker nerve fibers. For example, in patients with headache, the infraorbital nerve acu-reflex point (trigeminal V2) invariably becomes sensitized before the supraorbital nerve acu-reflex point (trigeminal V1), and this is explained by the fact that the infraorbital nerve is bigger than the supraorbital nerve (Fig. 7-3). However, nerve

size may not be the only factor that dictates the pathophysiologic dynamics of the acu-reflex points when other anatomic determinants are involved.

Feature 2: Depth of the Nerve

More acu-reflex points are formed along superficial nerve trunks than along deeper ones. The superficial nerve receptors become sensitized more easily than receptors of nerves located deep in the tissue. For example, the sciatic nerve is the biggest nerve trunk in the human body, but only a few acu-reflex points can be attributed to this big nerve in the gluteal and thigh region because there the nerve lies deep beneath the thick gluteal and hamstring muscles. As the sciatic nerve enters the posterior compartment of the thigh and popliteal fossa and reaches the leg, it emerges superficially and forms branches. More acu-reflex points are found along

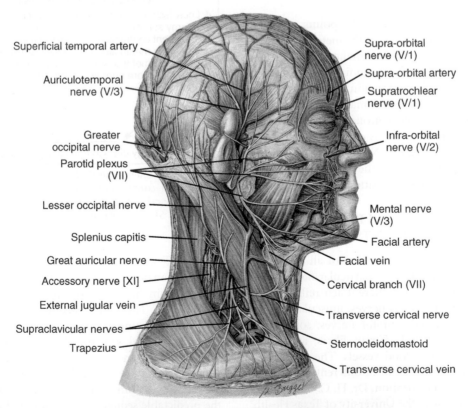

FIGURE 7-3 Acu-reflex points associated with thicker nerves become sensitized faster than those associated with thinner nerves. Thus for example, the infraorbital nerve is sensitized faster than the supraorbital nerve.

this nerve's branches in the leg. The same principle is applicable to other nerve trunks.

The pattern of acu-reflex point formation is the same in the upper extremity and the lower extremity. Nerve trunks in the upper limbs are located either deep beneath the muscles or inside the neurovascular compartment. As a result, only a few acu-reflex points are formed in the upper arm. On their way to the forearm, nerve trunks emerge closer to the surface, and therefore more acu-reflex points appear in this region. This is why more acu-reflex points are formed below than above the elbows and knees.

How acu-reflex point formation is affected by the depth of a nerve is illustrated as follows: The deep radial nerve is derived from the brachial plexus and courses through the upper arm without forming any important acu-reflex points. When it emerges from the deep fascia to the superficial fascia in the forearm, it forms the most important acu-reflex point in the body (H1 deep radial nerve) (Fig. 7-4).

Superficial acu-reflex points become sensitive more often than deeply located acu-reflex points because of the abundance of sensory receptors around the location where they are formed. An interesting neurologic fact is that the limbs below the elbows and knees occupy larger areas in the sensory gyrus in the brain. Therefore the acu-reflex points below elbows and knees also occupy a larger part of the cortical representation in the postcentral sensory gyrus in the brain. This may explain why acu-reflex points below elbows and knees contain more sensory receptors and why needling stimulation of these points may induce a stronger reaction and activity in the brain.

Feature 3: Penetration of Deep Fascia

The term *fascia* is rather loosely applied in anatomy. Most fasciae are connective tissue layers and are arranged in sheets or tubes between or around anatomic structures. Superficial fascia is a padding that is connected with the dermis and located above the deep fascia. Deep fascia lies under the superficial fascia and often forms the outer connective layer or covering of the structures underneath, such as blood vessels, nerves, or muscles. Acupuncture points are formed at locations where a nerve trunk passes through deep fascia and emerges close to the surface (Fig. 7-5).

Feature 4: Passage Through Bone Foramina

Acu-reflex points are found at bone foramina where nerve trunks emerge to distribute cutaneously. The cutaneous branches of the trigeminal nerves (V) give rise to this kind of acu-reflex point at the infraorbital (V2), supraorbital (V1), and mental (V3) foramina. (see Fig. 7-3).

Feature 5: Neuromuscular Attachments

Acu-reflex points are formed at the loci where nerve trunks enter the muscle. Muscular nerve trunks contain afferent (sensory) fibers, efferent (motor) fibers, and sympathetic fibers. Two acu-reflex points formed in this way can be found at the centers of the supraspinous and infraspinous fossae, where the suprascapular nerve enters the supraspinatus and infraspinatus muscles (Fig. 7-6). In this example, one nerve forms two attachments with two muscles, but the infraspinatus attachment is more superficial because the muscle is thinner; therefore this locus (H8, infraspinatus) usually becomes sensitive before the supraspinatus point, inasmuch as the latter lies deeper below the round, thick supraspinatus muscle.

In theory, each muscle has at least one neuromuscular attachment. However, most similar attachments do not form acu-reflex points because the attachments are located deep in the muscle masses and do not become sensitive very frequently.

Feature 6: Concomitant Blood Vessels

Arteries and veins course along the nerve trunks to form neurovascular bundles to reach the muscle attachments. Acu-reflex points associated with neurovascular bundles tend to become sensitive more readily than do acu-reflex points associated only with cutaneous nerves, because the cutaneous nerves are not accompanied by concomitant blood vessels.

The deep radial nerve is a clear example of how an acu-reflex point is formed by concomitant blood vessels and nerves. At the lateral surface of the proximal portion of the forearm, the deep radial nerve is buried inside the intermuscular septum between the muscles of the brachioradialis and the extensor radialis longus. Both the deep radial nerve and the lateral antebrachial cutaneous nerves are located at a similar depth and have similar size, except that the

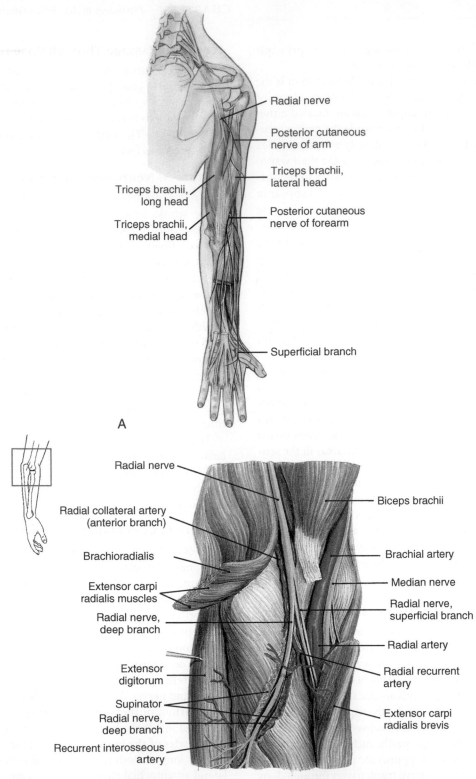

A

B

FIGURE 7-4 Radial nerve forms an important acu-reflex point (H1) at the site in the forearm where it penetrates the fascia.

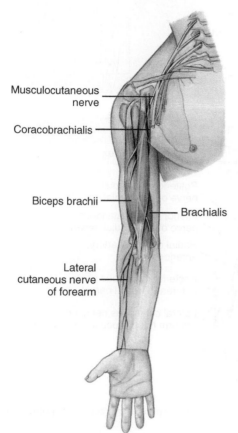

Musculocutaneous nerve

Coracobrachialis

Biceps brachii

Brachialis

Lateral cutaneous nerve of forearm

FIGURE 7-5 The lateral antebrachial cutaneous nerve, a branch of the musculocutaneous nerve, forms an acu-reflex point (H9) at the lateral side of the elbow where it penetrates the fascia.

deep radial nerve is associated with rich concomitant blood vessels. The acu-reflex point H1 (deep radial) appearing in this location always becomes sensitive before the acu-reflex point H9 (lateral antebrachial cutaneous) associated with lateral antebrachial cutaneous nerve (see Fig. 7-4).

The physiologic role of blood vessels in forming acu-reflex points is unknown. More sensory receptors are presumably formed where the nerve innervates the smooth muscles of the blood vessel.

Feature 7: Nerve Fiber Composition

A cutaneous nerve contains only afferent (sensory) and postganglionic sympathetic fibers, whereas a muscular nerve contains these two types of fibers as well as efferent (motor) fibers connecting to the skeletal muscles. Thus the cutaneous and muscular nerves differ in fiber composition.

When all other anatomic features are similar, acu-reflex points associated with nerve trunks containing more nerve fibers are more likely to become sensitized than are those with fewer nerve fibers.

The afferent (sensory) fibers provide sensory receptors attached to the blood vessels, muscle fibers, muscle spindles, muscle tendons, and skin. The sensory fibers collect sensory information from all these structures.

The efferent (motor) fibers innervate skeletal muscles and smooth muscles. The postganglionic sympathetic fibers innervate glands in the skin and internal organs. The motor fibers activate muscle contraction, and the sympathetic fibers control the activities of the glands and internal organs.

Feature 8: Bifurcation Points

Acu-reflex points are found at locations where a large nerve trunk branches into two or more smaller branches. For example, acu-reflex points are found in the distal portions of the four limbs, particularly in the dorsal surfaces of the hand and foot (Fig. 7-7).

Feature 9: Sensitive Ligamentous Structures

Sensitive loci can become acu-reflex points. Sensitive ligamentous structures include ligaments, muscle tendons, bone retinacula, thick fascial sheets, joint capsules, and collateral ligaments. They are all formed by dense fibrous connective tissue and are sensitive to pressure, palpation, and stretching because of rich afferent nerve receptors in the tissues. For example, a number of sensitive or even painful points can be found on the collateral ligaments when the knee hurts.

Feature 10: Suture Lines of the Skull

Acu-reflex points are formed along the suture lines of the skull. The acu-reflex points can be palpated along the coronal suture, sagittal suture, lambdoidal suture, and other sutures. Such acu-reflex points appear at the nasion, fontanelle, bregma, and pterion. When chronic headache is not adequately treated, sensitive points eventually appear at these locations.

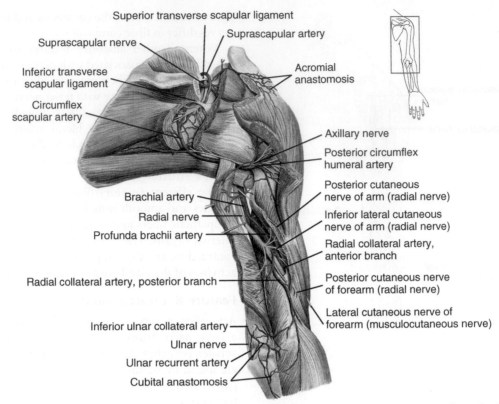

Superior transverse scapular ligament

Suprascapular nerve

Suprascapular artery

Inferior transverse
scapular ligament

Acromial
anastomosis

Circumflex
scapular artery

Axillary nerve

Posterior circumflex
humeral artery

Posterior cutaneous
nerve of arm (radial nerve)

Brachial artery

Inferior lateral cutaneous
nerve of arm (radial nerve)

Radial nerve

Profunda brachii artery

Radial collateral artery,
anterior branch

Radial collateral artery, posterior branch

Posterior cutaneous nerve
of forearm (radial nerve)

Lateral cutaneous nerve of
forearm (musculocutaneous nerve)

Inferior ulnar collateral artery

Ulnar nerve

Ulnar recurrent artery

Cubital anastomosis

FIGURE 7-6 The suprascapular nerve innervates both the infraspinatus and supraspinatus. An acu-reflex point is formed at the site of neuromuscular attachment.

Summary of the Anatomic Features of Acu-Reflex Points

The 10 basic neuroanatomic features of acu-reflex points provide a solid foundation for understanding the nature of their structural configuration, pathophysiologic dynamics, and clinical importance for evaluating and selecting points during treatment, through the use of the INMARPS.

Other structures could also contribute to the formation of acu-reflex points. Japanese researchers, for example, have suggested a close association between some acu-reflex points and lymphatic channels.[10]

Each acu-reflex point can have one or more of the 10 basic anatomic features. As discussed previously, the neural configurations of the points were numbered according to their relative propensity to become sensitive. Acu-reflex points with lower numbers (e.g., site of the nerve trunk, numbered 1) usually become sensitive earlier and faster than acu-reflex points with higher numbers (e.g., suture lines of the skull, numbered 10).

Thus the deep radial nerve acu-reflex point on the forearm (H1, deep radial, with feature 1) always becomes sensitive before the superficial radial nerve point on the hand (H12, superficial radial, with feature 8). The former should be selected for needling first because it sends more therapeutic signals.

All sensitive acu-reflex points, no matter where they appear, are invariably formed in association with sensory nerves. Sensory nerves are extensively distributed in the structures of the soft tissue such as skin, muscles, ligaments, joint capsules, fascias, blood vessels, and bones.

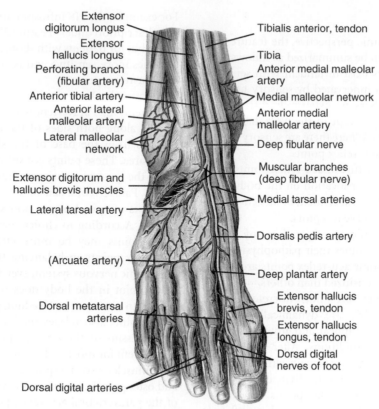

Extensor digitorum longus

Extensor hallucis longus

Perforating branch (fibular artery)

Anterior tibial artery

Anterior lateral malleolar artery

Lateral malleolar network

Extensor digitorum and hallucis brevis muscles

Lateral tarsal artery

(Arcuate artery)

Dorsal metatarsal arteries

Dorsal digital arteries

Tibialis anterior, tendon

Tibia

Anterior medial malleolar artery

Medial malleolar network

Anterior medial malleolar artery

Deep fibular nerve

Muscular branches (deep fibular nerve)

Medial tarsal arteries

Dorsalis pedis artery

Deep plantar artery

Extensor hallucis brevis, tendon

Extensor hallucis longus, tendon

Dorsal digital nerves of foot

FIGURE 7-7 Bifurcation of the deep fibular nerve on the dorsal surface of the foot, where an acu-reflex point (H5) is formed.

The sensitiveness of acu-reflex points arises from pathologic conditions affecting either peripheral nerve fibers or central neurons. Peripheral nerve fibers could be sensitized to form sensitive points by the chemicals leaking from damaged tissues. The neurons in the spinal cord could become sensitized by sustained stimulation of nerve impulses from peripheral receptors, as would occur in cases of chronic pain or cumulative trauma.[12]

Chronic pain is not like prolonged acute pain because the pain mechanisms involved are different. Acute pain is the warning signal of tissue injury that is locally restricted, whereas chronic pain is a disease that involves both peripheral and central sensitization.

Some sensitive points may indicate local damage in the affected area, but the local damage could at the same time produce distant pain by the mechanism of referred pain. An example of referred pain is angina pectoris, in which acu-reflex points palpated on the medial side of the left arm, the upper back, and the lower jaw are found to be sensitive.

Sensitive points may represent any type of damage of the tissue innervated by sensory nerves. For example, five acu-reflex points in the lumbar area and lower limbs are usually sensitive in the case of lower back pain, but the cause of the sensitivity could be any of several factors: nerve damage; infection or inflammation of the dura of the nerve roots; muscle contraction (mostly big muscles such as the erector spinae, although sometimes small muscles may be involved); pathologic problems with fascias, joint capsules, or ligaments; herniated discs; bone fracture; arthritis; infections; tumors; emotional disorders; and mechanical abnormalities between vertebrae.

SUMMARY

From a neuroanatomic perspective, the features of acu-reflex points can be summarized as follows:

1. Acu-reflex points exist in tandem with sensory nerves or tissues innervated by sensory nerves. Sensory nerve fibers are extensively distributed all over the body, except in the nails, hair, and part of the cornea. Where there are sensory nerve fibers, there are acu-reflex points.
2. The anatomic structure of acu-reflex points varies according to their location on the body, but the common structural element of all acu-reflex points is sensory nerve receptors.
3. The neuroanatomic configuration of acu-reflex points determines their pathophysiologic dynamics; thus some acu-reflex points are more likely to become sensitized than others.
4. Acu-reflex points are not discrete, static points; instead, they are dynamically changing structures. They appear and grow in certain pathophysiologic conditions. After healing is completed, some of them remain, although with reduced sensitivity, and some disappear.
5. The sensitivity of acu-reflex points may indicate injury to peripheral tissues, such as inflammation of the nerves, muscles, ligaments, joint capsules, and bones, or it may indicate that the sensitized neurons in the central nervous system have provoked sensitivity in the periphery.
6. The pattern according to which sensitized acu-reflex points appear is related to the anatomic distribution of the peripheral nerve trunks (on the limbs) and nerve fibers. Thus acu-reflex points on the arm or leg become sensitive in a linear pattern along the nerve trunk, primarily along the cutaneous nerves, whereas acu-reflex points on the back or face become sensitive in an area that follows the nerve endings of different nerve branches.

Pathophysiologically, there are three types of acu-reflex points:

1. Homeostatic acu-reflex points (HAs)
2. Symptomatic acu-reflex points (SAs)
3. Paravertebral acu-reflex points (PAs)

Each type of acu-reflex point has its own particular pathologic mechanism. However, the way each type has been defined is not absolute. A homeostatic acu-reflex point can also be a symptomatic point.

For example, the H8 infraspinatus acu-reflex point (see description under "Feature 5") is a homeostatic point, but for patients with shoulder pain, this point becomes more sensitive and is clearly a symptomatic acu-reflex point.

Paravertebral acu-reflex points merit special attention. Paravertebral acu-reflex points are located along both sides of the spine on the back muscles from the base of the skull down to the sacral area. These points consist of the nerve fibers from the posterior primary rami of the spinal nerves. Paravertebral acu-reflex points are closer to the roots of spinal nerves and sympathetic trunk ganglia. According to clinical evidence, these acu-reflex points may be more effective than other acu-reflex points in balancing the activity of the autonomic nervous system, even though every acu-reflex point in the body does balance autonomic activity to some extent. Needling paravertebral acu-reflex points also relaxes the back muscles, which eases pressure on the vertebral joints. This function is of benefit for most of the symptoms related to the back muscles and the spine, such as radiculopathy and osteoporosis. Sometimes a particular grouping of the paravertebral acu-reflex points may become sensitive, in which case the points in this section can also be regarded as symptomatic points. For example, in a patient with a stomach ulcer, sensitive points are palpable around the xiphoid process in front, but sensitive points may also appear on one or both sides of the spine from T7 to T12.

From a clinical perspective, paravertebral acu-reflex points do not have exact locations as homeostatic acu-reflex points and symptomatic acu-reflex points do, because the cutaneous branches of neighboring spinal nerves overlap each other. To achieve maximal results from needling, it is better to needle all the neighboring spinal nerves. For example, if postherpetic pain is related to spinal nerves from T5 to T6, needling is recommended from T4 to T7.

References

1. Barlas P, Walsh DM, Baxter GD, et al: Delayed onset muscle soreness: effect of an ischemic block upon mechanical allodynia in humans, *Pain* 87:221–225, 2000.
2. Crenshaw AG, Thornell LE, Friden J: Intramuscular pressure, torque and swelling for exercise-induced sore vastus lateralis muscle, *Acta Physiol Scand* 152:265–277, 1994.

3. Stauber WT, Clarkson DM, Fritz VK, et al: Extracellular matrix disruption and pain after eccentric muscle action, *J Applied Physiol* 69:868–874, 2002.

4. Trappe TA, Carrithers JA, White F, et al: Titin and nebulin content in human skeletal muscle following eccentric resistance exercise, *Muscle Nerve* 25:289–292, 2002.

5. Proske V, Morgan DC: Muscle damage from eccentric exercise: mechanisms, mechanical signs, adaptation and clinical application, *J Physiol* 537:333–345, 2001.

6. Rocabado M, Iglarsh AZ: *Musculoskeletal approach to maxillofacial pain*, Philadelphia, 1991, Lippincott, pp 136–137.

7. Jarrell J, Robert M: Myofascial dysfunction and pelvic pain, *Can J CME (Feb)* 107–116, 2003.

8. Weiss JM: Pelvic floor myofascial trigger points: manual therapy for interstitial cystitis and the urgency-frequency syndrome, *J Urol* 166:2226–2231, 2001.

9. Wiygul RD, Wiygul JP: Interstitial cystitis, pelvic pain, and the relationship to myofascial pain and dysfunction: a report on four patients, *World J Urol* 20:310–314, 2002.

10. Hetrick DC, Ciol MA, Rothman I, et al: Musculoskeletal dysfunction in men with chronic pelvic pain syndrome type III: a case-control study, *J Urol* 170:828–831, 2003.

11. Zermann DH, Ishigooka M, Doggweiler R, et al: Chronic prostatitis: a myofascial pain syndrome? *Infect Urol* 12:84–92, 1999.

12. Shah JP, Philips T, Danoff J, et al: Novel microanalytical technique distinguishes three clinically distinct groups: (1) subject without pain and without myofascial trigger points; (2) subject without pain with myofascial trigger points; (3) subject with pain and myofascial trigger points [Abstract], *Am J Phys Med Rehabil* 83:231, 2004.

13. Weinstein A, Britchkov M: Lyme arthritis and post–Lyme disease syndrome, *Curr Opin Rheumatol* 14:383–387, 2002.

14. Plotnikoff GA, Guigley JM: Prevalence of severe hypovitaminosis D in patients with persistent nonspecific musculoskeletal pain, *Mayo Clin Proc* 78:1463–1470, 2003.

15. Thompson PD, Clarkson P, Karas RH: Statin-associated myopathy, *JAMA* 289:1681–1690, 2003.

16. Gerwin RD, Gambel J, Shannon S, et al: A comparison of two possible perpetuating factors in a military and civilian population [Abstract], *J Musculoskel Pain* 9(Suppl 5): 83, 2001.

17. Gambel J, Shannon S, Rubertone ML, et al: Comparison of biochemical markers between active duty U.S. service members with chronic myofascial pain and matched controls [Abstract], *J Musculoskel Pain* 9(Suppl 5):85, 2001.

18. Gunn CC: *Gunn approach to the treatment of chronic pain: intramuscular stimulation for myofascial pain of radiculopathic origin*, ed 2, Edinburgh, 1996, Churchill Livingstone.

19. Simons DG: Referred phenomena of myofacial trigger points. In Vecchiet L, Albe-Fessard D, Lindblom U, editors: *Pain research and clinical management: new trends in referred pain and hyperalgesia*, vol 27, Amsterdam, 1993, Elsevier, Chap 28.

20. Dung HC: *Anatomical acupuncture*, San Antonio, Tex, 1997, Antarctic Press, Chap 5.

Neuroanatomy of Acu-Reflex Points

ANATOMIC SURVEY OF HOMEOSTATIC ACU-REFLEX POINTS

The human nervous system develops in segments, and acu-reflex points (ARPs) are distributed all over the body according to the neural segments. The head segments are fused together and expand to form the cerebral hemispheres and brainstem. Twelve pairs of cranial nerves exit these segments.

The spinal nerves arise from the segments of the spinal cord. Each segment gives rise to both sensory and motor nerve roots on each side of the body (Fig. 8-1). Through all the segments of the spinal cord, motor systems tend to be more ventral and sensory systems more dorsal. Because of this scheme, dorsal nerve roots convey mainly afferent sensory information into the dorsal spinal cord, whereas ventral nerve roots carry mainly efferent motor signals from the ventral spinal cord to the periphery. The segments and nerve roots of the spinal cord are named according to the level at which they exit the bony vertebral canal: cervical, thoracic, lumbar, and sacral nerve roots.

A spinal nerve divides into two primary rami: the dorsal (posterior) ramus and the ventral (anterior) ramus. The short (posterior) ramus, with its two end branches, innervates the muscles and skin of the back. The ventral (anterior) primary ramus travels within the body wall to innervate the skin and muscles of the lateral and anterior parts of the body (Fig. 8-2).

During development, the bony vertebral canal increases in length faster than the spinal cord; as a result, the spinal cord ends at the level of the first or second lumbar vertebral bones (L1 or L2). Below this level, the spinal canal contains a collection of nerve roots known as the *cauda equina*. The sensory and motor nerve roots join together a short distance outside the spinal cord and form a mixed sensory and motor spinal nerve.

The distribution of ARPs follows the same segmental scheme as do the peripheral nerves. After exiting from the spinal cord, many fibers of nerve roots, both sensory and motor, are mixed to form a mesh that is called the *plexus* (Fig. 8-3).

Facial ARPs are formed by cranial nerves. Clinically important cranial nerves that form the facial points are the trigeminal nerves (Fig. 8-4) and facial nerve (Fig. 8-5). Neck ARPs are innervated by cervical plexus from C1 to C5 (Fig. 8-6).

Arms and legs, because of their importance in movement, provide much more signal flow to the central nervous system and therefore require more neural control and coordination than do muscles of the chest and abdomen. Therefore the enlarged segments of C5 to T1 give rise to the brachial plexus

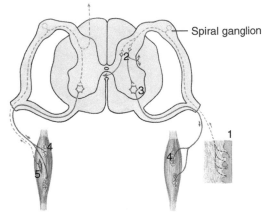

1 = Skin
2 = Interneurons
3 = Motoneuron of anterior horn
4 = Motor end-plate
5 = Muscle spindle

FIGURE 8-1 Reflex at the spinal cord. *Left,* Monosynaptic reflex: bineuronal reflex: patellar tendon and Achilles tendon reflex. *Right,* Polyneuronal reflex: abdominal and plantar reflex.

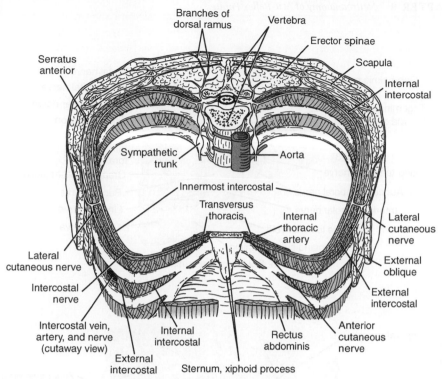

FIGURE 8-2 Diagram of a section of a spinal nerve. A spinal nerve divides into two primary rami: the dorsal (posterior) ramus and the ventral (anterior) ramus. The short dorsal primary ramus with its two end branches innervates the muscles and skin of the back. The ventral primary ramus travel within the body wall to innervate the skin and the muscles on the lateral and anterior parts of the body.

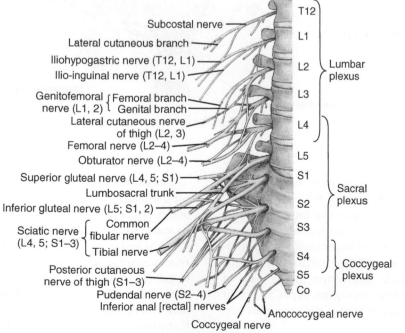

FIGURE 8-3 The lumbosacral and coccygeal plexus.

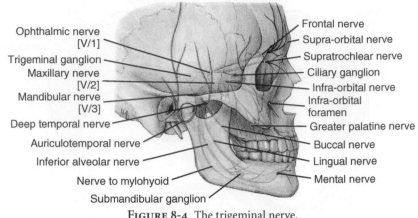

Ophthalmic nerve [V/1]
Trigeminal ganglion
Maxillary nerve [V/2]
Mandibular nerve [V/3]
Deep temporal nerve
Auriculotemporal nerve
Inferior alveolar nerve
Nerve to mylohyoid
Submandibular ganglion

Frontal nerve
Supra-orbital nerve
Supratrochlear nerve
Ciliary ganglion
Infra-orbital nerve
Infra-orbital foramen
Greater palatine nerve
Buccal nerve
Lingual nerve
Mental nerve

FIGURE 8-4 The trigeminal nerve.

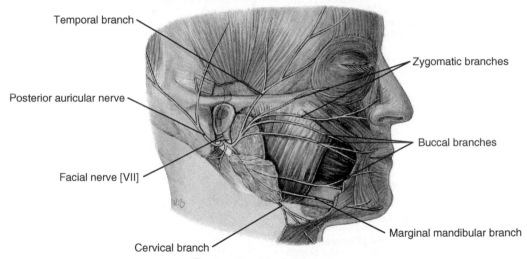

Temporal branch
Posterior auricular nerve
Facial nerve [VII]
Cervical branch

Zygomatic branches
Buccal branches
Marginal mandibular branch

FIGURE 8-5 The facial nerve.

for the arm (Fig. 8-7) and lumbosacral plexus from T12 or L1 to S3 for the leg (Fig. 8-8).

In addition to the sensory and motor pathways, the peripheral nervous system includes some specialized neurons involved in controlling such autonomic functions as heart rate, peristalsis, sweating, and smooth muscle contraction in the walls of blood vessels, bronchi, sex organs, pupils, and other areas. These neurons are part of the autonomic nervous system.

The autonomic nervous system provides the tissue-, organ-, and system-level integration of the body's physiologic processes to achieve homeostasis and to support the activities of human behavior. With the endocrine system, the autonomic nervous system coordinates the continuous adjustments in blood chemistry, respiration, circulation, digestion, reproductive status, body temperature, elimination of metabolic wastes, and immune responses that protect homeostasis. The autonomic nervous

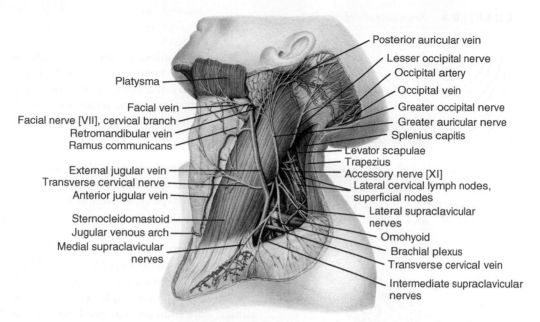

FIGURE 8-6 The cervical plexus. Acu-reflex points are formed by greater auricular nerve, lesser occipital nerve, transverse cervical nerve, and supraclavicular nerves.

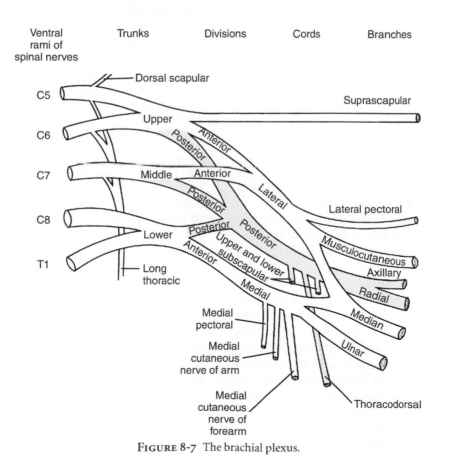

FIGURE 8-7 The brachial plexus.

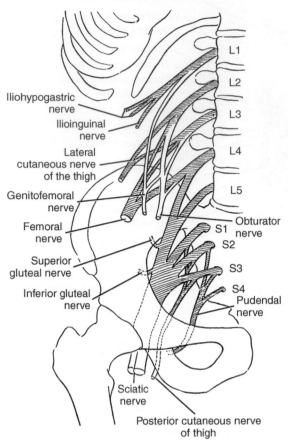

Iliohypogastric nerve
Ilioinguinal nerve
Lateral cutaneous nerve of the thigh
Genitofemoral nerve
Femoral nerve
Superior gluteal nerve
Inferior gluteal nerve
L1
L2
L3
L4
L5
S1
S2
S3
S4
Obturator nerve
Pudendal nerve
Sciatic nerve
Posterior cutaneous nerve of thigh

FIGURE 8-8 The lumbosacral plexus.

system also actively coordinates the function of skeletal muscles involved in behavior.

Impairment of the autonomic nervous system results in a loss of ability to mobilize physiologic responses and adaptations to challenges to homeostasis.

The autonomic nervous system has two major divisions. The sympathetic division arises from thoracic and lumbar spinal nerves T1 to L2 (the thoracolumbar division; Fig. 8-9). It releases the neurotransmitter norepinephrine onto target organs and is involved in such stress-related activities as the "fight or flight" response with its functions, such as increased heart rate and blood pressure, bronchodilation, and increased pupil size. The parasympathetic division, in contrast, arises from the cranial nerves and from sacral spinal levels

S2 to S4 (the craniosacral division). It releases acetylcholine onto target organs and is involved in more sedentary and energy-conserving functions, such as increasing gastric secretions and peristalsis, slowing the heart rate, and decreasing pupil size (Fig. 8-10).

The sympathetic and parasympathetic pathways are controlled by higher centers in the hypothalamus and limbic system, as described in previous chapters, as well as by afferent sensory information from the body. According to data from research with functional magnetic resonance imaging, acupuncture needling causes responses in both the hypothalamus and the limbic system. The molecular interpretation of those responses is still incompletely understood, but clinical data indicate that needling helps restore homeostasis.

The enteric nervous system is considered a third autonomic division; it consists of a neural plexus lying within the walls of the gut that is involved in controlling peristalsis and gastrointestinal secretions.

In the following description, the general anatomy of each nerve is described first, and then the focus is on the 24 primary homeostatic ARPs.

CUTANEOUS AND MUSCULAR ACU-REFLEX POINTS

A cutaneous sensory nerve innervates a large skin area; for example, the lateral antebrachial cutaneous nerve on the forearm innervates the skin surface along a pathway that extends from elbow to wrist. When this nerve is stimulated, the sensation can propagate along the entire zone (Fig. 8-11). A muscular nerve specifically innervates a particular muscle. When a muscular nerve is stimulated, the sensation and muscular response may be limited to only the particular muscle. However, when a needle is inserted into an ARP, it punctures the skin and distinct layers of muscle and fasciae. Thus the result is complex and includes both cutaneous and muscular responses.

Of the 24 primary ARPs, some are cutaneous nerve points, some are muscular nerve points,

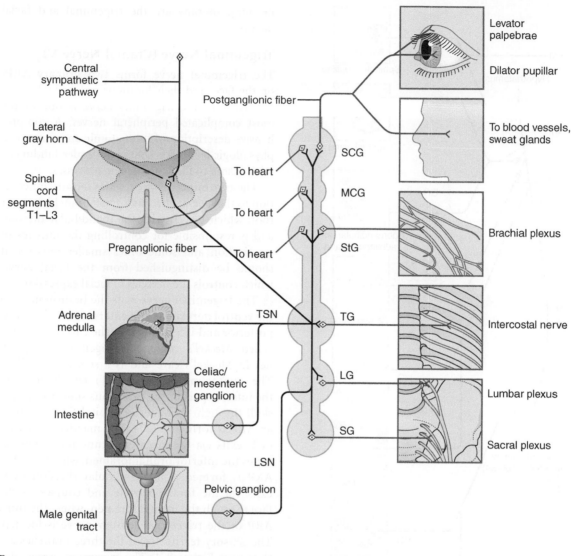

FIGURE 8-9 General plan of the sympathetic nervous system. Preganglionic neurons are located in the lateral gray horn of the spinal cord. *LG,* Lumbar ganglion; *LSN,* lumbar splanchnic nerve; *MCG,* middle cervical ganglion; *SCG,* superior cervical ganglia; *SG,* sacral ganglia; *St.G,* stellate ganglia; *TG,* thoracic ganglia; *TSN,* thoracic splanchnic nerve.

and some points are neither cutaneous nor muscular (e.g., the H1 deep radial nerve point, which is formed at the branching of the deep radial nerve).

The 24 primary homeostatic ARPs are depicted in Figure 8-12. Neural origins and segmentations of ARPs are listed in Table 8-1.

HOMEOSTATIC ACU-REFLEX POINTS ON THE FACE: THE TRIGEMINAL NERVE AND THE FACIAL NERVE

Anatomic Survey

All facial ARPs are related to cranial nerves. The most clinically important cranial nerves in

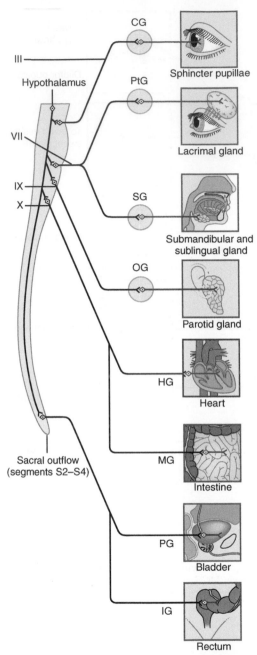

FIGURE 8-10 General plan of the parasympathetic nervous system. Preganglionic neurons are located in the lateral gray horn of the spinal cord. *CG,* Ciliary ganglion; *HG,* heart ganglia; *IG,* intramural ganglia; *MG,* myenteric ganglia; *OG,* otic ganglion; *PG,* pelvic ganglion; *PtG,* pterygopalatine ganglion; *SG,* submandibular ganglion.

needling therapy are the trigeminal and facial nerves.

Trigeminal Nerve (Cranial Nerve V)

The trigeminal nerve forms two primary ARPs on the face, and their locations are easily defined. Nevertheless, the trigeminal nerve is one of the most complicated peripheral nerves. A comprehensive description of its anatomic and functional physiologic features is helpful for understanding its relationship to facial pathologic processes.

The trigeminal nerve provides sensory innervation to the face. It also has a small branchial motor root, which travels with the mandibular division and is responsible for controlling the muscles of mastication and some other smaller muscles. It should be distinguished from the facial nerve, which controls the muscles of facial expression.

The trigeminal nerve exits the brainstem from the ventrolateral pons and enters a small fossa just posterior and inferolateral to the cavernous sinus called *Meckel's cave.* The trigeminal ganglion lies in Meckel's cave and is a sensory ganglion. The ophthalmic division (V1) travels through the inferior part of the cavernous sinus to exit the skull through the superior orbital fissure, where an ARP is formed (H23). The maxillary division (V2) exits via the foramen rotundum and penetrates the inferior orbital foramen, where another ARP is formed. The mandibular division (V3) exits via the foramen ovale and courses to the face through the mental foramen, where the third ARP of the trigeminal sensory nerve is located. The sensory territories of the three branches are shown in Figure 8-4. The trigeminal nerve also conveys touch and pain sensation for the nasal sinuses, the inside of the nose and mouth, and the anterior two thirds of the tongue.

The trigeminal nuclei receive general somatic sensory inputs from the nerve's own input and from other cranial nerves. Smaller inputs from the facial nerve (VII), glossopharyngeal nerve (IX), and vagus nerve (X) convey sensation for part of the external ear.

The trigeminal nuclear complex runs from the midbrain to the upper cervical spinal cord and contains three nuclei: the mesencephalic, main sensory,

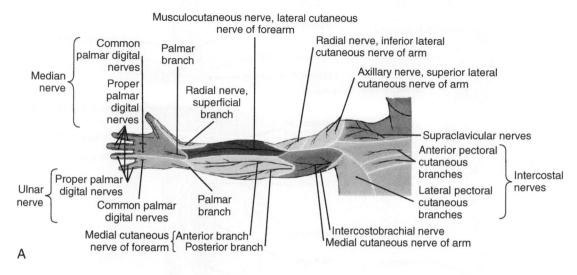

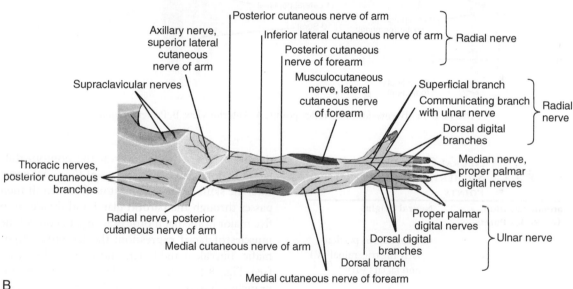

FIGURE 8-11 Cutaneous nerves of the upper limb. **A,** Anterior view. **B,** Posterior view.

and spinal trigeminal nuclei. The mesencephalic nucleus is the only one in which primary sensory neurons lie within the central nervous system instead of in a peripheral ganglion. This nucleus conveys proprioceptive input from the muscles of mastication and probably from the tongue and extraocular muscles. The other two nuclei serve as major sensory systems for fine and touch, pressure, pain, and temperature.

Facial Nerve (Cranial Nerve VII)

The facial nerve controls the muscles of facial expression. However, a smaller branch of the facial nerve, the nervus intermedium, carries fibers for the parasympathetic nervous system (tears and salivation), taste, and general somatosensory functions.

The facial nucleus is located in the branchial motor column, more caudally in the pons than is the trigeminal motor nucleus. The nerve exits

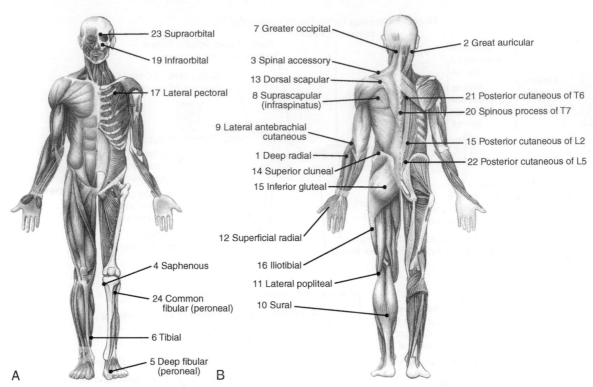

FIGURE 8-12 Twenty-four acu-reflex points. **A,** Anterior view. **B,** Posterior view.

TABLE 8-1	NEURAL ORIGIN AND SEGMENTATION OF ACU-REFLEX POINTS
Anatomic Location of Acu-Reflex Points	**Neural Origins**
Face	Cranial nerves, particularly the trigeminal (V) and facial (VII)
Neck	
Lateral and anterior neck	Cervical plexus (C1–C4), anterior rami
Posterior neck (paravertebral acu-reflex points)	C1–C8, posterior rami
Torso	
Lateral and anterior	Anterior rami of T1–T12
Posterior (paravertebral acu-reflex points)	Posterior rami of T1–S4
Shoulder and upper limb	Brachial plexus (C5–T1), anterior rami
Low back, hip, and lower limb	Lumbosacral plexus (L2–S3), anterior rami

the brainstem ventrolaterally at the pontomedullary junction. The main portion of the facial nerve exits the skull at the stylomastoid foramen. It then passes through the parotid gland and divides into five major branchial motor branches to control the muscles of facial expression: the temporal, zygomatic, buccal, mandibular, and cervical branches (see Fig. 8-5). Other smaller branchial motor branches innervate the stapedius and occipitalis muscles, the posterior belly of the digastric muscle, and the stylohyoid muscle.

The preganglionic parasympathetic fibers of the facial nerve arise from the superior salivatory nucleus and travel in two small branches off the main trunk of the facial nerve. At the genu of the facial nerve, the greater petrosal nerve branches to reach the sphenopalatine (pterygopalatine) ganglion, where postganglionic parasympathetic neurons innervate the lacrimal glands and nasal mucosa. The chorda tympani leaves the facial nerve and exits the skull at the petrotympanic fissure just medial and posterior to the temporomandibular joint. The chorda tympani then joins the lingual nerve (a branch of the trigeminal nerve) to reach the submandibular ganglion, where postganglionic parasympathetic pathways arise to supply the submandibular and submaxillary salivary glands.

A small branch of the facial nerve provides general somatic sensation near the external auditory meatus, and the glossopharyngeal nerve (IX) and vagus nerve (X) also innervate this region. The somatosensory fibers for trigeminal, facial, glossopharyngeal, and vagus nerves all synapse in the trigeminal nuclei.

About 20 muscles of facial expression are known. Each muscle has at least one neuromuscular attachment point. Thus when practitioners treat facial conditions such as sinusitis or Bell's palsy, the affected muscles in each case should be carefully detected. Because all neuromuscular attachments of the muscles of facial expression can become sensitized if the muscles are affected, these points can be used for needling therapy.

H19 Infraorbital (Cutaneous)

This ARP is located exactly on the infraorbital foramen (Fig. 8-13). The infraorbital nerve, a cutaneous nerve from the maxillary branch (V2) of the trigeminal nerve, passes the foramen and innervates the facial skin. To avoid hematoma when needling in this area, the practitioner should use 38- or 36-gauge needles (0.18- or 0.20-mm diameter, respectively). The depth for needling ranges from 2 to 5 mm.

The H19 infraorbital ARP is always the first ARP on the face to become sensitive because the infraorbital nerve is the biggest cutaneous nerve on the face. In addition to homeostatic decline, all symptoms related to the face and the head may further sensitize this point. Thus the sensitivity and size of the point provide useful information on the severity or chronicity of the symptom. Common symptoms that may sensitize this ARP are cranial neuralgias; all kinds of headache; facial, myofascial, and temporomandibular disorders; dental and intraoral pain; ocular and periocular pain; pain in the ear;

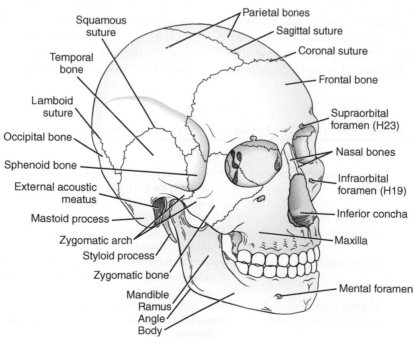

FIGURE 8-13 The infraorbital and supraorbital nerve.

sinusitis; cold; allergy; and facial paralysis. The H19 infraorbital ARP should be used for all these symptoms. Pain caused by cancer of the head and neck also sensitizes this point.

H23 Supraorbital (Cutaneous)

This ARP is formed right on the supraorbital notch, which is the passage for the supraorbital nerve (see Fig. 8-13). This cutaneous nerve from the ophthalmic branch (V1) of the trigeminal nerve extends to the top of the head. The method of needling this point is similar to that for the H19 infraorbital.

The supraorbital nerve is smaller than the infraorbital nerve; therefore the H23 supraorbital becomes sensitive after the H19 infraorbital. For example, the H19 infraorbital point is always sensitive in a patient with a slight headache. If the headache lingers on, the H23 supraorbital point becomes sensitive, too. If the headache continues further, other points in the face—such as the mental nerve (V3), the zygomaticofacial nerve (V2), and the zygomaticotemporal nerve—also become sensitive. The more sensitive points there are, the more chronic and more severe the symptom is and the more treatments are needed.

In treatment of patients with facial problems such as temporomandibular pain, chronic sinus pain, or facial paralysis, other points innervated by the facial nerve (VII) should be carefully palpated and selectively needled according to the individual symptom.

Other Facial Acu-Reflex Points

The trigeminal nerve contains both sensory (afferent) nerves and motor (efferent) nerves and is responsible for general sensation in the skin of the face and the front of the head, as well as for controlling the muscles of chewing (mastication). Muscles of mastication and muscles of facial expression are the two kinds of facial muscle. Two important muscles of mastication, the temporalis and masseter muscles, are innervated by the motor nerves of the trigeminal nerve. The ARPs formed in those two muscles are essential in treating some headaches and facial symptoms such as temporomandibular joint syndrome and facial paralysis.

The five branches of the complicated facial nerve innervate the 20 known muscles of facial expression and other structures, including the tongue (Table 8-2). Injury to the facial nerve or some of its branches leads to paresis (weakness) or paralysis (loss of voluntary movement) of all or some of the facial muscles on the affected side. The injuries may be caused by chilling of the face, inflammation, middle ear infection, fractures, and tumor. Proper needling of the affected muscles helps reduce inflammation and accelerates healing in many facial symptoms, including Bell's palsy.

TABLE 8-2   NERVES THAT FORM THE IMPORTANT FACIAL ACU-REFLEX POINTS

Nerve	Functional Categories	Functions
Trigeminal nerve	General somatic sensation	Sensations of touch, pain, temperature, joint position, and vibration for the face, mouth, anterior two thirds of tongue, nasal sinuses, and meninges
	Branchial motor	Muscles of mastication and tensor tympani muscle
Facial nerve	Branchial motor	Muscles of facial expression, stapedius muscles, and part of digastric muscle
	Parasympathetic	Parasympathetic function to lacrimal glands, and submaxillary, submandibular, and all other salivary glands except parotid gland
	Visceral sensory (special)	Taste from anterior two thirds of tongue
	General somatic sensory	Sensation from a small region near the external auditory meatus

ACU-REFLEX POINTS FORMED BY THE CERVICAL PLEXUS

The neck is one of the most important parts of the body in acupuncture therapy. Because of its critical involvement in both postural and physiologic homeostasis, it should be examined in every case and treated in most cases. The cervical plexus is not given particular attention in most anatomy textbooks, but its importance here cannot be overemphasized. This nerve plexus is described briefly here in order for readers to understand its anatomic scheme. Some of the most important neck ARPs are illustrated as well (see Fig. 8-6).

The branches of the cervical plexus are as follows:

- Cutaneous: lesser occipital, greater auricular, transverse cutaneous, and supraclavicular nerves
- Muscular branches to the neck muscles:

  Prevertebral muscles: sternocleidomastoid (proprioceptive; arising from C2 and C3), levator scapulae (arising from C3 and C4), and trapezius (proprioceptive; arising from C3 and C4)

  Omohyoid, sternohyoid, and sternothyroid muscles (arising from C1 to C3)

  Thyrohyoid and geniohyoid (arising from C1)
- Phrenic nerve to diaphragm: C3 to C5

The ventral primary rami of spinal nerves of C1 through C4, with a small contribution from C5, form the cervical nerve plexus. The nerves of the cervical nerve plexus innervate most of the anterior and lateral muscles of the neck, and its sensory fibers supply sensation to most of the neck and some part of the head. Readers should understand the innervation of this plexus because it is connected to many pathologic conditions of the neck and other physiologic systems.

The network of the cervical nerve plexus is formed by communications between the ventral rami of C1 through C5 (see Fig. 8-6). The plexus lies deep to the internal jugular vein and the sternocleidomastoid muscle. Cutaneous branches from the plexus emerge around the middle of the posterior border of the sternocleidomastoid to supply the skin of the neck and scalp, between the auricle and external occipital protuberance. The ventral rami of C2 to C4 of the cervical nerve plexus give rise to the great auricular, lesser occipital, transverse cervical, supraclavicular, and phrenic nerves.

After the communicating branches from C2 and C3, the main trunk of the great auricular nerve curves over the middle point of the posterior border of the sternocleidomastoid muscle and ascends vertically toward the parotid gland. It supplies branches to the skin of the neck and then divides into anterior and posterior branches, which supply the skin on the inferior part of the auricle on both anterior and posterior surfaces and an area extending from the mandible to the mastoid process.

The lesser occipital nerve, arising from C2 and sometimes C3, ascends a short distance along the posterior border of the sternocleidomastoid muscle before dividing into several branches that supply the skin of the neck and scalp posterior to the ear and the superior part of the auricle.

The transverse cervical nerve, arising from C2 and C3, curves around the posterior border of the sternocleidomastoid muscle near its middle point, too, and then passes transversely across it. Its branches supply the skin over the anterior triangle of the neck.

The supraclavicular nerve arises from C3 and C4 as a single trunk, which divides into medial, intermedial, and lateral branches. The small branches from this nerve travel to the skin of the neck and then penetrate the deep fascia just superior to the clavicle to supply the skin over the anterior aspect of the chest and shoulder. The medial and lateral supraclavicular nerves also supply the sternoclavicular and acromioclavicular joints.

The phrenic nerve, arising from C3 to C5, curves around the lateral border of the scalenus anterior muscle and then descends obliquely across its anterior surface deep to the transverse cervical and suprascapular arteries. The phrenic nerve enters the thorax by crossing the origin of the internal thoracic arteries between the subclavian artery and vein. The phrenic nerve is the only motor nerve that supplies the diaphragm.

H2 Great Auricular (Cutaneous)

The great auricular nerve is the site of one of the most important ARPs in the human body. Its location is crucial for the balance of head weight and therefore to the balance of the entire head. The importance of this nerve can be understood from its relation to the homeostasis of both mechanical posture and systemic physiology. However, the vasculature related to this point challenges clinicians because of safety concerns.

This point is located just behind the earlobe and on the anterior border of the sternocleidomastoid muscle. It is one of the four branches of the cervical nerve plexus. Four cutaneous branches from the cervical plexus emerge around the middle of the posterior border of the sternocleidomastoid muscle (Fig. 8-14).

The greater auricular nerve curves over and ascends obliquely toward the earlobe and the angle of the mandible. This nerve bundle surfaces through the investing fascia just below the earlobe and divides into branches to supply the skin on the inferior part of the ear and the area extending from the mandible to the mastoid process.

The H2 greater auricular ARP is sensitive in almost every patient. However, needling this point often causes bleeding because the external jugular vein descends just beside the greater auricular nerve. If the external jugular vein is prominent throughout its course, this is a sign that venous pressure is elevated owing to heart problems; in such cases, to avoid an accident such as a venous air embolism, this point should not be needled. A fine needle of gauge 36 or 38 (0.20- or 0.18-mm diameter) may be used to needle this point, with a needling depth of about 5 to 8 mm.

Other Neck Acu-Reflex Points

Several ARPs on the neck are formed by three other nerves derived from the cervical plexus: (1) the lesser occipital nerve, for which an ARP is located on the insertions between the sternocleidomastoid and the trapezius muscles on the occipital bone; (2) the transverse cervical nerve, which curves around the middle of the posterior border of the sternocleidomastoid and then passes transversely to the anterior border of the same muscle (several ARPs are formed over the anterior triangle of the neck); and (3) the

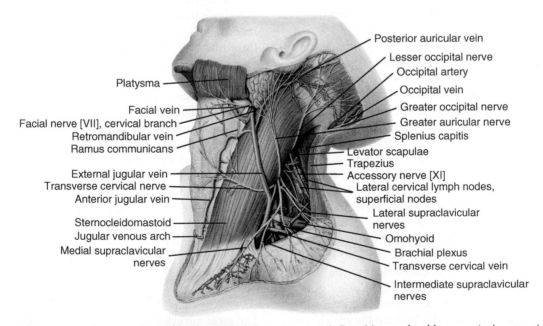

FIGURE 8-14 Acu-reflex points formed by the cervical plexus (C1 to C4). Practitioners should pay particular attention to the great auricular nerve, accessory nerve, and transverse cervical nerve.

supraclavicular nerve, which divides into medial, intermedial, and lateral branches. These nerves send small branches to the skin of the neck and then emerge from deep fascia just superior to the clavicle to supply the skin over the anterior aspect of the chest and shoulder. When needling sensitive ARPs in this area, a practitioner should always pay attention to the direction and depth of the needling so as not to puncture the lung.

H3 Spinal Accessory (Muscular)

This point contains both spinal and accessory nerves, as indicated by its name. The spinal accessory nerve (XI) originates both from cranial roots (nucleus ambiguus in medulla) and from spinal roots (C1 to C6), and it contains both afferent (sensory) and efferent (motor) fibers. A branch of the spinal accessory nerve enters the trapezius muscle, in the middle of the upper front edge, at the point over the shoulder bridge. This point is a neuromuscular attachment point. The H3 spinal accessory ARP appears sensitive in more than 98% of the population. The author uses a needle of no more than 2.5 cm in length and inserts the needle perpendicularly to the skin. Practitioners should be extremely careful when needling this point because the apex of the lung is just below this point (see Fig. 8-14).

Another branch of the spinal accessory nerve also innervates the sternocleidomastoid muscle.

ACU-REFLEX POINTS FORMED BY THE BRACHIAL PLEXUS

The brachial plexus enters the upper limb to provide both sensory and motor functions, which include the following:

- Sensory innervation to the skin and joints
- Motor innervation to the muscles
- Influence over the diameters of the blood vessels via the sympathetic vasomotor nerves
- Sympathetic secretomotor supply to the sweat glands

The brachial plexus arises just lateral to the scalenus anterior muscle. The ventral rami of C5, C6, C7, and C8 and the greater part of T1, in addition to a communicating loop from C4 to C5 and one

from T2 (sensory) to T1, form the five roots, three trunks, six divisions (three anterior and three posterior), three cords, and five terminal branches (see Fig. 8-7).

The anterior divisions form the lateral and medial cords, which give rise to their peripheral nerves innervating anterior or flexor muscles of the upper extremity. The posterior divisions form a posterior cord, which gives rise to its peripheral nerves innervating the posterior or extensor muscles of the upper extremity. With this 5-3-6-3-5 scheme, it is easier to understand the logical configuration of the brachial plexus.

The five roots form the three trunks: superior, middle, and inferior. The superior trunk consists of jointed ventral rami of C5 and C6 fibers. The middle trunk contains C7 fibers. The inferior trunk contains joint C8 and T1 fibers. Each of the three trunks splits into two branches: the anterior and posterior divisions for flexor (preaxial) and extensor (postaxial) muscles, respectively.

The three cords—the lateral, medial, and posterior—are formed by the six divisions. The anterior divisions from the superior and middle trunks, composed of C5, C6, and C7 fibers, unite to form the lateral cord. The anterior division from the inferior trunk, composed of C8 and T1 fibers, forms the medial cord. The posterior divisions from all three trunks, composed of C5 through C8 fibers, unite to form the posterior cord.

The cords then divide and reunite into branches that become peripheral nerves. The posterior cord branches into the axillary and radial nerves. The medial cord, after receiving a branch from the lateral cord, terminates as the ulnar nerve. One branch of the lateral cord becomes the musculocutaneous nerve; the other branch unites with one from the medial cord to form the median nerve.

The brachial plexus extends from the neck into the axilla, situated partly in the neck and partly in the axilla. The supraclavicular part (rami and trunks with their branches) is in the posterior triangle of the neck, and its infraclavicular part (cords and their branches) is in the axilla (Fig. 8-15). Peripheral nerves innervating muscles of the shoulder and a few muscles of the upper arm exit directly from various components of the plexus.

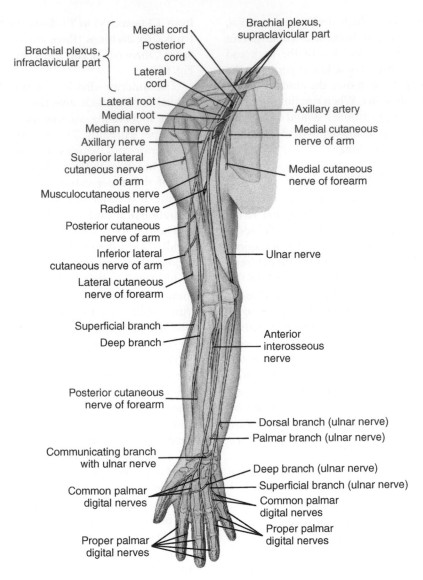

FIGURE 8-15 The brachial plexus.

A general survey of upper limb anatomy is necessary to better understand the innervation and configuration of the brachial plexus. The upper limb is the organ of manual activity. It consists of two parts: the shoulder (junction of the arm and the trunk) and the free arm. The free arm includes four parts: the arm (brachium, between the shoulder and the elbow), the forearm (antebrachium, between the elbow and the wrist), the wrist (carpus), and the hand (manus). The bones of the upper limb are the clavicle (collar bone) and the scapula (shoulder blade) in the shoulder; the humerus in the arm; the radius and ulna in the forearm; the eight carpal bones in the wrist; the five metacarpal bones in the hand; and the 14 phalanges in the digits (fingers) of one hand. More than 50 big and small muscles are attached to the bones of the upper limb.

The shoulder girdle and its muscles, such as the pectoralis, rhomboid, supraspinatus, and infraspinatus muscles, in the anterior and posterior walls of the thorax are considered as belonging to the upper limb. With the exception of a small area of skin on the shoulder, the brachial plexus supplies the innervation to the skin of all those regions and all of the muscles of the upper limb.

The anterior divisions innervate two pectoral muscles in the anterior thoracic region, muscles of the anterior compartment in the brachium, muscles in the medial compartment of the antebrachium, and intrinsic muscles on the palms of the hands. The posterior divisions innervate the levator scapulae, the rhomboid major and minor, the supraspinatus and infraspinatus in the shoulder and posterior thoracic regions, muscles in the posterior compartment of the brachium, and muscles in the lateral compartment of the antebrachium.

The cutaneous branches from the plexus have similar configuration. The cutaneous nerves from the anterior division include the medial brachial cutaneous, the medial antebrachial cutaneous and the lateral antebrachial cutaneous nerves. The posterior divisions give off branches of the posterior brachial cutaneous, the posterior antebrachial cutaneous, and the superficial radial nerve. All of the ARPs attributed to the brachial plexus are formed along these nerves, and so the points can be named according to nerves innervating the points.

HOMEOSTATIC ACU-REFLEX POINTS ON THE UPPER LIMB

The musculature of the arm is simple because it moves one joint. The arm is divided into two compartments: anterior and posterior, separated from one another by the humerus and the medial and lateral intramuscular septa. Large flexor and extensor muscles occupy them. Between these muscles, the brachial artery accompanied by the median nerve and ulnar nerve approaches the elbow in the anterior compartment on the medial side of the arm. Neither nerve gives off any branches in the arm; both innervate only the forearm and hand. Emerging from the axilla, the musculocutaneous and radial nerves course through the flexor and extensor compartments, respectively (Fig. 8-16).

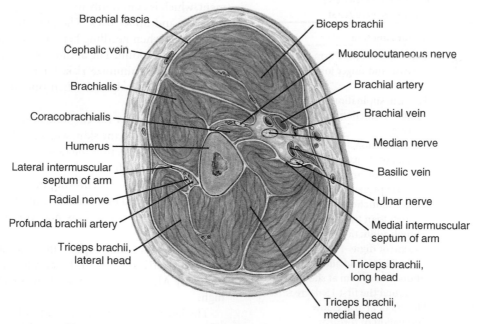

FIGURE 8-16 The flexor and extensor compartments of the upper arm.

Nearly 20 muscles are contained in the forearm. The forearm, which also consists of anterior (flexor) and posterior (extensor) compartments, is much more complex than the arm because it contains the prime movers for several joints. These muscles are packed into layers in each compartment. After entering the forearm, the radial, median, and ulnar nerves pass down to the hand beneath the superficial muscles of the anterior compartment (Table 8-3). They give off most of their branches to the superficial muscles in the region of the elbow. A deep branch of the median nerve, the anterior interosseous nerve, innervates the deep muscles anteriorly. The deep branch of the radial nerve and its posterior interosseous branch supply the remaining muscles in the back of the forearm. The radial and ulnar nerves descend to the wrist, accompanied by the arteries to the wrist in the anterior compartment.

The upper limb has six primary homeostatic ARPs: the lateral pectoral nerve on the chest, the dorsal scapular and suprascapular nerves on the shoulder, the lateral antebrachial cutaneous and deep radial nerve on the forearm, and the superficial radial nerve on the hand.

As emphasized previously, each ARP contains a main peripheral nerve that is responsible for the dynamic physiology of the point. In addition, different nerves also innervate different tissues at different layers of the same point. Only the major nerves that affect the physiology of the primary homeostatic ARPs are discussed as follows.

Preaxial Innervation

Two primary homeostatic ARPs are formed by two terminal branches: the lateral pectoral nerve, directly derived from the proximal lateral cord supplying the pectoralis major muscle, and the lateral antebrachial cutaneous nerve, derived from the muscular cutaneous nerve, which innervates the skin on the lateral elbow.

H17 Lateral Pectoral (Muscular)

As one of the small terminal branches of the lateral cord, the lateral pectoral nerve (arising from C5 to C7) pierces the clavipectoral fascia and enters the pectoralis major muscle at a spot about 4 to 5 cm inferior to the middle point of the clavicular bone.

An ARP is formed at this neuromuscular attachment, which is commonly needled for symptoms of the chest and upper back. The practitioner should be cautious when needling here because the lung is just below this point. The author uses specific techniques here to minimize risk. First, the pectoralis major muscle is palpated. Then one of two techniques is applied:

1. In thin patients, a 1.5-cm-long needle is inserted perpendicular to the skin, with care that the needle does not puncture the lung.
2. In patients with a well-developed pectoralis major muscle, a 4.0-cm-long needle is directed horizontally and inferiorly. The needle must stay outside the rib cage so as not to puncture the lung.

The author has developed an additional new method, electrical vacuum therapy, to replace needling any ARP when the risk of pneumothorax is high.

The lateral pectoral nerve sends a branch laterally to the medial pectoral nerve, which supplies the

TABLE 8-3	THE FIVE IMPORTANT NERVES IN THE ARM
Nerve	**Motor Function**
Radial nerve	Extension of entire arm, forearm, wrist, and finger joints below the shoulder
	Forearm supination
	Thumb abduction in plane of the palm
Median nerve	Thumb flexion and opposition
	Flexion of digits 2 and 3
	Wrist flexion and abduction
	Forearm pronation
Ulnar nerve	Finger adduction and abduction other than the thumb
	Thumb adduction
	Flexion of digits 4 and 5
	Wrist flexion and adduction
Axillary nerve	Abduction of arm at shoulder beyond the first 15 degrees
Musculocutaneous nerve	Flexion of arm at elbow
	Supination of forearm

pectoralis minor muscle and forms another ARP. The lateral pectoral nerve is so named because it arises from the lateral cord of the brachial plexus. Note that the H17 lateral pectoral ARP is located medially on the pectoralis major muscle, whereas the medial pectoral nerve is on the pectoralis minor muscle lateral to the H17 lateral pectoral ARP.

H9 Lateral Antebrachial Cutaneous (Cutaneous)

This ARP is located at the lateral end of the skin crest at the elbow joint and is easy to detect when the forearm is flexed at a 90-degree angle (Fig. 8-17). The musculocutaneous nerve (arising from C5 to C7) from the lateral cord of the brachial plexus courses

along the lateral side of the arm and pierces the deep fascia at the lateral edge of the cubital fossa to become the lateral antebrachial cutaneous nerve. An ARP is formed at the location where the nerve pierces the deep fascia.

Postaxial Innervation

The radial nerve branches into two nerves, the deep and superficial radial nerves on the forearm. At the branching location of each of these two nerves is a primary homeostatic ARP.

Two primary homeostatic ARPs on the posterior shoulder muscles are supplied by the posterior branches of the superior trunk from the brachial nerve plexus: the dorsal scapular nerve, and the suprascapular nerve.

H13 Dorsal Scapular (Muscular)

The dorsal scapular nerve branches from the ventral ramus of C5 and descends from the cervical region down to the medial border of the scapula. It innervates three muscles: the levator scapulae, the rhomboid major, and the rhomboid minor. This nerve enters the levator scapulae muscle approximately 1 cm superior to the base of the spine of the scapula (Fig. 8-18). The H13 dorsal scapular ARP is formed at this neuromuscular attachment.

The H13 dorsal scapular ARP is needled for all symptoms related to the head, neck, shoulder, arm, and upper back. All of the three muscles—the levator scapulae, rhomboid major, and rhomboid minor—are innervated by the dorsal scapular nerve and are sore or sensitive in most patients with these symptoms. These muscles should be treated in most patients. However, the needling is very tricky because the lung is directly under this ARP and under both the rhomboid muscles. The author suggests the following needling methods, but the practitioner should ensure that the needle is always outside the rib cage:

1. In a thinner patient, a 2.5-cm-long needle is directed horizontally and either inferiorly or laterally, to ensure entrance into the muscle but remaining outside the rib cage. If this is difficult, the alternative method is to needle this point perpendicularly with four or five 1.5-cm-long

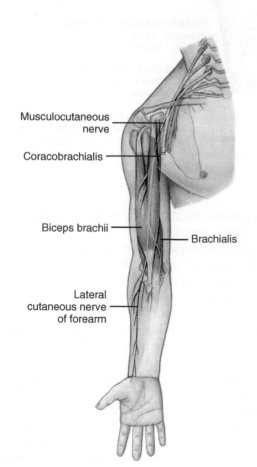

Musculocutaneous nerve

Coracobrachialis

Biceps brachii

Brachialis

Lateral cutaneous nerve of forearm

FIGURE 8-17 The musculocutaneous nerve and its branch, the lateral antebrachial cutaneous nerve.

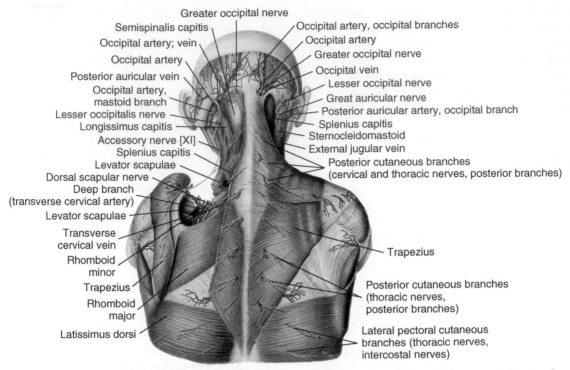

Greater occipital nerve
Semispinalis capitis
Occipital artery; vein
Occipital artery
Posterior auricular vein
Occipital artery, mastoid branch
Lesser occipitalis nerve
Longissimus capitis
Accessory nerve [XI]
Splenius capitis
Levator scapulae
Dorsal scapular nerve
Deep branch (transverse cervical artery)
Levator scapulae
Transverse cervical vein
Rhomboid minor
Trapezius
Rhomboid major
Latissimus dorsi

Occipital artery, occipital branches
Occipital artery
Greater occipital nerve
Occipital vein
Lesser occipital nerve
Great auricular nerve
Posterior auricular artery, occipital branch
Splenius capitis
Sternocleidomastoid
External jugular vein
Posterior cutaneous branches (cervical and thoracic nerves, posterior branches)

Trapezius

Posterior cutaneous branches (thoracic nerves, posterior branches)

Lateral pectoral cutaneous branches (thoracic nerves, intercostal nerves)

FIGURE 8-18 The dorsal scapular nerve branches from the ventral ramus of C5 and descends from cervical region down to the medial border of the scapula. It innervates three muscles: the levator scapulae, the rhomboid major, and the rhomboid minor. This nerve enters the levator scapulae muscle approximately 1 cm superior to the base of the spine of the scapula. The H13 dorsal scapular point is formed at this neuromuscular attachment. The muscle levator scapulae is cut away in this illustration to show the dorsal scapular nerve.

needles. This alternative method is less effective but safer in dealing with thin patients.

2. In patients with average musculature, a 2.5-cm-long needle is directed perpendicularly at this point.

3. For more effective treatment, the forearm of a patient is laid under the back with a 90-degree flexion in order to raise the scapula, and a 4-cm-long needle is directed laterally at this point. The same method can be used to needle both the rhomboid muscles and the subscapularis muscle, which lies on the costal surface of the scapula.

H8 Infraspinatus (Muscular)

The infraspinatus ARP (Fig. 8-19) is so named because it is located right on the infraspinatus muscle. However, the infraspinatus and the supraspina-

tus muscles are all innervated by the same nerve: the suprascapular nerve.

The suprascapular nerve receives fibers from C5 and C6 and arises from the posterior division of the superior trunk of the brachial plexus. It supplies the suprascapular and infrascapular muscles and the shoulder joint. This nerve descends down from the neck, sends a branch to the supraspinatus muscle, and curves around the scapular notch to reach the infraspinatus muscle. The nerve enters the infraspinatus muscle from underneath at the center of the infraspinatus fossa, and the ARP is formed at this neuromuscular attachment. It is easy to palpate this sensitive point, inasmuch as it is right in the center of the infrascapular fossa.

Although it is easy to find this point and safe to needle it because it is right on the scapular bone, caution is still needed. If a patient positions his or

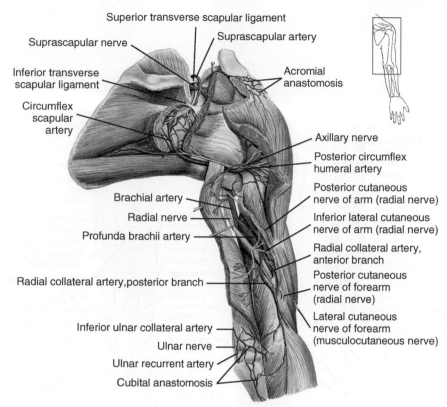

Superior transverse scapular ligament

Suprascapular nerve

Suprascapular artery

Inferior transverse
scapular ligament

Acromial
anastomosis

Circumflex
scapular
artery

Axillary nerve

Posterior circumflex
humeral artery

Brachial artery

Posterior cutaneous
nerve of arm (radial nerve)

Radial nerve

Inferior lateral cutaneous
nerve of arm (radial nerve)

Profunda brachii artery

Radial collateral artery,
anterior branch

Radial collateral artery, posterior branch

Posterior cutaneous
nerve of forearm
(radial nerve)

Lateral cutaneous
nerve of forearm
(musculocutaneous nerve)

Inferior ulnar collateral artery

Ulnar nerve

Ulnar recurrent artery

Cubital anastomosis

FIGURE 8-19 The infraspinatus acu-reflex point is so named because it is located right on the infraspinatus muscle. The infraspinatus and the supraspinatus muscles are all innervated by the suprascapular nerve.

her arms in a particular way, the scapula moves laterally, and the lung is exposed. For the sake of safety, practitioners must always make sure that the ARP is on the infraspinatus fossa of the bone.

Some patients have thick infraspinatus muscle, and so the needle can be directed perpendicular to the ARP and inserted all the way to the bone. For patients with a thin infraspinatus muscle, the needle can be tilted at a proper angle according to the thickness of the muscle.

H1 Deep Radial

This is the most important ARP because its sensitivity is evident in more than 99% of the population. The deep radial nerve (arising from C5 to C8 and from T1) is one of the terminal branches from the posterior cord of the brachial nerve plexus

(Fig. 8-20). This nerve provides the major nerve supply to the extensor muscles of the upper limb: triceps, anconeus, brachioradialis, and all the extensor muscles of the forearm. It also supplies cutaneous sensation to the skin of the extensor region, including the hand.

The radial nerve leaves the axilla and runs posteriorly, inferiorly, and laterally between the long and medial heads of the triceps muscle. It enters the radial groove in the humerus. The radial nerve penetrates the lateral intermuscular septum of the arm and divides into two terminal branches: the deep and the superficial radial nerves. The primary homeostatic ARP of the body is located at the branching spot, which is about 4 cm distal to the lateral epicondyle between the brachioradialis muscle and the extensor carpi radialis longus muscle.

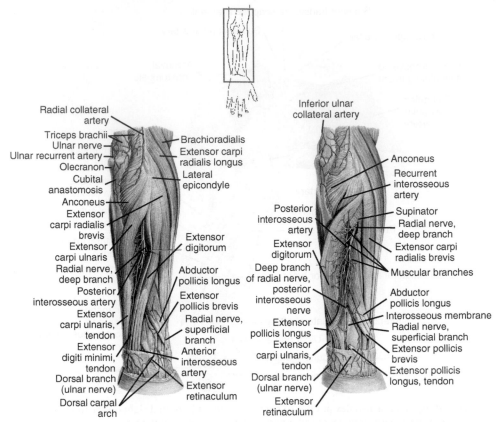

FIGURE 8-20 Deep branches from the radial nerve. An acu-reflex point is formed at the branching site.

There, the deep radial nerve is accompanied by the radial artery and vein and their tributaries. As the deep radial nerve runs distally to the wrist from this point, it sequentially gives off branches to nine muscles.

The H1 deep radial point is the first ARP to become sensitive in the human body. However, its clinical value is more in diagnosis. As discussed, the efficacy and prognosis of acupuncture therapy depends on the self-healing capability of the body. As homeostasis declines, the self-healing potential drops, and more points gradually become sensitive along the deep radial nerve distally from the H1 deep radial point. Thus the number of sensitive points appearing on the deep radial nerve provides quantitative information about the body's homeostasis and self-healing potential.

The H1 deep radial ARP can be needled all the way down to the bone below.

H12 Superficial Radial (Cutaneous)

After branching from the deep radial nerve just below the elbow, the superficial radial nerve runs under the brachioradialis muscle and emerges to the surface at the distal portion of the radius. This nerve starts branching first at the anatomic snuffbox and then on the web between the thumb and the index finger. The H12 superficial radial ARP is located on the second branching spot (Fig. 8-21).

HOMEOSTATIC ACU-REFLEX POINTS ON THE LOWER LIMB

The primary function of the lower limbs is locomotion, bearing weight, and maintaining equilibrium. The lower limb consists of four major parts: the hip, the thigh, the leg, and the foot. The lower limb has eight primary homeostatic ARPs: one on the hip, one on the thigh, five on the leg, and one on the foot.

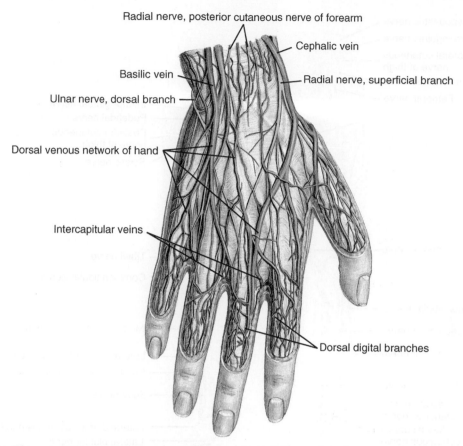

Radial nerve, posterior cutaneous nerve of forearm

Cephalic vein

Basilic vein

Radial nerve, superficial branch

Ulnar nerve, dorsal branch

Dorsal venous network of hand

Intercapitular veins

Dorsal digital branches

FIGURE 8-21 The superficial radial nerve runs under the brachioradialis muscle and emerges to the surface at the distal portion of the radius. This nerve branches first at the anatomic snuffbox and then on the web between the thumb and the index finger. The second branching spot is the site of the H12 superficial radial point.

The lower limb, including its bone, joints, muscles, and skin, is innervated by the nerves from both the lumbar nerve plexus and the sacral nerve plexus. All the spinal nerves have dorsal and ventral rami, as described previously, but only the ventral rami of the lumbar and sacral spinal nerves are interconnected to form the lumbar plexus and the sacral plexus. Collectively, they are called the *lumbosacral nerve plexus* (Fig. 8-22). Like the brachial nerve plexus, the lumbosacral plexus branches into anterior and posterior divisions. The posterior division has two major nerves: the femoral and the common fibular nerves. The anterior division likewise has two major nerves: the obturator and

the tibial nerves. The tibial nerve has two terminal branches: the medial plantar and the lateral plantar nerves.

In the leg region, the saphenous nerve is the longest branch of the femoral nerve. Branches from the tibial nerve (medial) and the common fibular nerve unite to form the sural nerve.

The lumbosacral nerve plexus supplies the lower limb. The lumbar part is located in the abdomen, and the sacral part in the pelvis. The major nerves that supply the lower limb are derived from the anterior rami of L2 to S3 spinal nerves. L1 and S4 usually supply only a limited area of skin in the inguinal (L1) and perianal (S4) region (see Fig. 8-8).

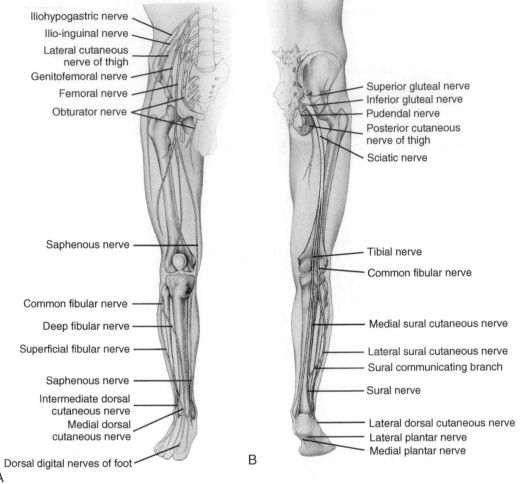

FIGURE 8-22 Nerves of the lower limb. **A,** Anterior view. **B,** Posterior view.

Only the terminal nerves that form the primary homeostatic ARPs in the lower limb are discussed in the following sections.

Lumbar Plexus

The lumbosacral plexus consists of the lumbar and sacral plexuses. Immediately after L2, L3, and L4 roots of the lumbar plexus split off from their spinal nerves and emerge from the intervertebral foramina, they are embedded in the psoas major muscle because this muscle is attached to the lateral surfaces and transverse process of the lumbar vertebrae. Within the psoas major muscle, the roots split into anterior and posterior divisions, which then reunite to form the branches of the lumbosacral

plexus. The posterior divisions emerge from the muscle along either its lateral or medial border. The femoral nerve, formed by the posterior divisions of L2, L3, and L4, descends from the plexus lateral to the psoas muscle. The anterior divisions of the same roots unite to form the obturator nerve, the other major branch of the lumbar part of the plexus. The obturator nerve leaves the psoas major medially. Only a portion of the L4 anterior ramus contributes to the lumbar plexus; the remaining smaller part, along with the L5 root, forms the lumbosacral trunk, which descends into the pelvis and joins the sacral plexus. The lumbosacral trunk and the obturator nerve enter the pelvis on the ala of the sacrum, medial to the psoas major muscle (see Fig. 8-8).

Sacral Plexus

The anterior rami of S1, S2, and S3 emerge from the anterior (pelvic) foramina of the sacrum and proceed laterally on the anterior surface of the piriformis muscle. The lumbosacral trunk joins the sacral roots and fuses with S1. The sacral nerve plexus lies in the posterior wall of the pelvic cavity (see Fig. 8-8).

All the roots, including L4 and L5 (contained in the lumbosacral trunk), split into anterior and posterior divisions. However, the separation of these divisions can be observed only through careful dissection of cadavers. The anterior and posterior divisions converge laterally to form the sciatic nerve. This large nerve trunk leaves the pelvis through the greater sciatic foramen. The sciatic nerve is actually composed of two nerves, the common fibular nerve and the tibial nerve, which usually separate from each other just above the knee (Table 8-4). Sometimes, however, these two nerves may exit independently from the plexus and leave the pelvis as separate nerves. The posterior divisions of L4, L5, S1, and S2 form the common fibular nerve, and the corresponding anterior divisions, plus the anterior division of S3, form the tibial nerve. The posterior division of S3 is represented in minor, cutaneous branches of the plexus.

H16 Inferior Gluteal (Muscular)

The H16 inferior gluteal ARP is located right in the center of the gluteal region (Fig. 8-23). The inferior gluteal nerve arises from the posterior divisions of

TABLE 8-4	IMPORTANT NERVES THAT HAVE PERIPHERAL BRANCHES IN THE LEG

Nerve	Motor Functions
Femoral nerve (L2–L4)	Leg flexion at the hip
Saphenous nerve	Leg extension at the knee
Obturator nerve (L2–L4)	Adduction of the thigh
Sciatic nerve (L4–S2)	Leg flexion at the knee
Tibial nerve (S1–S2)	Foot plantar flexion and inversion, toe flexion
Superficial fibular (peroneal) nerve (L5–S1)	Foot eversion
Deep fibular (peroneal) nerve (L5–S1)	Foot dorsiflexion, toe extension

the ventral rami of L5, S1, and S2. It leaves the pelvis through the inferior part of the greater sciatic foramen and under the piriformis muscle, accompanied by the gluteal artery. The nerve enters the gluteus maximus muscle deeply from underneath.

This ARP is sensitive in all patients with lower back pain, sciatica, or piriform muscle syndrome. Usually 7- to 10-cm-long needles are used for this ARP, inserted all the way to the bone.

In many patients with chronic lower back pain and lower limb pain, more sensitive points can be found around the H16 inferior gluteal ARP on the gluteus medius and minimus muscles. These sensitive points should be treated along with the H16 inferior gluteal ARP.

H18 Iliotibial (Cutaneous)

This ARP is located on the lateral surface of the thigh, about halfway between the hip and the knee on the iliotibial tract. The sciatic nerve may send cutaneous branches to innervate the iliotibial tract.

The H18 iliotibial point is used in treating lower back and lower limb problems. As symptoms become worse or chronic, more sensitive points appear on the iliotibial tract. These secondary or tertiary points should be palpated and needled to achieve better and faster results. The needling depth can be all the way to the bone.

H11 Lateral Medial Popliteal

The H11 lateral popliteal ARP is located on the lateral side of the tendon of the semitendinosus muscle, or on the medial side of the tendon of the biceps femoris. The sensitivity of these points can be evident in most patients on the lateral side, some on the medial side, or on both sides.

The innervation of these points is unclear, but it may be related to the innervation of the origin of the medial or lateral head of the gastrocnemius. These points are sensitive in 93% of the author's patients and may appear laterally or medially or on both sides, in which case they are still treated as one ARP. In patients with back or sciatic problems, this ARP is definitely sensitive. The author suggests directing a 4-cm-long needle perpendicularly at this point. Alternatively, the needle can be tilted slightly toward the midline of the popliteal fossa.

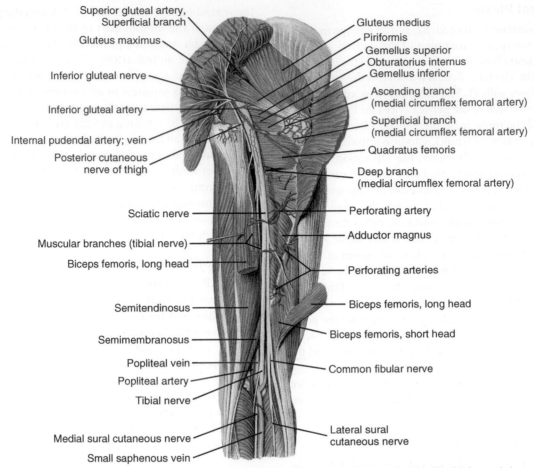

Superior gluteal artery,
Superficial branch

Gluteus maximus

Inferior gluteal nerve

Inferior gluteal artery

Internal pudendal artery; vein

Posterior cutaneous
nerve of thigh

Sciatic nerve

Muscular branches (tibial nerve)

Biceps femoris, long head

Semitendinosus

Semimembranosus

Popliteal vein

Popliteal artery

Tibial nerve

Medial sural cutaneous nerve

Small saphenous vein

Gluteus medius
Piriformis
Gemellus superior
Obturatorius internus
Gemellus inferior

Ascending branch
(medial circumflex femoral artery)

Superficial branch
(medial circumflex femoral artery)

Quadratus femoris

Deep branch
(medial circumflex femoral artery)

Perforating artery

Adductor magnus

Perforating arteries

Biceps femoris, long head

Biceps femoris, short head

Common fibular nerve

Lateral sural
cutaneous nerve

FIGURE 8-23 The inferior gluteal nerve, which innervates the gluteus maximus muscle. The iliotibial tract is innervated by cutaneous branches from the sciatic nerve. The popliteal acu-reflex point appears on the popliteal fossa, and the actual innervation is unclear.

Many patients may feel a tingling sensation moving along the peroneal nerve down to the ankle when this point is needled.

H4 Saphenous (Cutaneous)

The H4 saphenous point is easily found on the medial side of the knee below the medial condyle of the tibia (Fig. 8-24). This point is sensitive in almost every patient.

The H4 saphenous point is formed right at the site where the saphenous nerve emerges from the deep fascia. The saphenous nerve is a cutaneous branch of the femoral nerve that descends through the femoral triangle. It accompanies the

femoral artery and vein, and its branches supply innervation to the skin and fascia of the anterior and medial surfaces of the knee and leg as far as the medial malleolus.

The femoral nerve, from which the saphenous nerve branches, is the largest branch of the lumbar nerve plexus (arising from L2 to L4). The femoral nerve forms in the abdomen and enters the lower limb through the pelvis to the midpoint of the inguinal ligament. After passing distally in the femoral triangle, the femoral nerve divides into several terminal branches to supply innervation to the hip and knee joints and to the skin on the anteromedial side of the leg.

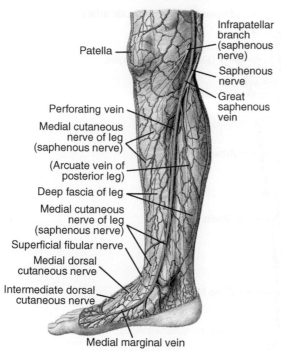

Patella

Infrapatellar branch (saphenous nerve)

Saphenous nerve

Great saphenous vein

Perforating vein

Medial cutaneous nerve of leg (saphenous nerve)

(Arcuate vein of posterior leg)

Deep fascia of leg

Medial cutaneous nerve of leg (saphenous nerve)

Superficial fibular nerve

Medial dorsal cutaneous nerve

Intermediate dorsal cutaneous nerve

Medial marginal vein

FIGURE 8-24 The saphenous nerve, a cutaneous branch from the femoral nerve.

Like the H1 deep radial ARP on the forearm, the H4 saphenous ARP is useful both for treatment and evaluation of health. As homeostasis declines, sensitivity develops gradually along the saphenous nerve distally from the H4 saphenous point. Thus the saphenous nerve provides quantitative information about healing potential and treatment prognosis. Information from both the H4 saphenous ARP and the H1 deep radial ARP constitutes the basis for quantitative evaluation of healing potential.

H24 Common Fibular (Peroneal)

The H24 common fibular ARP is just anteroinferior to the head of the fibula (Fig. 8-25). The common fibular nerve is one of the two terminal branches of the sciatic nerve. The finger-sized sciatic nerve, the largest nerve in the body, is formed by the ventral rami of L4 to S3. It leaves the pelvis through the greater sciatic foramen and runs inferiolaterally deep to the gluteus maximus. As it descends in the midline of the thigh, this nerve is overlapped posteriorly by the adjacent margins of the biceps femoris and semimembrano-

sus muscles. In the lower third of the thigh, it divides into the tibial and common fibular nerves.

The common fibular nerve enters the popliteal fossa along the medial border of the biceps muscle. It leaves the fossa by crossing superficially the lateral head of the gastrocnemius muscle. It then passes behind the head of the fibula, winds laterally around the neck of the bone, pierces the peroneus longus muscle, and divides into two terminal nerves: the superficial and deep fibular nerves. The H24 common fibular point is formed at the branching site.

This ARP is innervated by a terminal branch from the sciatic nerve; therefore it is needled to treat symptoms related to the lower back and sciatic nerve. Like the deep radial nerve and the saphenous nerve, the common fibular nerve has a linear course down the leg medial to the fibular bone. As the body's homeostasis declines, other sensitive points appear along the common fibular nerve distal from the H24 common fibular point.

H10 Sural (Cutaneous)

This ARP is located around the middle of the posterior aspect of the leg, between the two heads of the gastrocnemius muscle (Fig. 8-26). As mentioned previously, the sciatic nerve contains two nerves: the common fibular nerve and the tibial nerve. These two nerves separate before they enter the popliteal fossa. In the popliteal fossa, the common fibular nerve branches into the lateral sural nerve, and the tibial nerve branches into the medial sural nerve. These two branches descend and unite between the two heads of the gastrocnemius muscle to form the sural nerve. The sural nerve pierces the deep fascia around the middle of the posterior leg where the ARP is formed. The sural nerve is then joined by the fibular communicating branch of the common fibular nerve.

The sural nerve supplies the skin on the lateral and posterior part of the inferior one third of the leg. It enters the foot posterior to the lateral malleolus and supplies the skin along the lateral margin of the foot and the lateral side of the fifth digit.

H6 Tibial (Cutaneous)

This ARP is located on the medial aspect of the leg, about 6 to 8 cm above the medial malleolus. The tibial nerve is the larger terminal branch of the

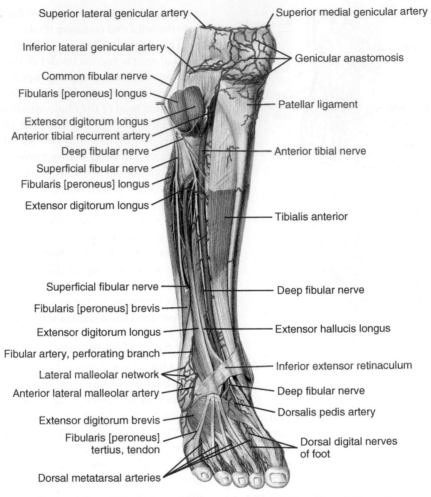

FIGURE 8-25 The common fibular nerve, a branch from the sciatic nerve.

sciatic nerve (L4 to S3). The tibial nerve descends through the middle of the popliteal fossa, straight down the median plane of the calf and deep to the soleus muscle, and supplies all muscles in the posterior compartment of the leg. In addition, the tibial nerve gives off a cutaneous branch to form the sural nerve (described in previous section). The tibial nerve comes close to the medial skin about 6 to 8 cm above the medial malleolus. This is where the very important H6 tibial ARP is formed. From this point, the tibial nerve courses down and passes deep

to the flexor retinaculum between the medial malleolus and calcaneus. Then the tibial nerve divides into the medial and lateral plantar nerves and the calcaneal branches, which supply the skin of the sole and heel (Fig. 8-27).

The H6 tibial ARP is sensitive in almost every patient. This point is very superficial in patients with thin leg muscles. For more effective needling in those patients, a 4-cm-long needle can be tilted downward to make better contact between the needle and tissues.

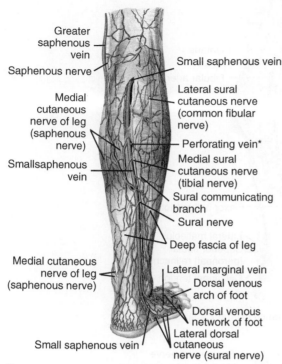

Greater
saphenous
vein
Saphenous nerve
Medial
cutaneous
nerve of leg
(saphenous
nerve)
Smallsaphenous
vein

Small saphenous vein
Lateral sural
cutaneous nerve
(common fibular
nerve)
Perforating vein*
Medial sural
cutaneous nerve
(tibial nerve)
Sural communicating
branch
Sural nerve
Deep fascia of leg

Medial cutaneous
nerve of leg
(saphenous nerve)

Lateral marginal vein
Dorsal venous
arch of foot
Dorsal venous
network of foot
Lateral dorsal
cutaneous
nerve (sural nerve)

Small saphenous vein

FIGURE 8-26 The sural nerve, a cutaneous branch from the sciatic nerve.

H5 Deep Fibular (Peroneal) (Cutaneous)

This ARP is located about 2 cm proximal to the web between the first and second toes. It appears sensitive in almost every patient.

As mentioned in the discussion of the H24 common fibular point, the deep fibular nerve is one of the two terminal branches of the common fibular nerve. The deep fibular nerve descends down the leg and gives off branches to the arteries, the ankle joint, and other articulations. This nerve becomes cutaneous approximately 2 cm proximal to the web between the first and second toes, where the ARP is formed (Fig. 8-28).

CUTANEOUS ACU-REFLEX POINTS OF THE TORSO

Every spinal nerve divides into two primary rami: posterior (dorsal) and anterior (ventral). The anterior primary ramus gives off two branches: the lateral cutaneous and the anterior cutaneous nerves. Each cutaneous nerve separates into two end branches to supply side and anterior parts of the same dermatome. Thus lateral ARPs and anterior ARPs are formed at each spinal nerve from T2 to T12 (Fig. 8-29).

HOMEOSTATIC ACU-REFLEX POINTS FORMED BY THE POSTERIOR RAMI OF THE SPINAL NERVES

All facial ARPs are formed on the cranial nerves, and all body ARPs are associated with the spinal nerves. Once the spinal nerve leaves the intervertebral foramen, it divides into two major branches: the anterior primary ramus and the posterior primary ramus.

The skin and muscles of the back are supplied in a segmental manner by the posterior rami of the 33 pairs of spinal nerves, 8 from cervical vertebrae (C1 to C8), 12 from thoracic vertebrae (T1 to T12), 5 from lumbar vertebrae (L1 to L5), 4 from sacral vertebrae (S1 to S4), and 4 (or 3 in some cases) from the coccygeal bones. The coccygeal spinal nerves are very small and are needled only in treating pain in the coccygeal region.

The posterior rami of C1, C6, C7, C8, L4, and L5 supply innervation to deep muscles but not to the skin. The posterior ramus of C2 ascends over the back of the head and supplies the skin of the scalp, and a very important ARP is formed there.

The posterior rami run downward and laterally and innervate a band of skin at a lower level than the intervertebral foramen from which they emerge. This can be understood from the scheme of dermatomes of the back. Skin nerve supply overlaps considerably.

As described, the posterior primary ramus of a spinal nerve goes to the back and divides into two terminal branches: the medial branch and the lateral branch. In the thoracic region, the medial branch supplies the skin and the lateral branch supplies the muscles, whereas in the lumbar area, the medial branch supplies muscles and the lateral branch supplies the skin. The posterior primary ramus also sends small branches to innervate the joints of the spine.

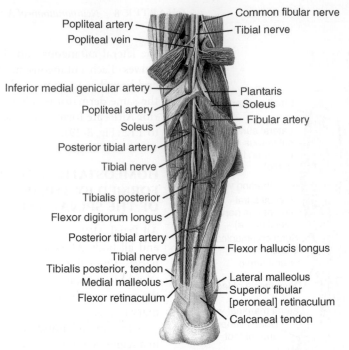

Common fibular nerve

Popliteal artery

Tibial nerve

Popliteal vein

Inferior medial genicular artery

Plantaris

Popliteal artery

Soleus

Soleus

Fibular artery

Posterior tibial artery

Tibial nerve

Tibialis posterior

Flexor digitorum longus

Posterior tibial artery

Flexor hallucis longus

Tibial nerve

Tibialis posterior, tendon

Lateral malleolus

Medial malleolus

Superior fibular [peroneal] retinaculum

Flexor retinaculum

Calcaneal tendon

FIGURE 8-27 The tibial nerve, a branch from the sciatic nerve.

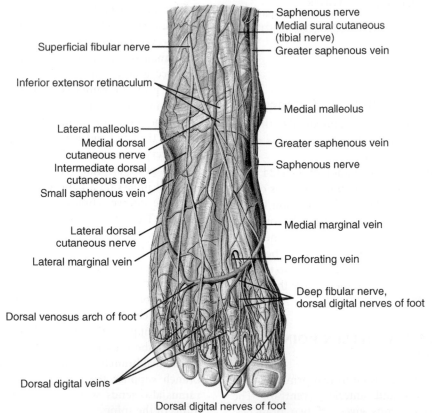

Saphenous nerve

Medial sural cutaneous (tibial nerve)

Superficial fibular nerve

Greater saphenous vein

Inferior extensor retinaculum

Medial malleolus

Lateral malleolus

Medial dorsal cutaneous nerve

Greater saphenous vein

Intermediate dorsal cutaneous nerve

Saphenous nerve

Small saphenous vein

Lateral dorsal cutaneous nerve

Medial marginal vein

Lateral marginal vein

Perforating vein

Deep fibular nerve, dorsal digital nerves of foot

Dorsal venosus arch of foot

Dorsal digital veins

Dorsal digital nerves of foot

FIGURE 8-28 The deep fibular nerve, a branch from the common fibular nerve.

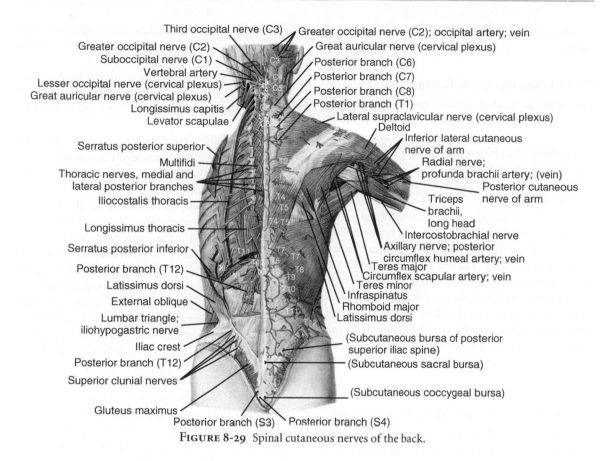

Third occipital nerve (C3)
Greater occipital nerve (C2)
Suboccipital nerve (C1)
Vertebral artery
Lesser occipital nerve (cervical plexus)
Great auricular nerve (cervical plexus)
Longissimus capitis
Levator scapulae

Serratus posterior superior
Multifidi
Thoracic nerves, medial and
lateral posterior branches
Iliocostalis thoracis

Longissimus thoracis

Serratus posterior inferior

Posterior branch (T12)

Latissimus dorsi

External oblique

Lumbar triangle;
iliohypogastric nerve

Iliac crest

Posterior branch (T12)

Superior clunial nerves

Gluteus maximus
Posterior branch (S3)

Greater occipital nerve (C2); occipital artery; vein
Great auricular nerve (cervical plexus)
Posterior branch (C6)
Posterior branch (C7)
Posterior branch (C8)
Posterior branch (T1)
Lateral supraclavicular nerve (cervical plexus)
Deltoid
Inferior lateral cutaneous
nerve of arm
Radial nerve;
profunda brachii artery; (vein)
Posterior cutaneous
Triceps   nerve of arm
brachii,
long head
Intercostobrachial nerve
Axillary nerve; posterior
circumflex humeal artery; vein
Teres major
Circumflex scapular artery; vein
Teres minor
Infraspinatus
Rhomboid major
Latissimus dorsi

(Subcutaneous bursa of posterior
superior iliac spine)
(Subcutaneous sacral bursa)

(Subcutaneous coccygeal bursa)

Posterior branch (S4)

FIGURE 8-29 Spinal cutaneous nerves of the back.

The posterior rami of the spinal nerve form the paravertebral ARPs. Sometimes paravertebral ARPs are physiologically different from both symptomatic and homeostatic points. The author selects and needles symptomatic and homeostatic ARPs because they are pathologically sensitive. Paravertebral ARPs are selected and needled because they are located close to the nerve roots of the symptomatic ARPs. Paravertebral ARPs are not necessarily sensitive during the needling session. In other words, both paravertebral ARPs and symptomatic ARPs are innervated by the spinal nerve fibers and share the same segmental organization. The stimulation of the paravertebral ARPs by needling will desensitize symptomatic ARPs through the physiologic segmental reflex. The relief of core muscle stress has also been shown to help the neuromuscular coordination of the limbs.

There is clinical evidence that very successful results have been obtained by needling only paravertebral ARPs in patients with complex regional pain syndrome.

To locate the paravertebral ARPs, the author starts with palpation of the midline (the spinous processes). The precise location of the ARPs is not critical because of overlapping innervation of the cutaneous segmentation of the spinal nerves, but locating a point at the same level as the spinous process of the corresponding vertebra is preferable because this point may be closer to the primary ramus of the spinal nerve. Both sides of the spine are needled to ensure that muscles on both sides are relaxed, which helps realign the vertebral joints and provides enough stimulation to the nerve endings. The points to be needled are usually 2 to 3 cm (about 1 inch) from the midline.

There are five primary homeostatic ARPs on the back.

H7 Greater Occipital (Cutaneous)

This ARP is located at the base of the occipital region, 2 or 3 cm from the midline (see Fig. 8-30). This ARP can be located easily because it is sensitive in more than 95% of the author's patients. The dorsal rami of the C2 spinal nerve form the greater occipital nerve. This nerve emerges between the posterior arch of the atlas (C1) and the lamina of the axis (C2), below the small inferior oblique muscle of the head. The greater occipital nerve surfaces to supply the skin of the occipital region and back of the skull (Fig. 8-30). The H7 greater occipital ARP is frequently used because many symptoms can be traced to problems of the neck, which are discussed in detail in later chapters. For effective treatment, the author usually uses 34-gauge (0.22-mm diameter) needles. The depth varies from 2 to 5 cm, depending on the thickness of a patient's neck tissues.

H20 Spinous Process of T7 (Cutaneous)

This ARP is located right on the spinous process of T7. This point is sensitive in 80% of the author's patients. The tissues of this ARP are innervated mainly by small branches from the posterior primary ramus of the seventh thoracic spinal nerve.

Two methods can be used to locate this ARP. The first method is to palpate the spinous process of C7, which is the most prominent process at the base of the neck. From C7, the practitioner can palpate down to T7. The second method is faster: This ARP is level with the inferior angle of the scapula, and so the practitioner can locate the scapula and its inferior angle first (Fig. 8-31).

It is still not clear neuroanatomically why this ARP becomes more sensitive than most other body points. T7, located at the lower edge of the scapula, may serve as a mechanical pivot between upper and lower thoracic spine. Because of the scapula, the intervertebral joints from T1 to T6 are less bendable. As a mechanical pivot, T7 is more vulnerable to mechanical wear. In addition, the center of the gravity of the head and shoulder girdle, including the upper limbs, is located just in front of T7, which makes it an important point of stress in maintaining posture.

Another possible reason why the spinous process of T7 can become sensitized earlier than other spinous processes is that the center of gravity of the upper limb and head is located just anterior to the body of the vertebra T7. This may create physical

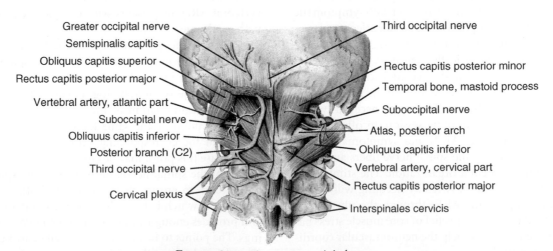

Greater occipital nerve
Semispinalis capitis
Obliquus capitis superior
Rectus capitis posterior major
Vertebral artery, atlantic part
Suboccipital nerve
Obliquus capitis inferior
Posterior branch (C2)
Third occipital nerve
Cervical plexus

Third occipital nerve
Rectus capitis posterior minor
Temporal bone, mastoid process
Suboccipital nerve
Atlas, posterior arch
Obliquus capitis inferior
Vertebral artery, cervical part
Rectus capitis posterior major
Interspinales cervicis

FIGURE 8-30 The greater occipital nerve.

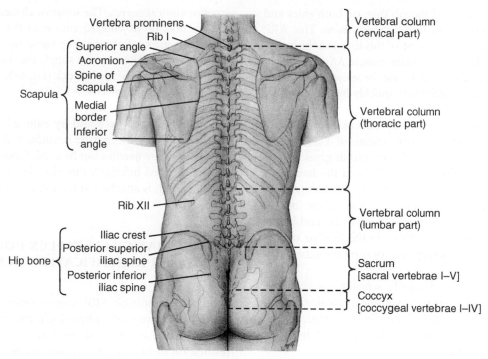

FIGURE 8-31 Skeletal markers for the H20 spinous process point of T7 and the H15 posterior cutaneous point of L2.

stress on the T7 level inasmuch as the muscles and ligaments have to maintain the postural balance of the upper part of the spine.

For needling this point, the author inserts a 5-cm-long needle diagonally into the ligament between the spinous processes of T7 and T8 until resistance is felt.

From T1 to T9, the spinous process of T7 is always the first point to become sensitive. The second sensitive spinous process is usually T5. As homeostasis declines, more sensitive points appear from T1 to T9. Thus the number of sensitive spinous processes from T1 to T9 provides quantitative information about the level of a person's homeostasis. Manual palpation of the spinous processes from T1 to T9 should be included in routine practice to estimate the healing potential of the patient.

H21 Posterior Cutaneous of T6 (Cutaneous)

This ARP is located about 3 cm laterally from the spinous process of C6. It is sensitive in 80% of the author's patients. This ARP is supplied by the cutaneous and medial branches of the posterior primary ramus of the T6 spinal nerve.

A 2.5-cm-long needle is tilted toward the midline and inserted to a depth of about 2 cm.

H15 Posterior Cutaneous of L2 (Cutaneous)

This ARP is sensitive in 90% of the author's patients. For most people, this ARP lies on the lateral border of the lower back muscle (erector spinae), at a level on the narrowest part of the waist. In patients with much subcutaneous fat, a practitioner can palpate the lowest edges of the rib cage on both sides and draw an imaginary line between them. This ARP lies on the crossing point of this line and the lateral border of the erector spinae muscle. An experienced practitioner can easily locate the spinous process of L2 and find this ARP very quickly by palpating the erector spinae muscle in the lumbar region.

This ARP is supplied by the cutaneous branch of the primary posterior ramus of L2 (see Fig. 8-31). Each posterior primary ramus gives off two terminal branches: the medial and the lateral. In the thoracic region, the medial branch is cutaneous and the lateral branch is muscular. In the lumbar region, the medial branch is muscular and lateral branch is cutaneous. Thus, in the lumbar region, palpation is important for locating the actual sensitive spot.

This point is extremely sensitive, especially in patients with lower back, leg, and gynecologic problems. A 4- to 5-cm-long needle is inserted, slightly tilted toward the midline. The depth of insertion varies from 3 to 5 cm.

H22 Posterior Cutaneous of L5 (Cutaneous)

To locate this point, it is better to locate the H15 posterior cutaneous ARP of L2 or the spinous process of L2, or both, first and then palpate down to locate the spinous processes of L4 and L5. This ARP is located about 3 cm from the spinous process of L5, right on the bulge of the erector spinae muscle. In some people, this point is closer to L4; in others, it is closer to L5. This point is innervated by the muscular branch of the posterior primary ramus of the spinal nerve of L5.

This is an important ARP in the treatment of lower back pain. The needling methods are the same as for the H15 posterior cutaneous ARP of L2, but the needle should be inserted perpendicularly downward.

H14 Superior Cluneal (Cutaneous)

This point is located at the highest point of the iliac crest. The iliac crest is palpated first in order to locate this ARP, which is sensitive in 90% of the patients. The lateral branches of the posterior primary rami of the first three lumbar nerves unite to form the superior cluneal nerves. The superior cluneal nerves take an oblique downward course to the buttock region and emerge from the deep fascia just superior to the iliac crest. These nerves supply the skin on the superior two thirds of the buttock (Fig. 8-32).

A 5- to 7-cm-long needle is inserted perpendicularly or downward just superior to the iliac crest. In case of severe lower back and leg pain, a large area around the iliac crest may be sensitive and painful, and three to five needles can be used. Some needles may be directed inferiorly into the gluteus medius muscle, which is attached to the external surface of the ilium.

SYMPTOMATIC ACU-REFLEX POINTS AND THEIR IDENTIFICATION IN EACH CASE

Needling homeostatic ARPs creates general stimulation, which improves physiologic and mechanical coordination and restores homeostasis. This restoration of homeostasis is nonspecific; in other words, the improvement in physiologic coordination is the same in every case regardless of the specific pathologic process. The specific pathologic process sensitizes a specific part of the body, and the ARPs related to that condition become sensitive. Thus homeostatic ARPs themselves are very often involved and become symptomatic. For example, the low back homeostatic H15, H14, H22, and H16 ARPs are always sensitive in patients with lower back pain. In these cases, homeostatic ARPs are also symptomatic ARPs.

The author needles local sensitive ARPs to desensitize them because these sensitized points usually are related to or generate pain. To understand the nature of symptomatic ARPs, practitioners need to understand the organization of a segment of the spinal cord. The body of a sensory neuron is housed in the dorsal (posterior) root ganglion, which is outside the spinal cord. This sensory neuron sends an axon (the peripheral nerve fiber) to the skin or muscle, or both, and to a dendrite centrally to the spinal cord gray matter.

The spinal cord gray matter contains different neurons and is divided into three parts: the dorsal (posterior) horn, the lateral horn, and the ventral

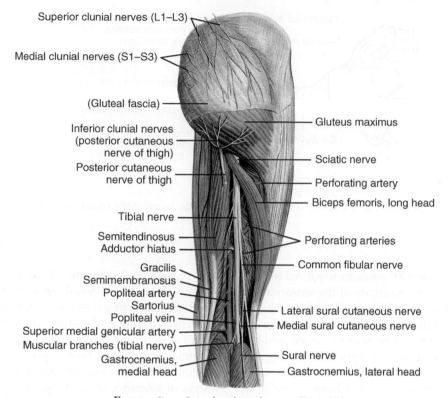

Superior clunial nerves (L1–L3)

Medial clunial nerves (S1–S3)

(Gluteal fascia)

Inferior clunial nerves (posterior cutaneous nerve of thigh)

Posterior cutaneous nerve of thigh

Tibial nerve

Semitendinosus
Adductor hiatus

Gracilis
Semimembranosus
Popliteal artery
Sartorius
Popliteal vein
Superior medial genicular artery
Muscular branches (tibial nerve)
Gastrocnemius, medial head

Gluteus maximus

Sciatic nerve

Perforating artery

Biceps femoris, long head

Perforating arteries

Common fibular nerve

Lateral sural cutaneous nerve
Medial sural cutaneous nerve

Sural nerve
Gastrocnemius, lateral head

FIGURE 8-32 Superior cluneal nerves (L1 to L3).

(anterior) horn. The neurons in the dorsal (posterior) horn connect with the dendrites from the sensory neuron of the dorsal root ganglion.

The dorsal horn neurons may inhibit, facilitate, or perform the relay of the sensory signals to the lateral horn and the ventral horn or to other segments of the spinal cord and to the brain. The processed signals from the dorsal horn neurons modulate the physiologic activities of the neurons of the lateral horn and the ventral horn.

The lateral horn neurons control the autonomic physiologic activities of internal organs, blood vessels, and glands. The ventral horn neurons are motor neurons, which control muscle activity.

The brain centers, after being activated by ascending signals from sensory neurons, may send signals to the segment to affect spinal cord neurons. Therefore the signals from the sensory nerve fibers influence lateral horn neurons, ventral horn neurons, other spinal segments, and the brain.

The lateral horn neurons regulate the autonomic activity of the organ systems (Fig. 8-33), blood vessels, joints, muscles, and skin. For example, the skin may become pale and cold as a result of vasoconstriction (constriction of the blood vessels). A muscle may show a diminished ability to stretch because of trophic changes caused by low blood circulation. Lack of sufficient blood circulation means low supplies of nutrition and oxygen to the joints. As a result of trophic changes of the ligaments, the joints will have a restricted range of motion.

The motor ventral horn controls muscle movement. It is important to keep in mind that the sensitized sensory fibers will in turn sensitize the motor neurons, which will cause muscle shortening or stiffness. The shortened muscles on the back can lead to blocked vertebral joints, resulting in stiffness of the neck and back, or to injuries to other shortened skeletal muscles and restrict the power of normal movement.

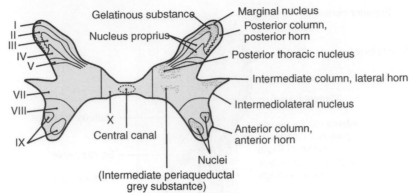

FIGURE 8-33 Organization of the spinal cord. The neurons of the lateral horn regulate the autonomic physiologic activities.

Every sensitive ARP contains sensitized sensory nerve fibers. If the sensitivity of the sensory nerve increases for an extended period of time, the sensitized nerve will sensitize the neurons in the lateral horn and anterior horn of the spinal cord in a retrograde direction. As a result of this retrograde sensitization from peripheral nerves, the anatomy, physiologic activities, and biochemical profile of the spinal cord will become abnormal.

This spinal sensitization causes increased sympathetic activity, which affects the motor nerves and the postganglionic nerves. This process leads to vasoconstriction and muscle tension. Once this vicious circle is established, the local nerve fibers become more sensitive, affect more nerve fibers and other soft tissues, and finally cause the local tissues to react abnormally to mechanical, thermal, and chemical stimuli.

This peripheral pathologic phenomenon is known as *hyperalgesia* (pain) or *hyperesthesia* (discomfort). Local points are rendered sensitive by the acute onset of diseases or injuries or by chronic diseases. The disease- and injury-related sensitive points are defined as symptomatic, segmental, or local ARPs according to their physiologic nature. For example, injuries of the upper limb, such as tennis elbow or carpal tunnel syndrome, create sensitive points on the upper limb. These points are called *symptomatic* points if the symptoms of the injuries are discussed.

These sensitive points of the upper limb can be traced, through the pathway of their peripheral nerve, to spinal segments C5 to T1. These same points are called *segmental points* if the emphasis is on their neural origin in spinal segments.

The appearance of symptomatic points is a very individual process because no two patients are identical in terms of body types, genetic makeup, medical history, onset of injury or illness, lifestyle, or tolerance of needling. The appearance of symptomatic points in each case is thus a unique process.

How, then, does a practitioner locate the symptomatic points in each patient? To decide which symptomatic ARPs should be needled in current treatment, a practitioner needs to obtain the patient's medical history, especially data from medical examinations (including laboratory tests and imaging studies) and information about all the injuries sustained by the patient and related events. If the case is suitable for acupuncture therapy, visual examination should be performed first.

The first data are collected from the patient's description of the complaint and from the medical history. Then the physical data should be considered. The undressed patient stands in a relaxed way so that the practitioner can check posture, three-dimensional muscle balance, and spine structure. Such visual data may help reveal symptomatic points. Subsequently, the practitioner should perform a thorough examination of the body by manual palpation to see whether the self-presented data match the visual data. This process enables a practitioner to determine the following:

1. What structures are involved in the injury or are related to the symptoms
2. Where the symptomatic points are located
3. The physical and psychologic status of the patient (some patients are psychologically or physically less tolerant of needling)
4. The possible outcome of treatment

It is not clinically difficult to relate particular symptomatic points to their corresponding spinal segments. The reason is simple. Symptoms may vary from one case to another, but each symptom is related to spinal nerves of one or two portions of the spinal cord. The spinal cord can be divided into five portions: cervical (C1 to C7), upper back (C7 to T7), middle back (T5 to L2), lower back (T12 – L5), and sacral (L5 to S4). (Because the innervation of neighboring spinal areas always overlaps, there is some overlapping between these portions.) Cervical paravertebral points should be selected when any head or face problems are addressed. In the treatment of any upper limb problems, the paravertebral points of C5 and T1 should be needled. Lumber and sacral paravertebral points should be considered in in the treatment of any problems associated with lower back and lower limbs, including lower back pain and gynecologic, urinary, and large intestine problems. The paravertebral points of the neck and upper back should be needled to improve symptoms related to muscle balance and posture, heart disease, respiratory symptoms such as cough, asthma, and blood pressure. Stomach, small intestine, and gall bladder functions are related to the spinal segments of the middle back. For each treatment, two to seven points on each side of the spine may be needled. The number of paravertebral points selected depends on the severity of the symptoms and on the body's physical or pathologic tolerance of needling.

PRINCIPLES OF USING SPINAL SEGMENTATION IN ACUPUNCTURE THERAPY

The innervation of skin, muscles, bones, and even viscera is segmented in terms of spinal nerves. By understanding the basic principles of this spinal segmentation, the practitioner can select the proper paravertebral ARPs to match particular symptomatic ARPs.

HOW TO SELECT PARAVERTEBRAL ACU-REFLEX POINTS

The principles of selecting the paravertebral ARPs to match the symptomatic ARPs according to spinal segmentation are described in the following sections. In most cases, these principles are simple and obvious. For example, for symptoms of the upper limb, paravertebral ARPs from C4 to T1 are needled. For lower limb disorders, paravertebral ARPs along L2 to S3 are needled. Paravertebral ARPs along T1 to T7 are needled for problems of the upper back and chest, and paravertebral ARPs from T8 to L1 are needled for problems of the abdominal region.

Segmentation of the Body Structure

The following description of body segmentation is aimed to help practitioners to relate symptomatic and segmental points to their corresponding spinal segments. For purposes of clinical acupuncture, the precise segment is not critical because the innervated field of one spinal nerve overlaps with the innervated fields of both neighboring spinal nerves.

The segmental innervations of the skin, muscles, viscera, and bones are referred to as *dermatome*, *myotome*, *viscerotome*, and *sclerotome*, respectively. The description of the segmentation of the neural supply is intended simply as an aid to understanding the segmental relationship between local points and their corresponding spinal segmentation.

Segmental Innervation of the Skin: Dermatomes

In the trunk, cutaneous segmentation is arranged in regular bands from T2 to L1 (Fig. 8-34).

A few body marks can help practitioners remember the dermatomes: T2 is at the sternal angle, T10 at the level of the umbilicus, and L1 in the region of the groin. As mentioned previously, there is

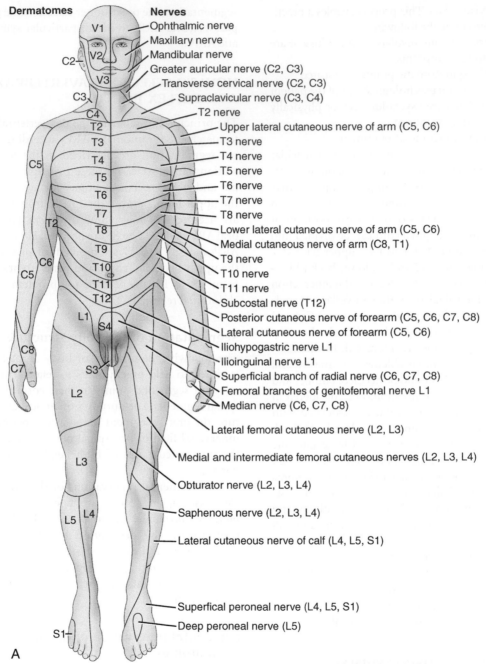

Dermatomes

Nerves

- Ophthalmic nerve
- Maxillary nerve
- Mandibular nerve
- Greater auricular nerve (C2, C3)
- Transverse cervical nerve (C2, C3)
- Supraclavicular nerve (C3, C4)
- T2 nerve
- Upper lateral cutaneous nerve of arm (C5, C6)
- T3 nerve
- T4 nerve
- T5 nerve
- T6 nerve
- T7 nerve
- T8 nerve
- Lower lateral cutaneous nerve of arm (C5, C6)
- Medial cutaneous nerve of arm (C8, T1)
- T9 nerve
- T10 nerve
- T11 nerve
- Subcostal nerve (T12)
- Posterior cutaneous nerve of forearm (C5, C6, C7, C8)
- Lateral cutaneous nerve of forearm (C5, C6)
- Iliohypogastric nerve L1
- Ilioinguinal nerve L1
- Superficial branch of radial nerve (C6, C7, C8)
- Femoral branches of genitofemoral nerve L1
- Median nerve (C6, C7, C8)
- Lateral femoral cutaneous nerve (L2, L3)
- Medial and intermediate femoral cutaneous nerves (L2, L3, L4)
- Obturator nerve (L2, L3, L4)
- Saphenous nerve (L2, L3, L4)
- Lateral cutaneous nerve of calf (L4, L5, S1)
- Superfical peroneal nerve (L4, L5, S1)
- Deep peroneal nerve (L5)

A

FIGURE 8-34   Adult dermatome pattern. **A,** Anterior view. **B,** Posterior view.

Nerves   **Dermatomes**

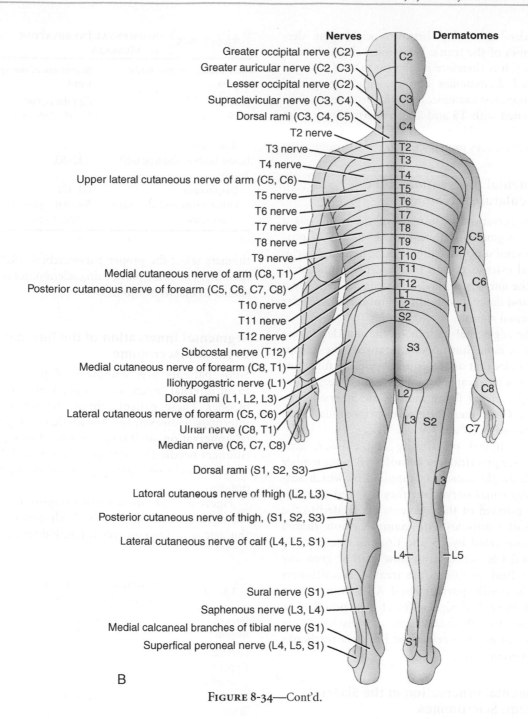

Greater occipital nerve (C2)
Greater auricular nerve (C2, C3)
Lesser occipital nerve (C2)
Supraclavicular nerve (C3, C4)
Dorsal rami (C3, C4, C5)
T2 nerve
T3 nerve
T4 nerve
Upper lateral cutaneous nerve of arm (C5, C6)
T5 nerve
T6 nerve
T7 nerve
T8 nerve
T9 nerve
Medial cutaneous nerve of arm (C8, T1)
Posterior cutaneous nerve of forearm (C5, C6, C7, C8)
T10 nerve
T11 nerve
T12 nerve
Subcostal nerve (T12)
Medial cutaneous nerve of forearm (C8, T1)
Iliohypogastric nerve (L1)
Dorsal rami (L1, L2, L3)
Lateral cutaneous nerve of forearm (C5, C6)
Ulnar nerve (C8, T1)
Median nerve (C6, C7, C8)

Dorsal rami (S1, S2, S3)
Lateral cutaneous nerve of thigh (L2, L3)
Posterior cutaneous nerve of thigh, (S1, S2, S3)
Lateral cutaneous nerve of calf (L4, L5, S1)

Sural nerve (S1)
Saphenous nerve (L3, L4)
Medial calcaneal branches of tibial nerve (S1)
Superfical peroneal nerve (L4, L5, S1)

B

FIGURE 8-34—Cont'd.

considerable overlap between neighboring dermatomes of the trunk. For clinical simplicity and efficacy, it is therefore important to treat both the affected dermatomes and the neighboring dermatomes. For example, if postherpetic neuralgia is associated with T5 and T6, the dermatomes from T4 to T7 should be needled together, including paravertebral ARPs from T4 to T7.

Segmental Innervation of the Musculature: Myotomes

The innervation of muscles of the trunk has a strictly segmental pattern from T1 to L1. The posterior rami supply the thoracic and lumbar muscles (spinal extensors), and their anterior rami innervate the intercostal muscles, abdominal flank muscles, and the rectus abdominis muscle in a regular segmental manner.

The segmental pattern of the muscles in the limbs is more functionally arranged. The groups of muscles that act for similar primary functions are often innervated by adjacent spinal nerves. For example, elbow flexor muscles are innervated by C5 and C6, whereas the elbow extensor muscles are innervated by C7 and C8.

For clinical practicality and efficacy, acupuncture practitioners do not need to remember which single muscle is supplied by which single segmental nerve, but they do need to know what portion of the segments are related to the particular muscles. For example, elbow flexors are innervated by C5 and C6, and extensors by C7 and C8. When any elbow pain or even any upper limb problems are treated, practitioners simply needle paravertebral ARPs from C4 to T1. Table 8-5, designed for clinical practicality, lists segmental innervation of muscles. More details of myotomes may be found in textbooks of neuroanatomy.

Segmental Innervation of the Skeletal System: Sclerotomes

Some patients seek acupuncture therapy for pain felt in the bones. One common example is the pain on the shin bone (tibia). Recognizing segmental supply by the spinal nerves (Table 8-6) helps prac-

TABLE 8-5	SEGMENTAL INNERVATION OF MUSCLES
Musculature of the Body Region	**Segments of the Spinal Cord**
Face	Cranial nerves
Neck	Cervical plexus C1–C4
Upper limb (including shoulder)	C5–T1
Lower limb (including hip)	T12–S3
Trunk:	
Diaphragm	C1–C5
Other trunk and abdominal muscles	Regular segmental pattern from C5 to S2

titioners select the proper paravertebral ARPs for needling. The principle of using sclerotomes is very similar to that of myotomes.

Segmental Innervation of the Internal Organs: Viscerotome

Some patients may complain of pain related to an internal organ such as the kidney or gall bladder. These patients should be referred to internists. However, the knowledge of segmental innervation of internal organs helps practitioners needle the correct paravertebral ARPs to relieve pain or muscle spasm of the internal organs.

Figure 8-35 shows that most important internal organs are innervated by both cervical and thoracic spinal nerves (including kidneys). Thus

TABLE 8-6	SEGMENTAL INNERVATION OF THE SKELETAL SYSTEM
Bones of the Body Region	**Segments of the Spinal Cord**
Cervical vertebrae	C1–C8
Upper limb (including shoulder)	C4–T1
Lower limb (including hip)	T12–S3
Trunk	
Costae	Regular pattern from T1 to T12
Thoracic and lumbar vertebrae	Regular segmental pattern from T1 to L5

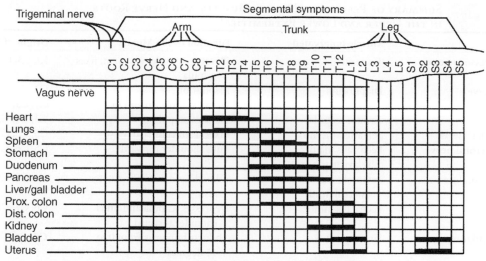

FIGURE 8-35 Segmentation of the internal organs.

it is important to needle the cervical paravertebral ARPs when treating disorders of these organs.

SUMMARY

Changes in homeostasis, chronic diseases, and acute injuries convert latent ARPs into passive ARPs. There are three types of ARPs: symptomatic, homeostatic, and paravertebral. From a pathophysiologic viewpoint, two types of ARP are considered: symptomatic and homeostatic. As homeostasis declines, homeostatic ARPs appear nonsegmentally all over the body in a predictable pattern and sequence. Symptomatic ARPs are segmentally associated with external injuries or internal diseases. The third type, paravertebral ARPs, helps balance the activities of the autonomic nervous system. For effective treatments, the three types of ARP should be properly combined.

The 24 homeostatic ARPs are used to treat *all* symptoms because needling these points improves homeostasis. All the other homeostatic ARPs may develop in some patterns related to these 24 homeostatic ARPs. When practitioners know the locations of the 24 homeostatic ARPs, they are able to predict where to find other homeostatic ARPs in which needling is necessary for the particular treatment.

Symptomatic ARPs are used to treat specific symptoms. Their appearance is usually local and segmental and less predictable. A practitioner should carefully palpate the patient's body to locate these points for each treatment.

Paravertebral ARPs should be selected to facilitate the therapeutic efficacy of the symptomatic ARPs that are being used. The paravertebral ARPs and symptomatic ARPs should be innervated by the spinal nerves of the same spinal segments.

In pain, acute symptoms sensitize only peripheral neurons, whereas chronic diseases sensitize both peripheral and central neurons. Acute symptoms can be easily desensitized with a few local treatments. Chronic diseases necessitate more holistic treatment to desensitize both peripheral and central neurons; in such cases, the pain symptoms are likely to reappear as a result of resensitization, even after some improvement is achieved.

Table 8-7 is a summary of the peripheral nerves and their muscular innervation.

TABLE 8-7	SUMMARY OF PERIPHERAL NERVES, MUSCLES, AND NERVE ROOTS IN THE UPPER AND LOWER EXTREMITIES*		
Nerve	**Muscle Innervated**	**Function of the Muscle**	**Origin of Nerve**
Spinal accessory nerve	Trapezius	Elevates shoulder and arm; fixes scapula	XI, C3, C4
Phrenic nerve	Diaphragm	Inspiration	C3, C4, C5
Dorsal scapular nerve	Rhomboid	Draws scapula up and in	C4, **C5**, C6
	Levator scapulae	Elevates scapula	C3, C4, C5
Long thoracic nerve	Serratus anterior	Fixes scapula on arm raise	C5, C6, C7
Lateral pectoral nerve	Pectoralis major (clavicular head)	Pulls shoulder forward	C5, C6
Medial pectoral nerve	Pectoralis major (sternal head)	Adducts and medially rotates arm	C6, C7, C8, T1
	Pectoralis minor	Depresses scapula and pulls shoulder forward	C6, C7, C8
Suprascapular nerve	Supraspinatus	Abducts humerus from 0 to 15 degrees	**C5**, C6
	Infraspinatus	Externally rotates humerus	**C5**, C6
Subscapular nerve	Subscapularis	Internally rotates humerus	C5, C6
	Teres major	Adducts and internally rotates humerus	C5, C6
Thoracodorsal nerve	Latissimus dorsi	Adducts and internally rotates humerus	C6, C7, C8
Axillary nerve	Teres minor	Adducts and internally rotates humerus	C5, C6
	Deltoid	Adducts humerus beyond 15 degrees	**C5**, C6
Musculocutaneous nerve	Biceps brachii	Flexes and supinates arm and forearm	C5, C6
	Brachialis	Flexes forearm	C5, C6
Radial nerve	Triceps	Extends forearm	C6, **C7**, C8
	Brachioradialis	Flexes forearm	C5, **C6**
	Extensor carpi radialis (longus and brevis)	Extend wrist; abduct hand	C5, **C6**
Posterior interosseus nerve (branch of radial nerve)	Supinator	Supinates forearm	C6, C7
	Extensor carpi ulnaris	Extends wrist; adducts hand	**C7**, C8
	Extensor digitorum (communis)	Extends digits	**C7**, C8
	Extensor digiti quinti	Extends digit 5	**C7**, C8
	Abductor pollicis longus	Abducts thumb in plane of palm	**C7**, C8
	Extensor pollicis (longus and brevis)	Extends thumb	**C7**, C8
	Extensor indicis proprius	Extends digit 5	**C7**, C8

*Boldface indicates the clinically important nerve root related to the primary acu-reflex points

TABLE 8-7	SUMMARY OF PERIPHERAL NERVES, MUSCLES AND NERVE ROOTS IN THE UPPER AND LOWER EXTREMITIES*—CONT'D		
Nerve	**Muscle Innervated**	**Function of the Muscle**	**Origin of Nerve**
Median nerve	Pronator teres	Pronates and flexes forearm	C6, C7
	Flexor carpi radialis	Flexes wrist; abducts hand	C6, C7
	Palmaris longus	Flexes wrist	C7, **C8**, T1
	Flexor digitorum superficialis	Flexes metacarpophalangeal and proximal interphalangeal joints	C7, **C8**, T1
	Lumbrical (I, II)	For digits 2 and 3, flex metacarpophalangeal joints; extend other joints	C8, **T1**
	Opponens pollicis	Flexes and opposes thumb	C8, **T1**
	Abductor pollicis brevis	Abducts thumb perpendicular to plane of palm	C8, **T1**
	Flexor pollicis brevis (superficial head)	Flexes first phalanx of thumb	C8, **T1**
Anterior interosseous nerve (branch of median nerve)	Flexor digitorum profundus (digits 2 and 3)	Flexes digits 2 and 3	C7, **C8**
	Flexor pollicis longus	Flexes distal phalanx of thumb	C7, **C8**
	Pronator quadratus	Pronates forearm	C7, C8
Ulnar nerve	Flexor carpi ulnaris	Flexes wrist; adducts hand	C7, **C8**, T1
	Flexor digitorum profundus (digits 4 and 5)	Flexes digits 4 and 5	C7, **C8**
	Lumbrical (III, IV)	For digits 4 and 5, flex metacarpophalangeal joints; extend other joints	C8, **T1**
	Palmar interossei	Adduct fingers; flex metacarpophalangeal joints; extend other joints	C8, **T1**
	Dorsal interossei	Abduct fingers; flex metacarpophalangeal joints; extend other joints	C8, **T1**
	Flexor pollicis brevis (deep head)	Flexes and adducts thumb	C8, **T1**
	Adductor pollicis	Adducts thumb	C8, **T1**
	Muscles of hypothenar eminence		
	Opponens digiti brevis	Internally rotates digit 5	C8, **T1**
	Abductor digiti minimi	Abducts digit 5	C8, **T1**
	Flexor digiti minimi	Flexes digit 5 at metacarpophalangeal joint	C8, **T1**
Superior gluteal nerve	Gluteus medius	Abducts and medially rotates thigh	**L4, L5**, S1
	Gluteus minimus	Abducts and medially rotates thigh	**L4, L5**, S1
	Tensor fasciae latae	Abducts and medially rotates thigh	**L4, L5**, S1
Inferior gluteal nerve	Gluteus maximus	Extends, abducts, and laterally rotates thigh; extends lower trunk	**L5, S1**, S2
Obturator nerve	Obturator externus	Adducts and outwardly rotates leg	**L2, L3**, L4
	Adductor longus	Adducts thigh	**L2, L3**, L4
	Adductor magnus	Adducts thigh	**L2, L3**, L4
	Adductor brevis	Adducts thigh	**L2, L3**, L4
	Gracilis	Adducts thigh	**L2, L3**, L4

(Continued)

TABLE 8-7	SUMMARY OF PERIPHERAL NERVES, MUSCLES AND NERVE ROOTS IN THE UPPER AND LOWER EXTREMITIES*—CONT'D		
Nerve	**Muscle Innervated**	**Function of the Muscle**	**Origin of Nerve**
Femoral nerve	Iliopsoas		
	Iliacus	Flexes leg at hip	L2, L3, **L4**
	Psoas	Flexes leg at hip	L2, **L3**, L4
	Quadriceps femoris		
	Rectus femoris	Extends leg at knee; flexes hip	L2, **L3, L4**
	Vastus lateralis	Extends leg at knee	L2, **L3, L4**
	Vastus intermedius	Extends leg at knee	L2, **L3, L4**
	Vastus medialis	Extends leg at knee	L2, **L3, L4**
	Pectineus	Adducts thigh	**L2, L3,** L4
	Sartorius	Inwardly rotates leg; flexes hip and knee	**L2, L3,** L4
Sciatic nerve	Adductor magnus	Adducts thigh	L4, L5, S1
	Hamstring muscles		
	Semitendinosus	Flexes knee; medially rotates thigh; extends hip	L5, **S1,** S2
	Semimembranosus	Flexes knee; medially rotates thigh; extends hip	L5, **S1,** S2
	Biceps femoris	Flexes knee; extends hip	L5, **S1,** S2
Tibial nerve (branch of sciatic nerve)	Triceps surae muscles		
	Gastrocnemius	Plantarflexes foot	S1, S2
	Soleus	Plantarflexes foot	S1, S2
Popliteus nerve	Tibialis posterior	Plantarflexes and inverts foot	L4, L5
	Plantaris	Spreads, brings together, and flexes proximal phalanges	L4, L5, S1
	Flexor digitorum longus	Flexes distal phalanges; aids plantar flexion	L5, **S1, S2**
	Flexor hallucis longus	Flexes great toes; aids plantar flexion	L5, **S1, S2**
	Small foot muscles	Cups sole	S1, S2
Superficial peroneal (fibular) nerve (branch of sciatic nerve)	Peroneus longus	Plantarflexes and everts foot	L5, S1
	Peroneus brevis	Plantarflexes and everts foot	L5, S1
Deep peroneal (fibular) nerve (branch of sciatic nerve)	Tibialis anterior	Dorsiflexes and inverts foot	L4, L5
	Peroneus tertius	Plantarflexes foot in pronation	L4, **L5**, S1
	Extensor digitorum longus	Extends phalanges; dorsiflexes foot	**L5**, S1
	Extensor hallucis longus	Extends first toe; aids dorsiflexion	**L5**, S1
	Extensor digitorum brevis	Extends toes	L5, S1

Modified from Devinsky O, Feldmann E: Examination of the cranial and peripheral nerves, New York, 1998, Churchill Livingstone.

Additional Readings

1. Dung HC: *Anatomical acupuncture*, San Antonio, Tex 1997, Antarctic Press, pp. 125-155.
2. Mens S, Simons DG: *Muscle pain*, Philadelphia, 2001, Lippincott Williams & Wilkins.
3. Kellgren HJ: The distribution of pain arising from deep somatic structures with charts of segmental pain areas, *Clin Sci* 4:35–46, 1939.
4. Dung HC, Clogston CP, Dunn JW: *Acupuncture: an anatomical approach*, Boca Raton, Fla, 2004, CRC Press.
5. Macdonald AJR: Acupuncture's non-segmental and segmental analgesic effects: the point of meridians. In Filshie J, White A, editors: *Medical acupuncture*, Churchill Livingston, 1998, Edinburgh, pp 93.
6. Simons DG, Travell JG, Simons LS: *Travell & Simons' myofascial pain and dysfunction: the trigger point manual, Volume 1: Upper half of body*, Philadelphia, 1999, Lippincott Williams & Wilkins, pp 59.
7. Simons DG, Travell JG, Simons LS: *Travell & Simons' myofascial pain and dysfunction: the trigger point manual, Volume 1: Upper half of body*, Philadelphia, 1999, Lippincott Williams & Wilkins, pp 58–69.
8. Nakatani Y, Yamashita K: *Ryodoraku acupuncture*, Osaka, 1977, Ryodoraku Research Institute.
9. Simons DG, Travell JG, Simons LS: *Travell & Simons' myofascial pain and dysfunction: the trigger point manual, Volume 1: Upper half of body*, Philadelphia, 1999, Lippincott Williams & Wilkins, p 71.
10. Jaffe LF: Extracellular current measurements with a vibrating probe, *Trends Neurosci* 8:517–521, 1985.
11. Ross R, Vogel A: The platelet-derived growth factor, *Cell* 14:203–210, 1978.

CHAPTER 9

Homeostatic Acu-Reflex Point System

SYSTEMIC PATTERN OF ACU-REFLEX POINT SENSITIZATION

From a physiologic perspective, there are two types of acu-reflex points (ARPs): homeostatic and symptomatic. Paravertebral ARPs, as clinically important ARPs, can be either homeostatic or symptomatic. According to both clinical experience and research, the sensitization of homeostatic ARPs follows an anatomically predictable pattern and sequence. This pattern of sensitization is found equally in all human beings for at least two reasons, according to current knowledge: First, homeostatic ARPs are neuroanatomically and pathologically dependent; second, the sensitization of homeostatic ARPs is related to human behavior: how we use our body to walk, to work, and to sit. If a person engages in special behavior such as the overuse of particular muscles in sports, a new pattern of ARP sensitization occurs and eventually causes the transformation of homeostatic ARPs into symptomatic ARPs. This phenomenon is examined in more depth in this chapter.

The anatomic configuration of ARPs, either homeostatic or symptomatic, varies in different parts of human body. As described in previous chapters, the common components of all ARPs are peripheral nerve fibers, which may include the sensory or postganglionic nerve fibers, or both, and motor nerve fibers such as muscle or tendon spindles. Secondary components include other soft tissues such as blood vessels, lymphatic vessels, and tendons or fasciae. The nerves at which the points form can be very different, according to their location; some are made of nerve endings, some are associated with big nerve trunks, and some contain a variety of different nerve fibers. The anatomic depths at which the points are formed are also varied. Ten anatomic features of ARP formation were discussed in detail in Chapter 8. All these features affect the formation, development, and appearance

of passive ARPs when homeostasis declines or central sensitization increases. As a whole, the sensitization of human homeostatic ARPs has a predictable pattern with regard to the locations and sequence of sensitization. This is very important in the pathophysiologic processes of the nervous system and has great clinical significance in both preventing and treating diseases and in slowing down the aging process.

SYMPTOMATIC PATTERN OF ACU-REFLEX POINT SENSITIZATION

When affected by particular pathologic factors, any sensory nerve fiber anywhere in the body may become sensitized. This is the random pattern of ARP formation. For example, diseased visceral organs above the diaphragm—such as the heart, lung, or esophagus—will sensitize ARPs on the upper part of the body and on the upper limbs, whereas the diseased visceral organs below the diaphragm will sensitize ARPs on the lower part of the body and on the lower limbs. Organs located on the level of the diaphragm—such as the stomach, liver, gall bladder, pancreas, and spleen—will sensitize ARPs on both upper and lower body and limbs. Liver disease may cause sensitization of liver ARPs on the right side of the body.

ARPs of both random and predictable pattern often coexist. For instance, the primary homeostatic H1 deep radial ARP is sensitized in all people, healthy and unhealthy alike. However, patients with neck, shoulder, elbow, wrist, and hand pain also exhibit sensitized random additional points around the H1 deep radial ARP. In such cases, the H1 point has become a symptomatic point.

ARPs have a dynamic physical and pathologic nature. They all have three phases: latent (nonsensitive), passive (sensitive), and active (oversensitive). The three phases reveal the quantitative and qualitative dynamics of an ARP: when affected by pathologic factors, the sensitivity and size of an ARP increase. With proper treatment, the sensitivity of an ARP is reduced, relieved, or even returned to normal. In the absence of proper treatment, or when the self-healing potential is impaired, an ARP grows in size and can become a permanent pathologic structure.

THE INTEGRATIVE NEUROMUSCULAR ACU-REFLEX POINT SYSTEM AS A CLINICAL GUIDANCE FOR TREATMENT

According to both clinical evidence and anatomic research, the most frequently used and therapeutically effective ARPs are associated with major peripheral nerves. The location of all ARPs can be clearly defined in terms of their neuroanatomic arrangement. With basic training in human anatomy, a clinician can easily locate each point.

ARPs become sensitive in association with certain anatomic structures and physiologic processes. For example, repetitive overuse or abuse injures particular muscles and soft tissues, which leads to the sensitization of specific ARPs. Thus these ARPs are specifically related to the abnormal condition. Direct needling of these symptomatic ARPs is more effective than indirect treatment of nonsymptomatic points in most cases, although sometimes indirect treatment also provide satisfactory results because of higher healing potential. Selecting specific symptomatic ARPs is therefore essential. The homeostatic ARP system, or the integrative neuromuscular acu-reflex point system (INMARPS), provides both physiologic and pathologic guidance for finding the most important symptomatic ARPs in every case. Thus it is important to understand the physiologic and pathologic implications of this system.

In the clinical setting, INMARPS provides important information: how healthy the person is or how the person will respond to any medical intervention. In addition, INMARPS provides reliable guidance for acupuncture treatment.

Needling is nonpharmaceutical and nonspecific therapy, and its efficacy depends partly on the health condition, or healing potential, in each case.

Health is defined in *Dorland's Illustrated Medical Dictionary*, 30th edition,[1] as "a state of optimal physical, mental, and social well-being; the popular idea that it is merely an absence of disease and infirmity is not complete." Physiologic health is definitely the foundation of physical and mental health. INMARPS is a quantitative system that can be used to more objectively define or measure the health condition of each individual.

All peripheral pathophysiologic factors are currently understood to interact with the central nervous system. Peripheral pathologic conditions or peripheral sensitization will lead to the sensitization of the neurons inside the central nervous system. These sensitized neurons then sensitize segmental peripheral nerves, and the sensitized ARPs are formed at the sensitized peripheral nerves. Thus the central sensitization represents peripheral physiologic health: The less healthy a person is, the more central sensitization exists, the more likely peripheral sensitization is to occur, and more sensitized ARPs will appear, in both quality (sensitivity) and quantity (the total numbers), on the entire body. Therefore the state of health can be measured by the number of sensitized or passive ARPs on the body. In this chapter, the concepts and method of measuring peripheral sensitization are introduced.

HISTORICAL REVIEW

The ancient Chinese practitioners noticed that pathologic insults created sensitized or painful spots on particular parts of the body surface. They traced these spots and formed the classic meridian charts, which included 361 meridian points and numerous nonmeridian points.

In the 1940s, Janet Travell independently discovered myofascial trigger points. It was noticed later that 80% of the trigger points matched the meridian acupuncture points.[1a] A. E. Sola, a military physician working in Lackland Air Force Base, San Antonio, Texas, in the 1950s, noticed that the young recruits developed sensitized spots in particular muscles after intensive training. He wrote, "These observations led to the question of the possible existence of latent trigger points in an asymptomatic individual, which upon being subjected to the physiological insult of strain, chronic fatigue, chilling, or other irritating stimuli, might serve as the source of clinical symptoms."[2] His observation reveals the dynamic physiology of these trigger points.

H. C. Dung, professor of human anatomy at the University of Texas Health Science Center at San Antonio, has studied the anatomy of acupoints and discovered systematic physiologic dynamics of these ARPs since the1970s.[3] Dung and the author collaborated in two books that introduced these concepts to Chinese acupuncture clinicians. Despite Dung's achievements, more research is needed to deepen the understanding of the systemic behavior of ARPs in the human body. The next section describes Dung's pioneer work in the 1970s to determine the distribution and sequence of sensitization of ARPs.

CHARTING THE ACU-REFLEX POINT SYSTEM

After careful research on classic acupuncture meridian points and modern trigger points, Dung selected 110 points from both systems according to neuromuscular anatomy. The selected points represent the different anatomic configurations, anatomic distribution, and clinical frequency of using these points. A checklist with all 110 points was made for recording the sensitivity of each point.

After the points were selected and the chart designed, 221 people with various pain symptoms were recruited for study (Table 9-1). Of these subjects, 130 (58.8%) were female and 91 (41.2%) were male. Patients between 40 and 69 years of age made up 63.8%. Only two patients were younger than 19 years of age. Some subjects were healthy young medical students. No attempt was made to differentiate the types of health problems present. All 110 points were palpated in each subject, and their sensitivities were recorded. All the subjects were examined by H. C. Dung himself. According to their own accounts, most of them suffered from soft tissue pain such as lower back pain, arthritis of various forms, joint pain, and headache.

If a point was sensitive in all the subjects, the sensitizing frequency of that point was described as 100%. If a point was sensitive in 70% of the patients, the frequency of that point was 70%. The data were processed to yield the percentage frequency of all 110 points. Thus the physical or physiologic pain of each patient was quantified by the number of sensitive ARPs.

In the following 30 years, these data were repeatedly applied to every patient at clinics in the United States, including Dung's, the author's, and a few other medical doctors' clinics. The pain quantified in each patient was compared with the results of treatment, and it was discovered that the fewer the sensitive points a patient had, the less treatments the patient needed and the longer the pain relief would last. This makes it possible to quantify, for each patient, the pain, the number of treatment sessions, and the prognosis.

	GENDER AND AGE DISTRIBUTION OF PATIENTS EXAMINED FOR PASSIVE ACU-REFLEX POINTS					
TABLE 9-1						
	FEMALE PATIENTS		**MALE PATIENTS**		**TOTAL PATIENTS**	
Age (Years)	No.	%	No.	%	No.	%
10–19	0	0	2	2.2	2	0.9
20–29	8	6.2	7	7.7	15	6.8
30–39	17	13.1	14	15.4	31	14.0
40–49	25	19.2	11	12.1	36	16.3
50–59	32	24.6	18	19.8	50	22.6
60–69	31	23.8	24	26.4	55	24.9
70–79	15	11.5	14	15.4	29	13.1
80–89	2	1.5	1	1.1	3	1.4
Total	130	100.0	91	100.0	221	100.0

Modified from Dung HC: *Anatomical acupuncture*, San Antonio, Tex, 1997, Antarctic Press, p 145.

From these empirical data—the number of sensitive ARPs they have—patients can be classified according to the level of their pain. As a clinical procedure, the quantification should be simple, quick, and reliable in its predictions.

There are two ways of classifying patients: the ABCD method or the 12-degree method. In the ABCD method, the 110 points are divided into four groups: A (points 0 to 24), B (points 25 to 50), C (points 51 to 80), and D (points 81 to 110). Patients of group A have fewer than 24 sensitive ARPs; those of group B, between 25 and 50; those of group C, between 51 and 80; and those of group D, more than 80. In the 12-degree method, each of the A, B, C, and D groups is divided into three subgroups; for example, of the patients in group A, those with fewer than 8 sensitive ARPs are classified as first degree, and those with 16 to 24 sensitive points are classified as third degree. Those with more than 100 sensitive ARPs have 12th-degree pain. In this book, the ABCD method is used (Tables 9-2 through 9-5 and Figs. 9-1 through 9-4).

The author and colleagues have developed a simple and reliable procedure to classify patients into ABCD groups. The procedure takes about 5 minutes and is introduced in this chapter.

A few words should be said about the research from which this method was derived. First, the pathophysiologic meaning of these empirical data needs to be explored further. Second, the developmental pattern of ARP sensitivity varies and is not exact point-like. When sensitivity starts to appear, it is restricted to a very specific location associated with a sensory nerve and can be regarded as a point. As the sensitivity develops, the sensitive area increases in size, becoming a big "point." If this "point" is located in the limbs, the continuous sensitization develops along the nerve trunk in a linear pattern; thus all the sensitive "points" on the same nerve trunk are connected, not discrete. If the sensitive "point" is located in the face or torso, it develops by increasing in area. Obviously, the difference in the patterns of development of sensitive points is related to the different innervation patterns of the peripheral nerve endings in the limbs and the face or torso (Figure 9-5).

ABCD GROUPING OR QUANTIFICATION OF PATIENTS: THE 16-POINT METHOD

The supply of energy is limited in every human body, and healing requires energy. The ABCD grouping is, in fact, a division into different energy levels, which provides the basis for predicting the response to and outcome of the treatment. Every pathologic condition, including peripheral sensitization and mental stress, consumes some energy. The more health problems a person has, the more slowly that any one of the problems will heal. For example, lower back pain heals much faster in a healthy person than in a person who has many health problems, with pain in several different parts of the body.

The nature of peripheral sensitization differs between chronic and acute cases. For example, a healthy person who suffers from acute lower back pain may have pain only in the lumbar area, whereas a patient with chronic lower back pain may also have pain in the upper back or legs, or both. With the same treatment, the first patient will recover in a few days, whereas the latter patient's recovery may take months. The healing of local pathologic conditions depends on the general health condition, or, in other words, the general level of healing energy in the body. The same lower back pain heals faster and better in a healthy and younger body. Thus it is important to know the general healing potential of the body in order to predict the outcome of each case.

The 110 acu-reflex point charts can be used to develop several methods of grouping patients because the homeostatic ARP system represents a regular pattern of sensitization. As a clinical principle, the grouping or quantification procedure should be simple, reliable, and reproducible. After more than a decade of clinical practice and teaching experience, the author and colleagues have used two points, H1 deep radial and H4 saphenous, for the purpose of quantification or grouping (Fig. 9-6). On each patient, H1 and its secondary, tertiary and nonspecific points are palpated on both upper limbs, and H4 and its secondary, tertiary, and nonspecific points are palpated on both lower limbs.

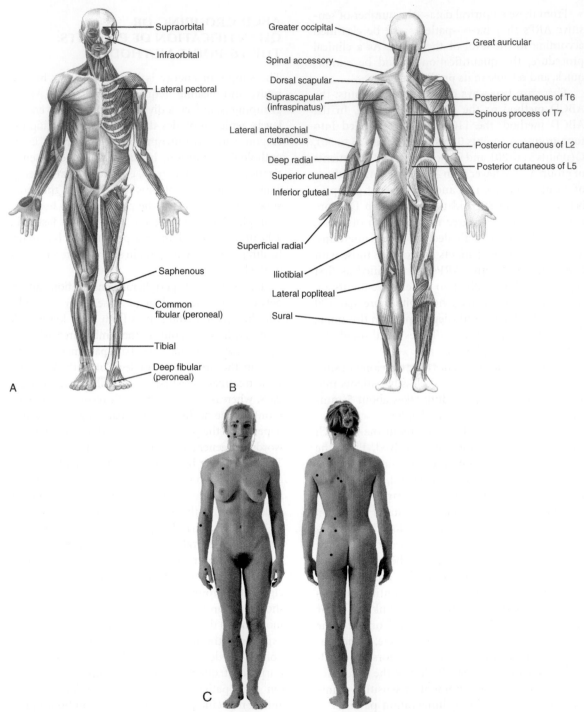

FIGURE 9-1 The primary 24 acu-reflex points. **A,** Anterior view. **B,** Posterior view. **C,** Surface anatomy of the primary homeostatic points.

TABLE 9-2	PRIMARY HOMEOSTATIC ACU-REFLEX POINTS		
Sequence	Name of Point	Frequency	%
1	Deep radial–I*	220	99.5
2	Great auricular	219	99.1
3	Spinal accessory–I	217	98.2
4	Saphenous–I	216	97.7
5	Deep fibular (peroneal)	215	97.3
6	Tibial	214	96.8
7	Greater occipital	213	96.4
8	Suprascapular (infraspinatus)	212	95.9
9	Lateral antebrachial cutaneous	211	95.5
10	Sural–I	209	94.6
11	Lateral or medial popliteal	207	93.7
12	Superficial radial	203	91.9
13	Dorsal scapular	201	91.0
14	Superior cluneal	198	89.6
15	Posterior cutaneous of L2	196	88.7
16	Inferior gluteal	195	88.2
17	Lateral pectoral	192	86.9
18	Iliotibial–I	185	83.7
19	Infraorbital	184	83.3
20	Spinous process of T7	178	80.5
21	Posterior cutaneous of T6	172	77.8
22	Posterior cutaneous of L5	168	76.0
23	Supraorbital	167	75.6
24	Common fibular (peroneal)	165	74.7

*The suffix "I" denotes the primary homeostatic point at the particular site.

The distance between two points is about the width of the thumbnail. A total of 16 ARPs are palpated. To estimate the general healing energy—that is, to classify a patient into A, B, C, or D groups—all the sensitive points must be added together (Table 9-6).

Because the sensitization develops linearly along the nerve trunk, what is measured is not isolated or discrete points but the extent of the development of sensitivity of the deep radial and saphenous nerves.

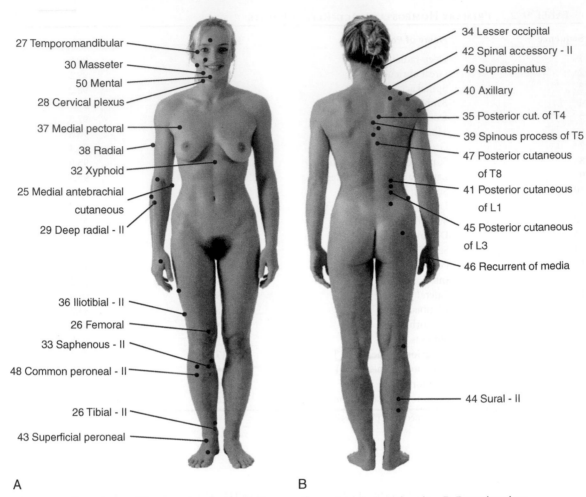

27 Temporomandibular
30 Masseter
50 Mental
28 Cervical plexus
37 Medial pectoral
38 Radial
32 Xyphoid
25 Medial antebrachial
      cutaneous
29 Deep radial - II

36 Iliotibial - II
26 Femoral
33 Saphenous - II
48 Common peroneal - II

26 Tibial - II
43 Superficial peroneal

34 Lesser occipital
42 Spinal accessory - II
49 Supraspinatus
40 Axillary
35 Posterior cut. of T4
39 Spinous process of T5
47 Posterior cutaneous
      of T8
41 Posterior cutaneous
      of L1
45 Posterior cutaneous
      of L3
46 Recurrent of media

44 Sural - II

A   B

FIGURE 9-2 The secondary homeostatic acu-reflex points. **A,** Anterior view. **B,** Posterior view.

TABLE 9-3   SECONDARY HOMEOSTATIC ACU-REFLEX POINTS

Sequence	Name of Point	Frequency	%
25	Medial antebrachial cutaneous	164	74.6
26	Tibial–II*	164	74.6
27	Temporomandibular	164	74.6
28	Cervical plexus	163	74.2
29	Deep radial–II	163	74.2
30	Masseter	162	73.6
31	Femoral	161	72.9
32	Xyphoid	160	72.4
33	Saphenous–II	156	70.6
34	Lesser occipital	152	68.8
35	Posterior cutaneous of T5	148	67.0
36	Iliotibial–II	147	66.5
37	Medial pectoral	146	66.1
38	Radial	143	64.7
39	Spinous process of T5	142	64.3
40	Axillary	138	62.4
41	Posterior cutaneous of L1	138	62.4
42	Spinal accessory–II	135	61.1
43	Superficial fibular (peroneal)	134	60.6
44	Sural–II	132	59.7
45	Posterior cutaneous of L3	128	57.9
46	Recurrent branch of median	123	55.7
47	Posterior cutaneous of T8	122	55.2
48	Common fibular (peroneal)–II	114	51.6
49	Suprascapular–II (supraspinatus)	111	50.2
50	Mental	110	49.8

*The suffix "II" denotes the secondary homeostatic point at the particular site.

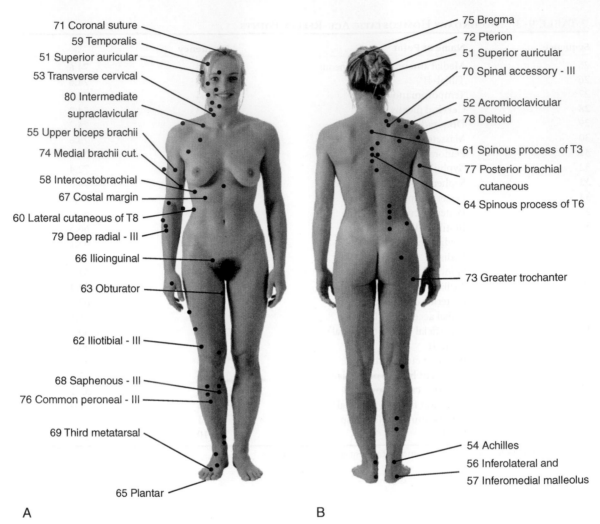

71 Coronal suture
59 Temporalis
51 Superior auricular
53 Transverse cervical
80 Intermediate
    supraclavicular
55 Upper biceps brachii
74 Medial brachii cut.
58 Intercostobrachial
67 Costal margin
60 Lateral cutaneous of T8
79 Deep radial - III
66 Ilioinguinal
63 Obturator
62 Iliotibial - III
68 Saphenous - III
76 Common peroneal - III
69 Third metatarsal
65 Plantar

75 Bregma
72 Pterion
51 Superior auricular
70 Spinal accessory - III
52 Acromioclavicular
78 Deltoid
61 Spinous process of T3
77 Posterior brachial
    cutaneous
64 Spinous process of T6
73 Greater trochanter
54 Achilles
56 Inferolateral and
57 Inferomedial malleolus

A   B

Figure 9-3 The tertiary homeostatic acu-reflex points. **A,** Anterior view. **B,** Posterior view.

TABLE 9-4	TERTIARY HOMEOSTATIC ACU-REFLEX POINTS		
Sequence	**Name of Point**	**Frequency**	**%**
51	Superior auricular	108	48.8
52	Acromioclavicular	108	48.8
53	Transverse cervical	108	48.8
54	Achilles	107	48.4
55	Upper biceps brachii	105	47.5
56	Inferolateral malleolus	104	47.1
57	Inferomedial malleolus	104	47.1
58	Intercostobrachial	102	46.2
59	Temporalis	102	46.2
60	Lateral cutaneous of T8	100	45.2
61	Spinous process of T3	95	43.0
62	Iliotibial–III*	93	42.1
63	Obturator	91	41.2
64	Spinous process of T6	83	37.6
65	Plantar	81	36.7
66	Ilioinguinal	79	35.8
67	Costal margin	78	35.3
68	Saphenous–III	76	34.4
69	Third metatarsal	73	33.0
70	Spinal accessory–III	72	32.6
71	Coronal suture	71	32.1
72	Pterion	71	32.1
73	Greater trochanter	70	31.7
74	Medial brachial cutaneous	69	31.2
75	Bregma	67	30.3
76	Common fibular (peroneal)	65	29.4
77	Posterior brachial cutaneous	63	28.5
78	Deltoid	63	28.5
79	Deep radial–III	61	27.7
80	Intermediate supraclavicular	61	27.7

*The suffix "III" denotes the tertiary homeostatic point at the particular site.

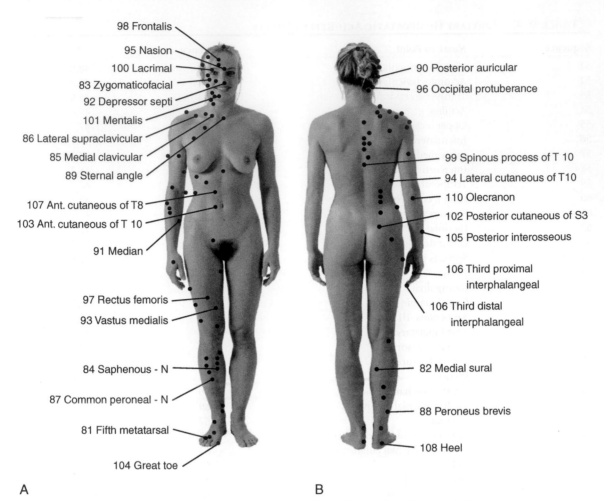

98 Frontalis
95 Nasion
100 Lacrimal
83 Zygomaticofacial
92 Depressor septi
101 Mentalis
86 Lateral supraclavicular
85 Medial clavicular
89 Sternal angle
107 Ant. cutaneous of T8
103 Ant. cutaneous of T 10
91 Median
97 Rectus femoris
93 Vastus medialis
84 Saphenous - N
87 Common peroneal - N
81 Fifth metatarsal
104 Great toe

90 Posterior auricular
96 Occipital protuberance
99 Spinous process of T 10
94 Lateral cutaneous of T10
110 Olecranon
102 Posterior cutaneous of S3
105 Posterior interosseous
106 Third proximal interphalangeal
106 Third distal interphalangeal
82 Medial sural
88 Peroneus brevis
108 Heel

A   B

FIGURE 9-4 The nonspecific homeostatic acu-reflex points. **A,** Anterior view. **B,** Posterior view.

TABLE 9-5	NONSPECIFIC ACU-REFLEX POINTS*		
Sequence	Name of Point	Frequency	%
81	Fifth metatarsal	60	27.1
82	Medial sural	58	26.2
83	Zygomaticofacial	55	24.9
84	Saphenous–N	51	23.1
85	Medial supraclavicular	48	21.7
86	Lateral supraclavicular	44	19.9
87	Common fibular (peroneal)–N	41	18.6
88	Fibular (peroneal) brevis	39	17.6
89	Sternal angle	37	16.7
90	Posterior auricular	35	15.8
91	Median–N	34	15.4
92	Depressor septi	32	14.5
93	Vastus medialis	28	12.7
94	Lateral cutaneous of T10	26	11.8
95	Nasion	24	10.9
96	Occipital protuberance	21	9.5
97	Rectus femoris	20	9.0
98	Frontalis	18	8.1
99	Spinous process of T10	17	7.6
100	Lacrimal	16	7.2
101	Mentalis	15	6.8
102	Posterior cutaneous of S3	14	6.3
103	Anterior cutaneous of T10	13	5.9
104	Great toe	12	5.4
105	Posterior interosseus	11	5.0
106	Third proximal interphalangeal	9	4.0
107	Anterior cutaneous of T8	8	3.6
108	Heel	7	3.2
109	Third distal interphalangeal	6	2.7
110	Olecranon	3	1.4

*The suffix "N" denotes the nonspecific homeostatic point at the particular site.

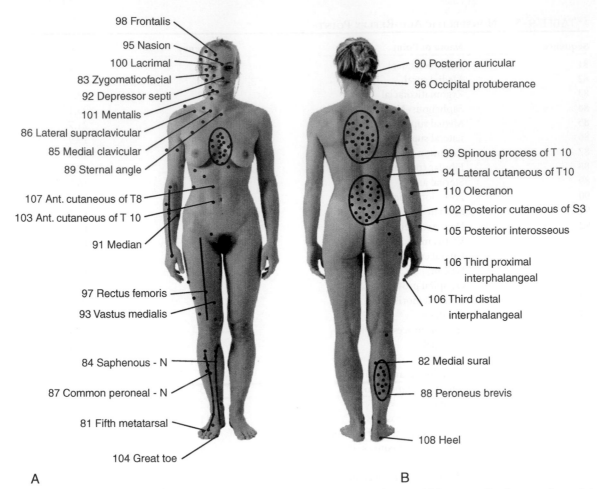

98 Frontalis
95 Nasion
100 Lacrimal
83 Zygomaticofacial
92 Depressor septi
101 Mentalis
86 Lateral supraclavicular
85 Medial clavicular
89 Sternal angle
107 Ant. cutaneous of T8
103 Ant. cutaneous of T 10
91 Median
97 Rectus femoris
93 Vastus medialis
84 Saphenous - N
87 Common peroneal - N
81 Fifth metatarsal
104 Great toe

90 Posterior auricular
96 Occipital protuberance
99 Spinous process of T 10
94 Lateral cutaneous of T10
110 Olecranon
102 Posterior cutaneous of S3
105 Posterior interosseous
106 Third proximal interphalangeal
106 Third distal interphalangeal
82 Medial sural
88 Peroneus brevis
108 Heel

A   B

FIGURE 9-5 As the acu-reflex points become more sensitized, the sensitized or sensitizing area of each acu-reflex point increases, and finally all the neighboring points become sensitized in a huge area (on the torso and face) or in a linear zone on the limbs. **A,** Anterior view. **B,** Posterior view.

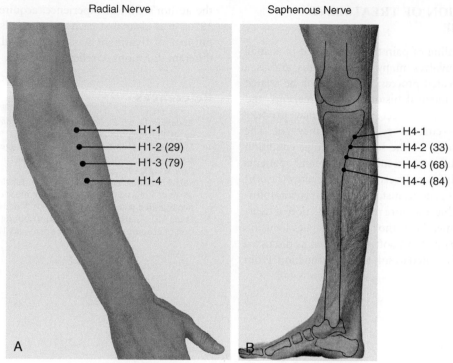

FIGURE 9-6   Acu-reflex points for evaluation on the arm (**A**) and the leg (**B**).

TABLE 9-6	ABCD GROUPING WITH 16-POINT METHOD
Group Classification	**Number of Sensitive Acu-Reflex Points**
A	0–4
B	5–8
C	9–12
D	≥13

TABLE 9-7   PAIN QUANTIFICATION AND PROGNOSIS

Characteristic	GROUP			
	A	**B**	**C**	**D**
Number of passive acu-reflex points found in a patient	<24	24–50	51–80	>80
Percentage of patient population	28%	34%	30%	8%
Number of treatments required for pain relief	4–8	8–16	16–32	>32
Time lapse before recurrence of the same pain	Years	Months to years	Weeks to months	Days to weeks

Modified from Dung HC: *Anatomical acupuncture*, San Antonio, Tex, 1997, Antarctic Press, p 226.

PREDICTION OF TREATMENT OUTCOME

Even the healing of pain that is confined to a small local area involves many body systems and is a very complicated process; the result will be related to personal medical history, genetic makeup, and social behavior. Correct treatment may produce two results—cure or relief—or it may fail. The same treatment for the same pathologic condition produces different results in different patients because of different levels of healing energy (health) and different genetic, historical, and behavioral situations. To achieve a more reliable prediction of treatment outcome, the author and colleagues focus on soft tissue pain. Most soft tissue pain, as discussed previously, is related to soft tissue dysfunction. From the author's clinical experience, acquired since the 1970s, it is clear that each group needs a different number of treatment sessions and will experience different durations of relief (Table 9-7).

References

1. Anderson D, ed: *Dorland's Illustrated Medical Dictionary*, ed 30, Philadelphia, 2003, Saunders.
1a. Melzack R, Stillwell DM, Fox EJ: Trigger points and acupuncture points for pain: correlations and implications, *Pain* 3:3–23, 1977.
2. Sola AE, Rodenberger ML, Gettys BB: Incidence of hypersensitive areas in posterior shoulder muscles; a survey of two hundred young adults, *Am J Phys Med* 34:585, 1955.
3. Dung HC: Anatomical features contributing to the formation of acupuncture points, *Am J Acupunct* 12:139, 1984.

Trigger Points and the Integrative Neuromuscular Acu-Reflex Point System

Trigger-point therapy was developed in modern times as a clinical technique for myofascial pain syndrome. A British physician was working as a young research assistant under Sir Thomas Lewis at University College Hospital in 1938, John Kellgren—later to become professor of rheumatology at Manchester University in the United Kingdom—observed that the pain in myalgia, or what is currently known as myofascial pain syndrome, originates in small, circumscribed, exquisitely tender points in muscle. He found that he could reproduce this spontaneously occurring pain by applying sustained pressure to these points and could alleviate it by injecting those points with procaine hydrochloride (Novocain). He also observed that this pain is not generally felt at the tender point itself but is referred to an area of the body some distance from it.[1] Kellgren's work prompted Janet Travell to study patients with musculoskeletal pain. She soon discovered that this referred pain is triggered by neural hyperactivity at the points in muscle and its surrounding fascia, Kellgren had referred to as "tender points"; she gave them the name *trigger points*. She introduced the terms *myofascial pain* and *zones of pain referral* and also named the disorder *myofascial pain syndrome*.

Later Travell and David G. Simons published their two-volume work, *Myofascial Pain and Dysfunction: The Trigger Point Manual*, which is now the classic clinical manual in trigger-point medicine. Although this book is authoritative in its field, Simons's observation[2] is noteworthy:

> "Despite the fact that an increasing number of clinicians and scientists believe that most common enigmatic unexplained musculoskeletal pain comes from trigger points, mainstream medicine has yet to accept or incorporate them as an integral part of its teaching, research and practice.

We are now becoming aware of several factors that may account for this slow progress.

Although the core of trigger points lies in skeletal muscle, all branches of the nervous system and several endocrine systems interact with them. In other words, trigger points are very complex."

Three factors appear to be critical:

> "1. There is no generally accepted account of the pathophysiology of trigger points, which prevents the establishment of authoritative diagnostic criteria, and this in turn inhibits research.
> 2. At present, there is no recognized laboratory test or imaging technique to serve as an objective standard for diagnosing trigger points. Diagnosis can be made only through physical examination and patient history.
> 3. In the absence of an established gold-standard diagnostic test, appropriate specific diagnostic tests and appropriate diagnostic criteria remain controversial and unresolved. This is in part because clinicians depend heavily on the history as well as the physical examination, but interrater reliability studies to date have addressed only the physical examination. These interrater reliability studies make it clear that for many clinicians it takes training and much experience to develop adequate skills for diagnostic reliability and therapeutic competence. Agreement on diagnostic criteria is also confounded by the many variations in structure and accessibility of some 500 individual muscles; no one examination applies to all muscles."[2] (p. 16)

Although these observations are still applicable today, an increasing number of clinicians of different medical disciplines are now successfully treating myofascial pain syndrome by using dry needling.

Another important clinical observation should be mentioned. In *Myofascial Pain and Dysfunction: The Trigger Point Manual*, Volume 1, Travell and Simons stated,

> "In comparative studies,[3,4] dry needling was found to be as effective as injecting an anesthetic solution such as procaine or lidocaine in terms of immediate inactivation of the trigger point. In the Hong study[3] of the response of trapezius muscle trigger points to 0.5% lidocaine or to dry needling, both groups experienced essentially the same amount of improvement immediately and 2 weeks later. However, within 2–8 hours, 42% of the lidocaine-injected patients and 100% of the dry-needled patients developed local soreness. The soreness of the patients treated by dry needling had significantly greater intensity and duration than the soreness of lidocaine-injected patients." (pp. 151–152)

These results indicate that the critical therapeutic factor in both cases is mechanical disruption by the needle. This is consistent with the understanding that disruption of the trigger-point knots of contraction by needling will terminate the local energy crisis and the sensitization of nearby nerves that it causes.

In the study by Hong[3] mentioned in this quotation, both the subjects who received lidocaine injections and those who received dry needling may have been subjected to the same size of syringe needles. In clinical practice, fewer patients experience postneedling soreness when finer acupuncture needles are used.

ETIOLOGY OF TRIGGER POINTS

Simons[2] suggested three major etiologic features of trigger points that explain the most widely recognized characteristics of their clinical pathophysiologic mechanisms. These features are related to one another in a positive feedback cycle that is self-perpetuating once it starts but can be interrupted at several points in the cycle in a number of ways. Although the understanding of the pathways between them are not well established,[5–8] substantial evidence supports this hypothesis. The three features are as follows:

- Increased acetylcholine release at the neuromuscular junction (motor plate)
- Increased tension of muscle fibers passing through the trigger point that produces a palpable taut band
- The presence of sensitizing substances in the muscle tissue of the trigger point that can produce pain

A brief description of these three features is provided below. The author believes that this account of the physiologic mechanisms of trigger points also describes the most common clinical features of most, if not all, acu-reflex points.

Acetylcholine Release

Research on the basic physiology of trigger points has revealed increased electrical activity at the motor endplate. This endplate "noise" is associated with greatly increased release of acetylcholine transmitter. Other pathophysiologic processes may also be responsible for these effects. For example, if an immune reaction were to block the normally prompt inactivation of acetylcholine by cholinesterase within the synaptic cleft, the acetylcholine receptors in the postjunctional membrane would continue to produce excessive levels of minute endplate potentials (endplate noise).

Calcitonin gene–related peptide inhibits the expression of cholinesterase in vertebrate experiments.[5] Such a process allows more acetylcholine to affect receptors in the postjunctional membrane, producing a result comparable to that caused by an increased release of acetylcholine. In addition, the peptide can induce expression of the acetylcholine receptor, which would also increase the number of minute endplate potentials.

Increased Fiber Tension

The specific mechanisms responsible for taut bands are still under investigation. Clinically, they are considered an essential feature of trigger points, and successful results have been achieved by needling them. Histologic studies have revealed increased tension in affected muscle fibers and evidence of disrupted contractile elements.[5] Local regions of hypercontracted fibers are observed as contraction knots or contraction discs that increase tension in those fibers. Shortened sarcomeres with adjacent regions of compensatory lengthening of the sarcomeres in those fibers are observed. Such a structure would further increase tension in the fiber because of the elastic resistance of sarcomeres to passive stretch, especially when elongated beyond their resting length. These observations help explain the increased physical tension and tissue distress in muscles that harbor trigger points. More research is needed to clarify the source of the increased tension that constitutes palpable taut bands.

Sensitizing Substances in Trigger Points

Researchers have demonstrated measurable quantities of sensitizing substances at trigger points. Shah and colleagues[6] made a study of the tissue milieu in the trigger points of nine subjects: three normal, three with latent trigger points, and three with active trigger points. They used a novel acupuncture-size microdialysis needle to sample both normal tissue and trigger points in upper trapezius muscles. The acupuncture needle contained in-and-out delivery tubes that ended at a dialyzer membrane set 0.2 mm from the open tip of the needle. The results are summarized in Table 10-1. These data convincingly indicate the physical and histopathologic milieu of a trigger point in the muscle, as distinct from normal tissue.

The significant difference in the levels of these substances between normal muscle tissue and trigger-point sites indicates that trigger points have demonstrable and complex histopathologic features. The significant histochemical difference found between latent and active trigger points provides a measurable clinical distinction between the

TABLE 10-1	Physiologic Comparison of Relative Amounts of Algogenic Substances Sampled by Microdialysis from Latent and Active Trigger Points
Measurement	**Active Trigger Points Compared with Latent Trigger Points and Normal Muscles**
Pressure pain threshold	↓ $P < 0.08$
pH	↓ $P < 0.03$
Substance P	↑ $P < 0.08$
Calcitonin gene-related peptide	↑ $P < 0.08$
Bradykinin	↑ $P < 0.08$
Serotonin	↑ $P < 0.08$
Norepinephrine	↑ $P < 0.08$
Tumor necrosis factor-α	↑ $P < 0.08$
Interleukin-1β	↑ $P < 0.08$

two types of point. All of this has advanced the understanding of the physiologic process of trigger-point formation and treatment.

INTERACTIONS OF MYOFASCIAL TRIGGER POINTS

The neuromuscular dysfunction of skeletal muscle seems to be the major clinical manifestation of trigger points, but their pathophysiologic processes are incredibly complex. In the context of pain and other internal problems, trigger points interact with all major components of the central nervous system, the endocrine system, and immune system. A muscle containing active trigger points becomes shorter and weaker. The affected muscle resists stretching, and any attempt to extend it results in pain. The physiologic processes of the muscle may change when trigger points develop. Changes such as gooseflesh, localized sweating, and intense coldness of the distal part of a limb have been observed. All these observations show that the development of trigger points in the muscles is not an isolated histologic structure.

How these points are interrelated to human physiologic systems and homeostasis is still not adequately understood. For example, trigger points often exist in clusters involving regional function. Lewit[8] recognized the tendency of trigger points to appear in chains of functionally related muscles, particularly the deep stabilizers of the lower torso and especially in the diaphragm and pelvic floor muscles. The importance of the core stabilizer muscles is now becoming recognized, but the diaphragm is often overlooked.[9] The surprising observation that trigger points in these core muscles are commonly found to be an important part of headache is a reminder that core systems are involved, as well as the trigger points of individual muscles. Evidence from research indicates the importance of treating core systems while working on peripheral problems such as those in the limbs.[9]

TRIGGER-POINT NOCICEPTORS

Myofascial pain syndrome develops as a result of the activation and sensitization of nociceptors at trigger-point sites in muscle. Two types of nociceptors are relevant in this discussion: cutaneous and muscular. In the skin there are high-threshold A∂-mechanothermal nociceptors and C-polymodal nociceptors. In muscle the corresponding nociceptors are group III and group IV, respectively.

Needling into the skin surface causes activation of cutaneous A∂-mechanothermal nociceptors, which in turn causes a transient pain and then activation of cutaneous C-polymodal nociceptors, which gives rise to a persistent, dull, aching, and sometimes burning or stinging pain. It is possible that the effect of trauma on muscle is similarly to activate A∂-mechanothermal (group III) and C-polymodal (group IV) nociceptors.

Because the persistent dull, aching type of pain present in myofascial pain syndrome is similar in every respect to the pain that arises when cutaneous nociceptors of C-afferent fibers are activated, however, it seems reasonable to relate that pain to the activation of C-afferent (group IV) nociceptors at trigger-point sites in muscle. This view is supported by the observation that the pain in this disorder may be eliminated by stimulating the cutaneous and subcutaneous A∂-mechanothermal nerve fibers with dry needles.

Although muscular trauma is the main etiologic factor for the development of passive and active trigger points, pathologic conditions of internal viscera may also cause the development of trigger points in skeletal muscles. Also, a muscle may suffer a direct injury and become acutely, chronically, or recurrently overloaded with sensitized trigger points. In addition, muscles may be subjected to repeated microtrauma such as the repetitive strain injury as found in patients with certain occupations. Some of these trauma or injuries can be prevented if attention is paid to regular maintenance of muscle health.

MYOFASCIAL TRIGGER-POINT SITES

Trigger points appear usually at sites associated with certain neural configurations, as discussed in previous chapters. They are often found in muscle bellies, especially in the region of muscular motor points where the nerves enter the muscles. Trigger points are also formed at muscle insertion sites because of physical stress and the rich innervation of dense connective tissues. Some trigger points, such as those in the sternocleidomastoid muscle, develop in the free borders of muscles where nerves penetrate the deep fascia and come up to the surface to give off branches.

Palpable taut bands are often detected in painful muscles, especially in the neck and upper back. These taut bands often harbor trigger points. Temporary pain relief is reported by patients when these trigger points in the taut bands are needled.

SOME MYOFASCIAL PAIN PATTERNS CAUSED BY TRIGGER POINTS

Some pain patterns caused by common trigger points are depicted in Figure 10-1. Keen attention should be paid to the relationship between the location of the trigger points, the types of pain that they are related to, and their neural innervation. Pain patterns are discussed as follows on a regional basis for convenience.

- Pain patterns in the head and face involve four muscles: the sternocleidomastoid, splenius capitis, temporalis, and masseter (Table 10-2).
- Pain patterns in the neck, shoulder, and upper limbs involve eight muscles: the scalene, trapezius, levator scapulae, infraspinatus, supraspinatus, subscapularis, deltoid, and pectoralis (Table 10-3).
- Pain patterns in the lumbar spine, hip, and lower limb involve 13 muscles: the gluteus maximus, gluteus medius, gluteus minimus, piriformis, vastus lateralis, vastus intermedius, vastus medialis, biceps femoris, gastrocnemius, soleus, peroneus longus, extensor digitorum longus, and tibialis anterior (Table 10-4).

The patterns of trigger points and those of homeostatic acu-reflex points match very well. Observant readers will see that the homeostatic acu-reflex point system provides a logical understanding of trigger-point pain patterns (Figs. 10-2 to 10-5).

Myofascial pain that is related to or caused by trigger points is a type of soft tissue pain. It is characterized by the development of sensitive or tender locations within muscles or other soft tissue, such as fascia, ligaments, or tendons, and these are known as trigger points.

Travell and Simons defined a myofascial trigger point (MTrP) as a "hyperirritable locus within a taut band of skeletal muscle, located in the muscle tissue or its associated fascia".[10] Sensitive MTrPs may arise a few days after an acute strain of a muscle, or their onset may be gradual, a cumulative effect of repeated overuse of a muscle. Some MTrPs are related to acute or chronic visceral diseases, such as those that can develop in the pectoral muscles as a result of heart disease, or in the abdominal muscles after gastroenteritis

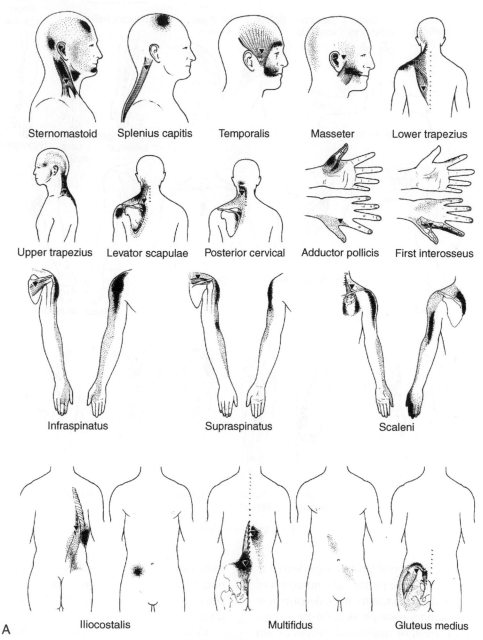

FIGURE 10-1 A and B, The most commonly found trigger points and their reference areas.

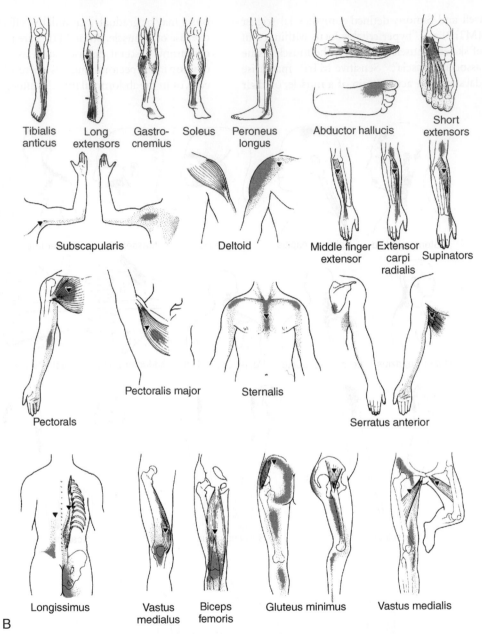

Tibialis anticus · Long extensors · Gastro-cnemius · Soleus · Peroneus longus · Abductor hallucis · Short extensors

Subscapularis · Deltoid · Middle finger extensor · Extensor carpi radialis · Supinators

Pectorals · Pectoralis major · Sternalis · Serratus anterior

Longissimus · Vastus medialus · Biceps femoris · Gluteus minimus · Vastus medialis

B

Figure 10-1—Cont'd.

or diarrhea. Constant mental tension, experienced as anxiety or stress, can cause prolonged contraction of the skeletal muscles, which results in the development of MTrPs. In addition, poor physical fitness or posture, emotional stress, or nutritional deficiency can perpetuate MTrPs. Some female patients complain of more painful MTrPs just before or during menstruation. Athletes experience more muscle tightness and consequently more sensitive MTrPs during and after training in cold weather.

Clinical symptoms related to MTrPs may include a deep ache or pain, stiffness of the muscles, and

Text continued on p. 159

TABLE 10-2   PAIN PATTERNS OF MAJOR TRIGGER POINTS IN THE HEAD AND NECK MUSCLES

Muscle	Origin	Insertion	Innervation	Main Function	Patterns of Referred Pain from Trigger Points of the Muscle
Sternocleidomastoid*	Lateral surface of mastoid process of temporal bone; lateral half of the superior nuchal line of occipital bone	*Sternal head:* attached to the anterior surface of the manubrium of sternum and lateral to jugular notch via a rounded tendon *Clavicular head:* superior surface of medial third of clavicle	Spinal root of accessory nerve (XI) and branches of cervical plexus (C2–C3)	*Unilateral action:* laterally flexes the neck, rotates the face to contralateral side *Bilateral action:* flexes the neck, facilitates inhalation	*Sternal division:* vertex; occiput; across the neck; over the eye, throat, and sternum Autonomic symptoms: eye and sinuses *Clavicular division:* frontal headache and earache; dizziness
Splenius capitis	Inferior half of ligamentum nuchae and spinous processes of superior six thoracic vertebrae	Lateral aspect of mastoid process and lateral third of superior nuchal line	Dorsal rami of C2–C4	Laterally flexes and rotates head and neck to same side; extends head and neck when acting bilaterally	Vertex of the head, occiput, and diffusely through the cranium, back of the orbit, sometimes down to the lower neck and shoulder
Temporalis	Floor of temporal fossa and deep surface of temporal fascia	Tip and medial surface of coronoid process and anterior border of ramus of mandible	Deep temporal branches of mandibular nerve (V3)	Elevates mandible, closing jaws; its posterior fibers revert mandible after protrusion	Temporal region (temporal headache), eyebrow, upper teeth; occasionally maxillary teeth and temporomandibular joint
Masseter†	Inferior border and medial surface of zygomatic arch Superficial parts, including superficial and intermediate layers	Lateral surface of ramus of mandible and its coronoid process	Mandibular nerve (V3) via masseteric nerve that enters its deep surface	Elevates and protrudes mandible to closing jaws; deep fibers revert it Superficial and deep layers have somewhat different functions	*Superficial layer:* Eyebrow, maxilla, anterior mandible, and upper or lower molar teeth *Deep layer:* region of temporomandibular joint and deep in the ear

*Sternal and clavicular divisions have different function.
†Superficial and deep layers have a different angulation of fiber direction.

TABLE 10-3 MAJOR PAIN PATTERNS FROM TRIGGER POINTS OF THE NECK, SHOULDER, AND UPPER LIMB

Muscle	Origin (Proximal or Medial Attachment)	Insertion (Distal or Lateral Attachment)	Innervation	Main Function	Patterns of Referred Pain from Trigger Points of the Muscle
Scalene					Referred pain can radiate from all three scaleni
Scalenus posterior	Posterior tubercles of transverse processes of C4–C6 vertebrae	External border of second rib	Cervical nerves of C7–C8	Flexes neck laterally; elevates second rib during forced inspiration	Upper vertebral of scapula
Scalenus medius	Posterior tubercles of transverse processes of C2–C7 vertebrae	Superior surface of first rib, posterior to groove for subclavian artery	Cervical nerves of C3–C8	Flexes neck laterally; elevates first rib during forced inspiration	Down the front and back of arm and radial forearm; may extend to thumb and index finger
Scalenus anterior	Anterior tubercles of transverse processes of C3–C6 vertebrae	Scalene tubercle on the inner border of first rib and ridge on the upper surface of first rib	Cervical nerves of C4–C6	Assists in elevating first rib; laterally flexes and rotates cervical part of the vertebral column	Pectoral region
Trapezius	Medial third of superior nuchal line; external occipital protuberance, ligamentum nuchae, spinous processes of C7–T12 vertebrae, lumbar and sacral spinous processes	Lateral third of clavicle, acromion, and spine of scapula	Spinal root of accessory nerve (XI) and C3 and C4	Scapula is elevated by superior fibers, retracted by middle fibers, and depressed by inferior fibers Superior and inferior fibers act together in superior rotation of scapula	*Upper fibers:* posterolaterally along neck, behind ear to temple *Lower fibers:* posterior side of neck and adjacent mastoid area; suprascapular and interscapular region
Levator scapulae	Posterior tubercles of transverse processes of C1–C4	Superior part of medial border of scapula	Dorsal scapular nerve (C5) and cervical plexus (C3–C4)	Elevates scapula and tilts its glenoid cavity inferiorly by rotating scapula	Concentrates in angle of neck and along vertebral border of scapula
Supraspinatus	Supraspinous fossa of scapula	Superior facet on greater tubercle of humerus	Suprascapular nerve (C4, C5, and C6)	Helps deltoid muscle abduct arm and acts with rotator cuff muscles	Mid-deltoid region; may extend down the arm, lateral epicondyle, and wrist

(Continued)

TABLE 10-3 MAJOR PAIN PATTERNS FROM TRIGGER POINTS OF THE NECK, SHOULDER, AND UPPER LIMB—CONT'D

Muscle	Origin (Proximal or Medial Attachment)	Insertion (Distal or Lateral Attachment)	Innervation	Main Function	Patterns of Referred Pain from Trigger Points of the Muscle
Infraspinatus	Infraspinous fossa of scapula	Middle facet on greater tubercle of humerus	Suprascapular nerve (C5 and C6)	Laterally rotates arm; helps hold humeral head in glenoid cavity of scapula	Deeply in anterior deltoid and shoulder joint; down the front and lateral aspect of arm and forearm; suboccipital and posterior cervical areas
Subscapularis	Subscapular fossa	Lesser tubercle of humerus	Upper and lower subscapular nerves (C5, C6, and C7)	Medially rotates and adducts arm; helps hold humeral head in glenoid cavity	Posterior deltoid area, medially over scapula, down posterior arm, wrist
Deltoid	Lateral third of clavicle, acromion and spine of scapula	Deltoid tuberosity of humerus	Axillary nerve (C5 and C6)	*Anterior fibers:* flexes and medially rotates arm *Middle fibers:* abducts arm *Posterior fibers:* extends and laterally rotates arm	Local region of affected deltoid muscle
Pectoral					
Pectoralis major	*Clavicular head:* anterior surface of the medial half of clavicle *Sternocostal head:* anterior surface of sternum, superior six costal cartilages, and aponeurosis of external oblique muscle	Lateral lip of intertubercular groove of humerus	Lateral and medial pectoral nerves *Clavicle head:* C5 and C6 *Sternocostal head:* C7, C8, and T1	Adducts and medially rotates humerus *Acting alone:* clavicular head flexes humerus; sternocostal head extends humerus	Anterior chest and breast, down ulnar aspect of arm to fourth and fifth fingers
Pectoralis minor	Ribs 3 to 5 near their costal cartilages	Medial border and superior surface of coracoid process of scapula	Medial pectoral nerve (C8 and T1)	Stabilizes scapula by drawing it inferiorly and anteriorly against thoracic wall	Front chest, front shoulder, down the ulnar side of arm, forearm, and fingers

TABLE 10-4 MAJOR PAIN PATTERNS FROM TRIGGER POINTS OF LOWER LIMB MUSCLES

Muscle	Origin (Proximal or Medial Attachment)	Insertion (Distal or Lateral Attachment)	Innervation	Main Function	Patterns of Referred Pain from Trigger Points of the Muscle
Gluteus maximus	External surface of ala of ilium, iliac crest, dorsal surface of sacrum and coccyx, and sacrotuberous ligament	Most fibers end in iliotibial tract; some fibers insert on gluteal tuberosity of femur	Inferior gluteal nerve (L5, S1, and S2)	Extends thigh and assists in its lateral rotation; steadies thigh and assists in raising trunk from flexed position	Medial, lateral, and inferior buttock
Gluteus medius	Lateral surface of ilium between anterior and posterior gluteus lines	Lateral surface of greater trochanter of femur	Superior gluteal nerve (L5 and S1)	Abducts and medially rotates thigh; steadies pelvis	Along the posterior crest of ilium, to sacrum, to posterior and lateral buttock, and to upper thigh
Gluteus minimus	Lateral surface of ilium between anterior and inferior gluteus lines	Anterior surface of greater trochanter of femur	Superior gluteal nerve (L5 and S1)	Abducts and medially rotates thigh; steadies pelvis	*Anterior fibers:* lower lateral buttock; down the lateral thigh, knee, and leg to the ankle. *Posterior fibers:* similar as for anterior fibers, but a more posterior or medial pattern
Piriformis	Anterior surface of sacrum and sacrotuberous ligament	Superior border of greater trochanter of femur	Branches from ventral rami of S1 and S2	Laterally rotates extended thigh and abducts flexed thigh; steadies femoral head in acetabulum	Sacroiliac region, posterior hip region, proximal two thirds of posterior thigh
Vastus lateralis	Greater trochanter and lateral lip of linea aspera of femur	Base of patella and, via patella ligament, to tibial tuberosity	Femoral nerve (L2, L3, and L4)	Extends leg at knee joint	Along lateral thigh from pelvis and greater trochanter to lateral knee region
Vastus medialis	Intertrochanteric line and medial lip of linea aspera of femur	Base of patella and, via patella ligament, to tibial tuberosity	Femoral nerve (L2, L3, and L4)	Extends leg at knee joint	Anteromedial aspect of knee; upper anteromedial aspect of thigh

(Continued)

TABLE 10-4 MAJOR PAIN PATTERNS FROM TRIGGER POINTS OF LOWER LIMB MUSCLES—CONT'D

Muscle	Origin (Proximal or Medial Attachment)	Insertion (Distal or Lateral Attachment)	Innervation	Main Function	Patterns of Referred Pain from Trigger Points of the Muscle
Vastus intermedius	Anterior and lateral surfaces of body of femur	Base of patella and, via patella ligament, to tibial tuberosity	Femoral nerve (L2, L3, and L4)	Extends leg at knee joint	Middle portion of anterior thigh
Biceps femoris	*Long head:* ischial tuberosity *Short head:* lateral lip of linea aspera and lateral supracondylar line	Lateral side of head of fibula; tendon is split at this site by fibular collateral ligament of knee joint	*Long head:* tibial division of sciatic nerve (L5, S1, and S2) *Short head:* common fibular division of sciatic nerve (L5, S1, and S2)	Flexes and rotates leg laterally; long head extends thigh	Back of the knee, may extend to up posterolateral area of thigh and up to the lower buttock
Gastrocnemius	*Lateral head:* lateral aspect of lateral condyle of femur *Medial head:* popliteal surface of femur, superior to medial condyle	Posterior surface of calcaneus via tendo calcaneus	Tibial nerve (S1 and S2)	Plantarflexes foot, raises heel during walking, and flexes knee joint	Over posterior ankle, calf, and back of knee and up to posterior thigh and midbelly of the muscle
Soleus	Posterior aspect of head of fibula; superior fourth of posterior surface of fibula; soleal line; and medial border of tibia	Posterior surface of calcaneus via tendo calcaneus	Tibial nerve (S1 and S2)	Plantarflexes foot and steadies leg on foot	Posterior and plantar surfaces of heel; over back of calf; distal Achilles tendon; sacroiliac joint
Fibularis (Peroneus) longus	Head and superior two thirds of lateral surface of tibia	Base of first metatarsal bone and medial cuneiform bone	Superficial fibular (peroneal) nerve (L5, S1, and S2)	Everts and weakly plantarflexes foot	Above, below, and posterior to the lateral malleolus
Extensor digitorum longus (Fig. 10-17)	Lateral condyle of tibia, superior three fourths of anterior surface of fibula, and interosseous membrane	Middle and distal phalanges of lateral four digits	Deep fibular (peroneal) nerve (L5 and S1)	Extends lateral four digits and dorsiflexes foot	On the muscle proper, dorsolateral aspect of foot, to the tips of middle three toes
Tibialis anterior	Lateral condyle and superior half of lateral surface of tibia	Medial and inferior surface of medial cuneiform bone and base of first metatarsal bone	Deep fibular (peroneal) nerve (L4 and L5)	Dorsiflexes and inverts foot	Anteromedial aspect of ankle and on the dorsal and medial surfaces of great toe

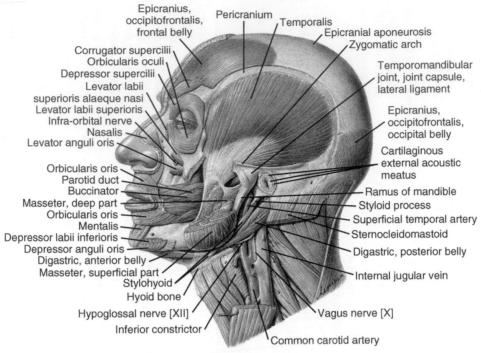

Epicranius, occipitofrontalis, frontal belly
Pericranium
Temporalis
Epicranial aponeurosis
Zygomatic arch
Corrugator supercilii
Orbicularis oculi
Depressor supercilii
Levator labii superioris alaeque nasi
Levator labii superioris
Infra-orbital nerve
Nasalis
Levator anguli oris
Temporomandibular joint, joint capsule, lateral ligament
Epicranius, occipitofrontalis, occipital belly
Cartilaginous external acoustic meatus
Orbicularis oris
Parotid duct
Buccinator
Masseter, deep part
Orbicularis oris
Mentalis
Depressor labii inferioris
Depressor anguli oris
Digastric, anterior belly
Masseter, superficial part
Stylohyoid
Hyoid bone
Ramus of mandible
Styloid process
Superficial temporal artery
Sternocleidomastoid
Digastric, posterior belly
Internal jugular vein
Hypoglossal nerve [XII]
Inferior constrictor
Vagus nerve [X]
Common carotid artery

FIGURE 10-2 Facial and masticatory muscles. Facial trigger points usually develop in these muscles.

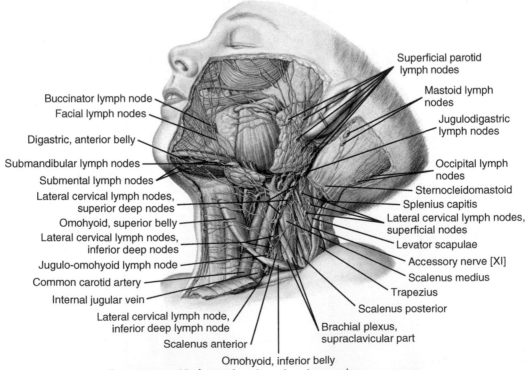

Superficial parotid lymph nodes
Mastoid lymph nodes
Jugulodigastric lymph nodes
Buccinator lymph node
Facial lymph nodes
Digastric, anterior belly
Submandibular lymph nodes
Submental lymph nodes
Lateral cervical lymph nodes, superior deep nodes
Omohyoid, superior belly
Lateral cervical lymph nodes, inferior deep nodes
Jugulo-omohyoid lymph node
Common carotid artery
Internal jugular vein
Lateral cervical lymph node, inferior deep lymph node
Scalenus anterior
Omohyoid, inferior belly
Occipital lymph nodes
Sternocleidomastoid
Splenius capitis
Lateral cervical lymph nodes, superficial nodes
Levator scapulae
Accessory nerve [XI]
Scalenus medius
Trapezius
Scalenus posterior
Brachial plexus, supraclavicular part

FIGURE 10-3 Neck muscles where the trigger points may appear.

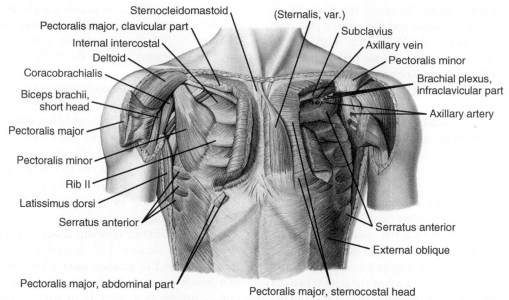

FIGURE 10-4 Muscles of the thorax where the trigger points develop but should be needled with caution.

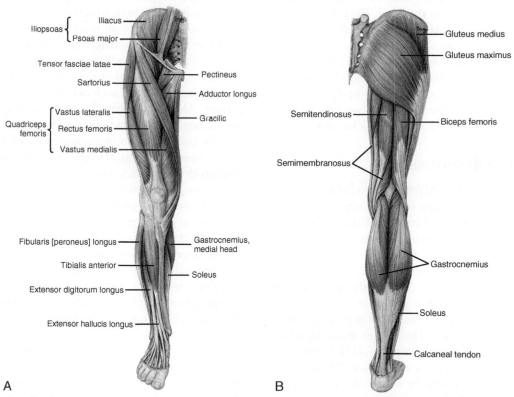

A   B

FIGURE 10-5 Muscles of the lower limb where some of the trigger points hide in deep tissues. **A,** Anterior view. **B,** Posterior view.

restriction of movement. The pain can be referred from the MTrPs to other areas, and the referred pain area may not even include the MTrPs; that is, the patient may feel pain only in the area of the referred pain, not in the MTrPs themselves. The pattern of pain referral is usually consistent for each muscle, and so the location of the relevant MTrPs can easily be determined. The author's primary homeostatic acu-reflex point system provides a road map for locating hidden MTrPs.

PALPATION

Palpation is the clinical technique used to locate MTrPs. A trigger point may be manifested as a taut band of varying size in a flat muscle such as the trapezius, infraspinatus, or rhomboideus muscle. The clinician can draw fingers across the patient's fibers to feel the taut band below the skin. When the taut band is identified, the clinician's thumb and the index finger can be used to gently lift the muscle off the underlying tissue and encircle it so as to find the most sensitive area on the band. The pain reported by the patient can then be reproduced by pressing the sensitive area for a few seconds.

In muscles that are thick, such as the gluteus maximus, or deep, such as the piriformis, the trigger points may not be accessible to palpation. The clinician may use the thumb or two fingertips to press the muscle to locate the sensitive area.

TWITCH RESPONSE

The development of MTrPs leads to tight or painful muscles and can reduce or even completely inhibit the response to neural control of muscle contraction. In athletes, any muscles that are overtrained respond more slowly to neural control, which impairs their physical performance.

Sometimes the tight fibers of the muscles relax suddenly when physical palpation or needling is applied to the sensitive area. This appears as a brief twitch under the skin. This sudden muscular relaxation, the local twitch response (LTR), produces enormous relief of muscular tension. Thus achieving LTR is considered by many clinicians to be a therapeutic goal of the treatment session.

To elicit the LTR, the needle should precisely touch or penetrate the sensitive tissue of the contracture within the muscle. In some muscles, the LTR is immediate. If straightforward needling does not elicit the desired response, the clinician can grasp the needling area with thumb and index finger while manipulating the needle with the other hand. Manipulation can be in a gentle piston-like motion up and down, while the needle is either rotated in alternate directions or withdrawn only as far as the subcutaneous layer and reinserted at a slightly different angle. This last procedure may be more painful than some patients can tolerate.

There are differing opinions about LTR as a therapeutic goal. Because LTR immediately provides enormous relief of tension, some clinicians believe that it is a necessity for healing muscle tightness. Others believe that relief from pain and tension can still be achieved with simple needling, without manipulating and producing LTR. Good clinical results have also been achieved by other needling techniques such as distant needling, scalp needling, and other styles of needling, often without producing noticeable LTR. In addition, the relief of soft tissue pain involves several distinct variables of muscle physiologic conditions, such as contracture, inflammation, blood and lymphatic microcirculation, trophic conditions, tissue adhesion, joint mechanics, and scar tissue. It seems that acute muscular injuries involve mostly fiber contracture and inflammation, whereas chronic muscle problems are affected by all the factors just mentioned. Thus the LTR does provide enormous and immediate relief for acute muscle pain, but it takes more time to achieve noticeable relief for chronic muscle pain, and the LTR may not be important for every session as long as the needling-induced lesion is made in the sensitive or painful area of the muscle. Patients who do not experience any LTR may nonetheless report relief of their pain a few hours or a day later.

The author believes that both views are based on clinical experience and that more research is therefore needed to illuminate the differences between them. Before clear data are available, however, a practitioner should probably know a variety of needling techniques so as to be able to select the proper technique for a particular condition to achieve the best results.

As described in previous chapters, homeostatic acu-reflex points gradually arise in symmetric, systemic, and predictable patterns. The pattern and sequence of this sensitization is universal in human beings. This universal sensitizing sequence also reflects the particular anatomic features of each homeostatic acu-reflex point. The development of the homeostatic acu-reflex point system is also related to the functional biomechanics of the human musculoskeletal system. For example, most of the 24 primary homeostatic acu-reflex points are related to the mechanical balance of the musculoskeletal core system, including the neck, upper spine, lumbar spine, and hips. These points are also related to visceral homeostasis. Acute muscle injuries or chronic mechanical imbalance sensitize both the primary homeostatic acu-reflex points and newly evolved trigger points. All the sensitized points are symptomatic points, and they arise usually as local and unilateral points.

TREATMENT AND PROGNOSIS

Direct needling into sensitive trigger points or sensitive tissue usually produces fast relief of the contracture of the affected muscle or muscles. In addition to local needling, systemic treatment is recommended according to the Integrative Neuromuscular Acureflex Point System (INMARPS). After a needling session, gentle physical therapy can help retrain the muscles for restoration of physiologic and functional homeostasis.

The prognosis of the treatment depends on both the healing potential of the body and the medical history of the injury. The method of evaluation of the healing potential was introduced in Chapter 9. In healthy patients or those with acute conditions, long-lasting relief can be achieved with a few treatments. Because MTrPs cannot dissipate perma-

nently, they will, in the majority of cases, revert to being latent MTrPs after treatment and may become active again in some months as a result of patient behavior and central sensitization. The author and colleagues have developed vacuum therapy, in which an area of negative pressure is created inside the muscles or around the trigger points. This negative pressure inside the tissue physically stretches the muscle fibers, reduces the adhesion between the tissue layers (micro-explosion), improves the blood and lymphatic microcirculation, and restores the biomechanical balance. Vacuum therapy greatly improves the effects of needling.

References

1. Kellgren JH: Observations on referred pain arising from muscle, *Clin Sci* 3:175–190, 1938.
2. Simons DG: New aspects of myofascial trigger points: etiological and clinical. In Pongratz DE, Mense S, Spaeth M, editors: *Soft tissue pain syndromes, clinical diagnosis and pathogenesis*, Binghamton, NY, 2004, Haworth Press, pp 15–21.
3. Hong CZ: Lidocaine injection versus dry needling to myofascial trigger point: the importance of the local twitch response, *Am J Med Rehabil* 73:256–263, 1994.
4. Jaeger B, Skootsky SA: Double blind, controlled study of different myofascial trigger point injection techniques [Abstract], *Pain* 4(Suppl):S292, 1987.
5. Mense S, Simons DG, Russel IJ: *Muscle pain: its nature, diagnosis, and treatment*, Philadelphia, 2001, Lippincott Williams & Wilkins.
6. Shah JP, Phillips T, Danoff J, et al: Novel microanalytical technique distinguishes three clinically distinct groups: (1) subjects without pain and without a myofascial trigger point; (2) subjects without pain with a myofascial trigger point; (3) subjects with pain and a myofascial trigger point [Abstract], *Am J Phys Med Rehabil* 83:231, 2004.
7. Lewit K: Incidence and possible role of myofascial trigger points in migraine [Abstract], *J Musculoskel Pain* 12(Suppl 9):31, 2004.
8. Akuthota V, Nadler SR: Core strengthening, *Arch Phys Med Rehabil* 85(Suppl 1):S86–S92, 2004.
9. Heiderscheit B, Sherry M: What effect do core strength and stability have on injury prevention and recovery? In MacAuley D, Best T, editors: *Evidence-based sports medicine*, London, 2007, Blackwell, pp 59–72.
10. Travell JG, Simons DG: *Myofascial pain and dysfunction: the trigger point manual* (vol 1), ed 2, Baltimore, 1999, Williams & Wilkins, p 5.

CHAPTER 11

Visceral Pain and Visceral-Somatic Reflexes

The purpose of this chapter is to describe the basic concepts of visceral pain and the referred hyperalgesia zones on the body surface, in order to enable clinicians to learn the pathophysiologic connection between surface acu-reflex points and visceral pathologic processes.

The homeostasis of a musculoskeletal system is always affected by both mechanical behavior and visceral pathophysiologic processes. Therefore restoration of visceral homeostasis is always a part of restoration of systemic homeostasis.

Visceral pain creates acu-reflex points on the skeletal muscles and joints, which impairs the musculoskeletal balance both in sports and in daily life. It is always necessary to balance visceral physiologic activities when musculoskeletal imbalance is treated.

Visceral pain is common clinically, but only since the 1990s have practitioners been able to improve the understanding of the qualities and mechanisms of this type of pain. Visceral pain is very different from somatic pain. A typical example is cancer pain: its pathologic processes and symptoms may not be correlated, and this complexity makes early diagnosis difficult.

Healthy visceral organs rarely give rise to conscious sensation. When diseased or inflamed, however, they become a source of overwhelming sensation that can monopolize conscious attention. Both visceral and somatic pain produce emotional responses, but visceral pain produces stronger emotional responses that may seem out of proportion to the perceived intensity of the pain. For example, nausea appears more commonly with visceral pain than with somatic pain. Sweating, dyspnea, and other autonomic responses can be extreme with some types of visceral pain, such as angina. Very extensive inflammation (as in ulcerative colitis) or tissue damage (as in gastric perforation) may produce little or no pain in some individuals, while barely discernible disease may produce intolerable pain in others.

Current research reveals these features of visceral pain[1]:
- It is diffuse and poorly localized.
- It is not linked to visceral injury.
- It is referred to other locations.
- It is accompanied by strong motor and autonomic reflexes.

These features are discussed briefly, but the focus of this chapter is on the referred hyperalgesia zones of major viscera.

DIFFUSE SPATIAL LOCALIZATION

A prominent clinical feature of visceral pain is that its clinical localization is unreliable. Visceral pain is deep and diffuse, and often the only localization possible comes with physical examination that stimulates the painful organs. Visceral pain projects sensation to the skeletal muscles on the body surface, but it may be felt in different areas at the same time or may migrate throughout a region even though the pathologic process is confined to a single organ. Unless highly recurrent, visceral pain is not normally perceived as localized to the organ itself; rather, it is perceived as emanating from somatic structures that receive afferent inputs at the same spinal segments as the afferent entry of the relevant viscera, as well as those that receive nonsegmental distribution. For this reason, visceral pain is classically described as being referred, and secondary somatic hyperalgesia, or referred hyperalgesia, may be present at skeletal muscles or joints.

UNCERTAINTY OF VISCERAL PATHOLOGIC PROCESSES

Some disorders, such as chronic pancreatitis, have definable pathology. Others, such as irritable bowel syndrome, noncardiac chest pain, and postcholecystectomy syndrome, appear to have no histopathologic basis for the discomfort and pain. The pain may be related to visceral inflammation or scar tissue that is not revealed by laboratory tests.

UNCERTAINTY OF TEMPORAL CORRELATION

During clinical examination, it was found that stimuli, noxious or otherwise, may be poorly correlated temporally with pain sensation. For example, in the case of esophageal stimulus, a sustained, relatively high intensity of sensation is perceived even after termination of the distending esophageal stimulus. Accordingly, hypersensitivity to natural visceral stimuli may be associated with discomfort and pain even in the absence of obvious visceral disease.[2] Tissue inflammation may be initiated after tissue injury.

REFERRED HYPERALGESIA

Hyperalgesia of a somatic area that is referred from diseased or inflamed viscera is a common clinical observation. It is particularly noticeable in conditions in which visceral pain occurs intermittently (e.g., dysmenorrhea), inasmuch as the referred hyperalgesia often continues during the pain-free periods. Patients report the experience of "tenderness" in the referral zone. Referred hyperalgesia has been quantified in patients with a variety of different visceral pain states and has also been measured in animal models of visceral pain.[3,4] Referred hyperalgesia is more pronounced in subcutaneous tissues than in the skin and, in most cases, is directly related to the duration and intensity of episodes of visceral pain.[5] The referral zone may also manifest trophic changes such as an increase in the thickness of the subcutaneous tissues and a reduction in muscle volume, which have been localized ipsilateral to painful organs.[6]

PERIPHERAL ORGANIZATION OF VISCERAL AFFERENT FIBERS

Sensation begins with the activation of receptors on the peripheral terminals of primary afferent nerve fibers. Visceral primary afferent fibers differ significantly from somatic primary afferent fibers in both number and pattern of distribution. Visceroreceptive afferent fibers are diffusely organized into web-like plexuses rather than forming distinct peripheral nerve entities. Afferent fibers with endings in a specific visceral site may have cell bodies in the dorsal root ganglia of 10 or more spinal levels in a bilaterally distributed manner. In contrast, somatic pain afferent fibers arise from a limited number of unilateral dorsal root ganglia. Individual visceroreceptive afferent fibers have been demonstrated to branch within the spinal cord and to spread over multiple spinal segments. Quantitative examination has revealed that spinal dorsal horn neurons with visceral inputs have multiple, convergent inputs from other viscera, from joints, from muscles, and from cutaneous structures. Together, these results suggest that visceral primary inputs are imprecisely organized, which would be consistent with imprecise localization by the central nervous system (CNS).

The clinical features of the referred hyperalgesia show that the referred zones from the diseased viscera form symptomatic acu-reflex points with more predictable zones of localization on the body surface (see "Referred or Reflex Zones of Major Viscera" section).

PRIMARY VISCERAL SENSORY AFFERENT FIBERS

Two types of polymodal visceral sensory receptors have been described in association with some viscera: low-threshold (about 75% to 80% of the afferent fibers) and high-threshold (about 20% to 25%) mechanoreceptors.

The low-threshold mechanoreceptors respond to mechanical stimuli in a physiologic range around, for example, distension of 5 mm Hg, whereas high-threshold receptors respond to a noxious intensity (60 to 80 mm Hg). These two types of receptors also respond to chemical and thermal stimuli; thus they are also chemonociceptive receptors. Accordingly, both low- and high-threshold mechanoreceptors can be activated and respond to chemical stimuli such as bradykinin, prostaglandins, and a group of inflammatory mediators.

CENTRAL TERMINATIONS
OF VISCERAL AFFERENT FIBERS

Most visceral sensory input to the CNS is not perceived consciously (Fig. 11-1). For example, much of the gastrointestinal vagal afferent input is associated with mucosal endings that sample the luminal contents and with secretory and motor events that do not reach conscious appreciation.

The cell bodies of vagal afferent fibers are in nodose ganglia, and the central terminals of these fibers are principally in the nucleus of the solitary tract in the dorsal medulla. A small portion of vagal afferent fibers continue either through the medulla or by another nonmedullary route and terminate in the first and second cervical segments of the spinal cord, where they may be involved in modulation of spinal nociceptive processing.[7]

Vagal afferent input to the CNS is not thought to contribute to visceral pain, but mechanosensitive vagal afferent fibers are sensitized when exposed to thermal or chemical stimuli such as hydrochloric acid, bile salts, or nerve growth factors, and these fibers may contribute to chemonociceptive input to the CNS. For example, intragastric instillation of hydrochloric acid leads to the expression of c-fos protein in the brainstem and stimulates visceromotor response to dilute the hydrochloric acid, whereas vagotomy blocks this visceromotor response.[8,9]

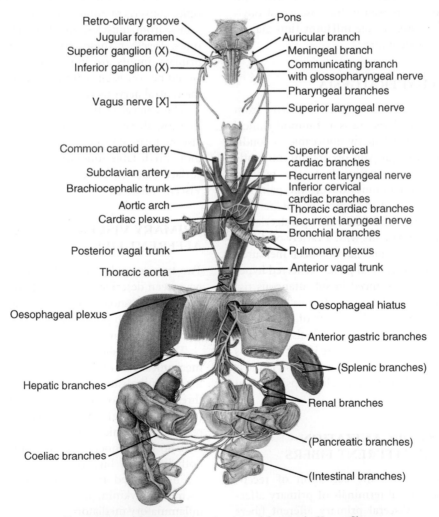

FIGURE 11-1 The central termination of the vagal afferent fiber.

The cell bodies of spinal visceral afferent fibers are in dorsal root ganglia, and the central terminals of these fibers are in laminae I and II, the superficial dorsal horn of the spinal cord, the intermediolateral cell column and sacral parasympathetic nucleus (pelvic nerve), and the lamina X (dorsal to the central canal) (see Fig. 11-1). Almost all second-order neurons in the spinal cord that receive visceral input also receive convergent somatic input from skin and muscle. This is considered the basis of referral of visceral sensation to somatic sensation. For example, a patient with myocardial ischemia feels pain in the left shoulder and upper arm and occasionally in the jaw, but not in the heart, the source of the pain. In addition to the convergence of somatic and visceral inputs on second-order spinal neurons, this kind of convergence is also common between, for example, bladder and colon and between colon and uterus.

In view of the physiologic activity of visceral afferent fibers, the diffuse character of visceral innervation and sensation, referral to somatic sites, and convergence of inputs from multiple viscera to the same spinal neurons, visceral pain is more challenging, both to patients and to physicians, than somatic pain.

In the past, it was demonstrated that the primary pathway for pain-related information from the dorsal horn of the spinal cord to the brain was via the anterolateral quadrant white matter of the spinal cord, within which are the spinothalamic, spinoreticular, spinomesencephalic, and spinohypothalamic tracts. More recent research demonstrated that a dorsal column pathway is also involved in visceral afferent inputs.[10]

Functional imaging during visceral stimulation has revealed consistency in the response from the brain. Rectal distension and urinary bladder distension both produce increased blood flow in select areas of the thalamus, hypothalamus, mesencephalon, pons, and medulla (Fig. 11-2).[11] Cortical responses include the anterior and midcingulate cortices, the frontal and parietal cortices, and the cerebellum.[12]

INTERACTIONS BETWEEN VISCERAL AND SOMATIC REFLEXES

Practitioners' knowledge of how needling acu-reflex points can induce balance in visceral physiology is developing fast, and this improved understanding of

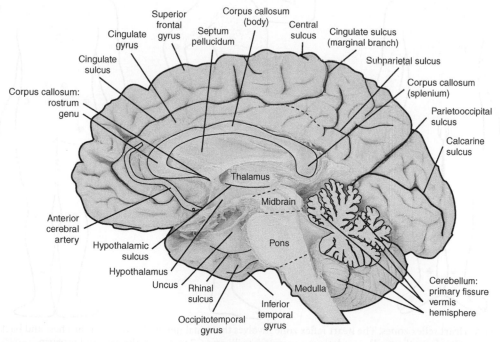

Figure 11-2 Median section of the brain to show the connection between the brain and some of the viscera (see text).

the interaction between reflex systems improves clinical practice. During electroacupuncture, low-frequency, low-intensity somatic afferent stimulation produces long-lasting reduction in blood pressure—increased by visceral afferent fibers—by as much as 40%.[13]

Acupuncture stimulates group III and IV somatic afferent fibers that provide input to both spinal and supraspinal centers in the CNS, as discussed in previous chapters. During acupuncture, polysynaptic input to the ventral hypothalamic arcuate nucleus, midbrain ventrolateral periaqueductal gray, and midline medullary (raphe) nuclei causes prolonged inhibition of sympathoexcitatory cardiovascular premotor neuronal activity and sympathetic outflow in the rostral ventrolateral medulla. Visceral afferent fiber–induced activity in bulbospinal glutaminergic neurons of the rostral ventrolateral medulla is inhibited by modulatory neuropeptides, including enkephalins and endorphins, nociceptin, and gamma-aminobutyric acid (GABA), released during low-level somatic stimulation.

These somatic visceral interactions have the capability of ultimately lowering elevated blood pressure and reducing demand-inducing myocardial ischemia.

REFERRED OR REFLEX ZONES OF MAJOR VISCERA

Most of the data from Chinese acupuncture literature on reflex zones are empirical, and further research is needed to confirm and refine these zones. In general, for the viscera that are anatomically above the diaphragm, such as the heart and lungs, acu-reflex points are projected to the upper part of the body and upper limbs (Figs. 11-3 and 11-4). For the viscera below the diaphragm, such as intestines or urogenital organs, acu-reflex points are projected to the lower part of body and lower limbs (Figs. 11-5 to 11-8). For an organ situated just level with the diaphragm, such as the stomach,

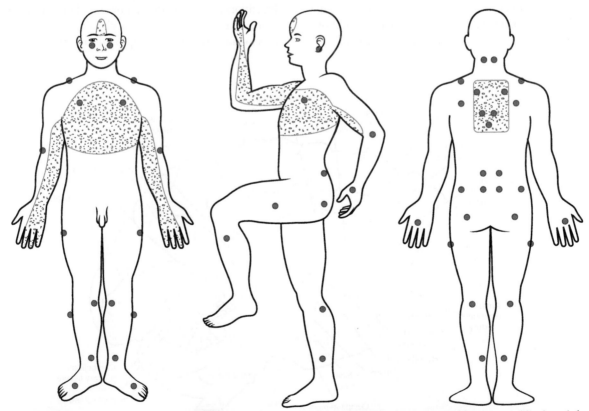

FIGURE 11-3 Heart reflex zones. The heart reflex zone involves the spinal nerves T1 to T7 on the chest and back and the cutaneous branches from the median and ulnar nerves (C5 to T1 and C7 to T1) on the arm and forearm.

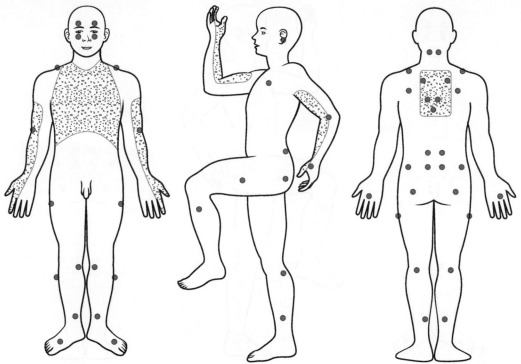

FIGURE 11-4 Lung reflex zones. The lung reflex zone involves the spinal nerves T1 to T7 on the chest and back, the musculocutaneous nerve, and its branches (C4 or C5 to C7).

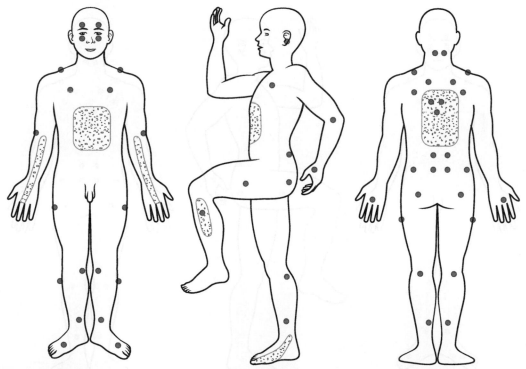

FIGURE 11-5 Stomach reflex zones. The stomach reflex zone involves the spinal nerves T3 to T5 or T6 on the front and T3 to T12 on the back and the medial cutaneous nerves (C5 to T1) on the arm and forearm.

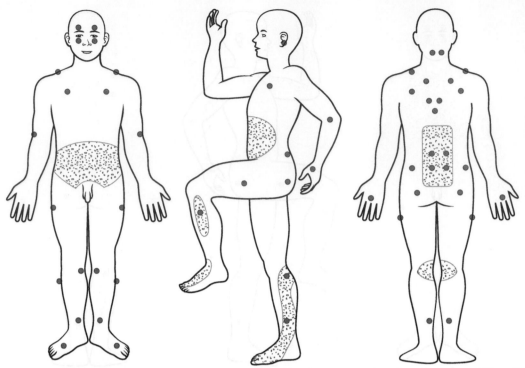

FIGURE 11-6 Intestine reflex zones. The small and large intestine reflex zone involves the spinal nerves T10 to S2 or S3 on the abdominal region and on the lower back, the iliohypogastric nerve (T12 to L1), the saphenous nerve (a branch from the femoral nerve [L1 or L2 to L4]), and the common fibular nerve (L4 to S2).

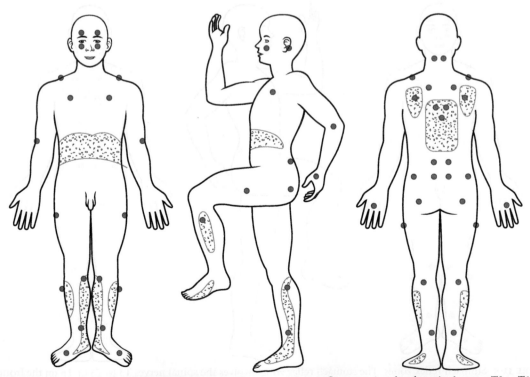

FIGURE 11-7 Liver, gall bladder, spleen, and pancreas reflex zones. These reflex zones involve the spinal nerves T3 to T12, the suprascapular nerve (C4 to C6), the saphenous nerve (L1 or L2 to L4), and the common fibular nerve (L4 to S2). The organs usually project reflex zones ipsilaterally; for example, the liver projects reflex zones only to the right side of the body.

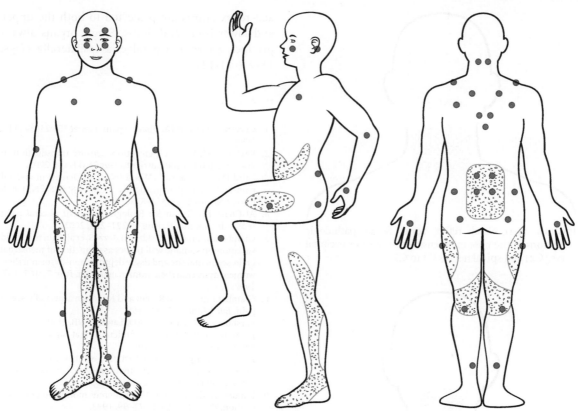

FIGURE 11-8 Urogenital reflex zones. This reflex zone involves the spinal nerves T10 to S2 or S3 on the back and T10 to L1 on the abdomen, the saphenous nerve (L1 or L2 to L4), and the sciatic nerve (L4 to S3).

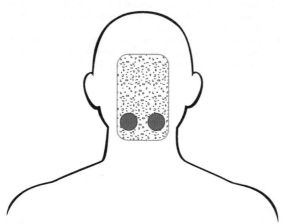

FIGURE 11-9 Optic reflex zone. Some pathologic conditions of the eyes may sensitize the greater occipital nerve (C2).

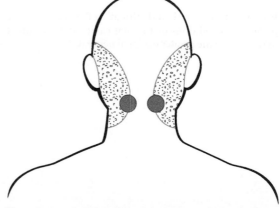

FIGURE 11-10 Otic reflex zone. Some pathologic conditions of the ears may sensitize the lesser occipital nerve (C2 to C3) and the greater auricular nerve (C2 to C3).

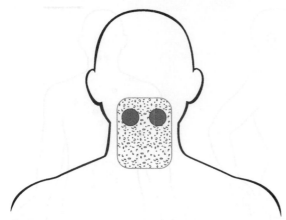

FIGURE **11-11** Nasal reflex zone. Some pathologic conditions of the nose may sensitize the greater occipital nerve (C2) and spinal nerves C3 to C7.

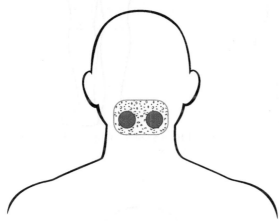

FIGURE **11-12** Oral and throat reflex zone. Some pathologic conditions of the oral cavity and the throat may sensitize the greater occipital nerve (C2).

acu-reflex points are projected to both the upper and lower body and limbs. Single organs always produce referred hyperalgesia ipsilaterally (Figs. 11-9 to 11-12).

References

1. Cervero F, Laird JMA: Visceral pain, *Lancet* 353:2145–2148, 1999.
2. Raybould H: Visceral perception: sensory transduction in visceral afferents and nutrients, *Gut* 51:i11–i14, 2002.
3. Laird JMA, Souslova V, Wood JN, et al: Deficits in visceral pain and referred hyperalgesia in Nav1.8(SNS/PN3) null mice, *J Neurosci* 22:8352–8356, 2002.
4. Al-Chaer ED, Traub RJ: Biological basis of visceral pain: recent developments, *Pain* 96:221–225, 2002.
5. Giamberardino MA, Berkley KJ, Iezzi S, et al: Pain threshold variations in somatic wall tissues as a function of menstrual cycle, segmental site and tissue depth in non-dysmenorrheic women, dysmenorrheic women and men, *Pain* 71:187–197, 1997.
6. Giamberardino MA: Recent and forgotten aspect of visceral pain, *Eur J Pain* 3:77–92, 1999.
7. Hirshberg RM, Al-Chaer ED, Lawand NB, et al: Is there a pathway in the posterior funiculus that signals visceral pain? *Pain* 67:291–305, 1996.
8. Lamb K, Kang Y-M, Gebhart GF, et al: Gastric inflammation triggers hypersensitivity to acid in awake rats, *Gastroenterology* 125:1410–1418, 2003.
9. Randich A, Gebhart GF: Vagal afferent modulation of nociception, *Brain Res Rev* 17:77–99, 1992.
10. Nauta HJW, Soukup VM, Fabian RH, et al: Punctate midline myelotomy for the relief of cancer pain, *J Neurosurg* 92:125–130, 2000.
11. Blok BFM: Central pathways controlling micturition and urinary continence, *Urology* 59:13–17, 2002.
12. Athwal BS, Berkley KJ, Hussain I, et al: Brain responses to changes in bladder volume and urge to void in healthy men, *Brain* 124:369–377, 2001.
13. Longhurst J: Acupuncture. In Robertson D, Low P, Burnstock G, et al: *Primer on the autonomic nervous system*, New York, 2004, Academic Press, pp 246–249.

CHAPTER 12

Pathomechanics of the Musculoskeletal System and Acu-Reflex Points

A clinician involved in rehabilitation treats patients with various disorders, and the goals of intervention include restoring normal function of the musculo-skeletal system or improving the patient's ability to move. For treatment of movement disorders to be effective in both athletes and other patients, the practitioner must understand the functional mechanisms of the movement and how the pathomechanics or imbalance of musculoskeletal system should be corrected. The essential factors that govern the movement of a structure are the composition of the structure and the forces applied to it. This chapter describes the basic functional anatomy and musculoskeletal mechanisms that are relevant to both athletic and daily activities. The physics involved in the biomechanics of musculoskeletal systems is omitted in this chapter, but readers are encouraged to learn and apply a physics-based understanding of human movement when treating patients, especially athletes.

In view of the unique mechanisms and effectiveness of dry needling therapy for soft tissue dysfunction and musculoskeletal pathomechanics, readers should keep in mind that all the muscles described in this chapter are very important in both examination and in treatment for improving movement or restoring normal function. The acu-reflex points often appear in the muscle bellies, neuromuscular attachments, and junction areas of origin and insertion. For visual convenience, the potential acu-reflex points are not labeled in the figures, but readers should know their locations.

To make the description concise, exact, and helpful for clinicians, a brief review of the musculoskeletal system (Fig. 12-1) is provided in the following section. Readers should compare the descriptions with the figures in this chapter.

FUNCTIONAL ANATOMY AND PATHOMECHANICS OF THE LOWER LIMB

The Hip

The hip is a very important joint in athletics. The muscles responsible for moving the hip joint originate from the pelvis and spinal column. Some of them pass over the knee joint. The hip bone has developed from three separate centers of ossification, which give rise to three bones: the ilium, ischium, and pubis. All the cavities, outgrowths, and spines have a specific musculoskeletal function. The most important bony marks are the iliac crest, anterior superior iliac spine, anterior inferior iliac spine, ischial tuberosity, and acetabulum.

The hip joint is a ball-and-socket joint. Certain extracapsular structures give strength to the joint and, in particular, prevent the leg from swinging outward and backward. Backward swinging is impeded by the powerful iliofemoral ligament, which is attached to the iliac part of the hip bone and passes downward to the femur. Outward swinging is restricted by the pubofemoral ligament (Fig. 12-2).

The major hip movements are abduction, adduction, flexion, extension, and medial and lateral rotation. The most important muscles that pass over the hip joint are described in the following sections. The anatomy and function of those muscles should be well understood because they are often involved in both local and systemic dysfunction of the musculoskeletal system in human movement. The muscles responsible for hip movements are listed in Table 12-1 for review and further discussion (Figs. 12-3 and 12-4).

The Hip Flexor Muscles

The iliac and psoas major muscles are responsible for powerful flexion at the hip joint. They have different points of origin but a common insertion point. When the iliopsoas muscle contracts, a flexion movement between the trunk and the legs can occur: If the legs are fixed, the trunk will move towards them, as in the last phase of a sit-up; if the trunk is fixed, the legs will move towards it, as when a person is hanging from a bar and bringing the knees up toward the chest. The iliopsoas is by far the most powerful hip flexor. It is forcefully engaged in hurdling, high jump, running, javelin throwing, and sit-ups. The enormous stress on this muscle is often overlooked.

The Hip Abductor Muscles

Two of the abductor muscles are attached to the greater trochanter. The gluteus medius and gluteus minimus have such a large area of origin that they can move the femur in all directions except adduction. These muscles are activated during walking and running. They serve to stabilize the hip joint when the corresponding foot alone is in contact with the ground. This stabilization is necessary in order to prevent the upper body from falling to the opposite side during walking. From the perspective of human mechanics and kinesiology, the hip abductor muscles together sustain about 1.5 to 2 times body weight to maintain the balance of single-limb stance. Meanwhile, the

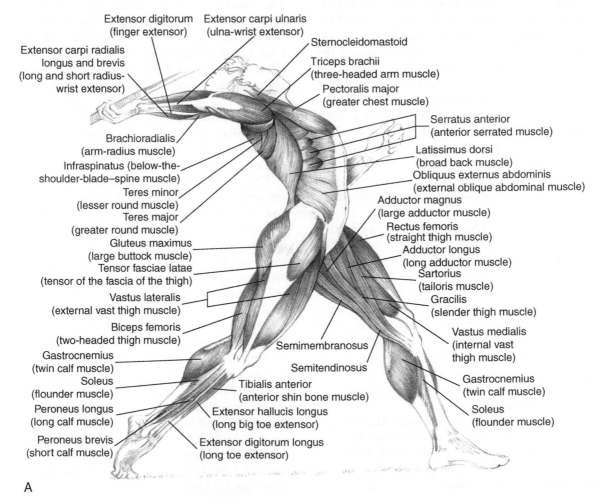

A

FIGURE 12-1 Review of skeletal muscles.

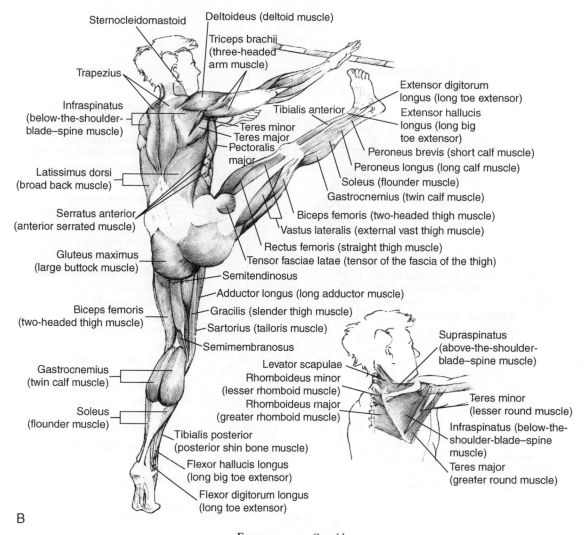

Sternocleidomastoid

Deltoideus (deltoid muscle)

Triceps brachii (three-headed arm muscle)

Trapezius

Infraspinatus (below-the-shoulder-blade–spine muscle)

Tibialis anterior

Extensor digitorum longus (long toe extensor)

Extensor hallucis longus (long big toe extensor)

Teres minor
Teres major
Pectoralis major

Peroneus brevis (short calf muscle)

Peroneus longus (long calf muscle)

Soleus (flounder muscle)

Gastrocnemius (twin calf muscle)

Latissimus dorsi (broad back muscle)

Serratus anterior (anterior serrated muscle)

Biceps femoris (two-headed thigh muscle)

Vastus lateralis (external vast thigh muscle)

Rectus femoris (straight thigh muscle)

Gluteus maximus (large buttock muscle)

Tensor fasciae latae (tensor of the fascia of the thigh)

Semitendinosus

Adductor longus (long adductor muscle)

Biceps femoris (two-headed thigh muscle)

Gracilis (slender thigh muscle)

Sartorius (tailoris muscle)

Semimembranosus

Levator scapulae

Rhomboideus minor (lesser rhomboid muscle)

Rhomboideus major (greater rhomboid muscle)

Supraspinatus (above-the-shoulder-blade–spine muscle)

Teres minor (lesser round muscle)

Infraspinatus (below-the-shoulder-blade–spine muscle)

Teres major (greater round muscle)

Gastrocnemius (twin calf muscle)

Soleus (flounder muscle)

Tibialis posterior (posterior shin bone muscle)

Flexor hallucis longus (long big toe extensor)

Flexor digitorum longus (long toe extensor)

B

FIGURE 12-1—Cont'd.

joint force on the head of the femur is about 2.5 times body weight.

The hip abductor muscles are subjected to great stress when a person runs uphill or downhill. During uphill running, the gluteus maximus is responsible for the powerful backward drive of the leg, which is necessary to raise the center of gravity. During downhill running, the gluteus medius and gluteus minimus stabilize the hip to control deceleration. The gluteus medius and gluteus minimus work eccentrically to restrain the upper body so that it does not fold medially at every step.

The gluteus maximus is used to swing the leg backward powerfully, and it can help straighten the knee. A part of the muscle is attached to the surface of the femur (at the gluteal tuberosity), which straightens the hip, and a part is inserted into a very strong, thick tendon, the iliotibial tract. This tendon band passes in front of the axis of motion of the knee and is inserted into the lateral tibial condyle. If the body is bent forward at the hip, the gluteus maximus can work with greater force because the distance between its origin and insertion becomes greater. Swinging the leg backwards

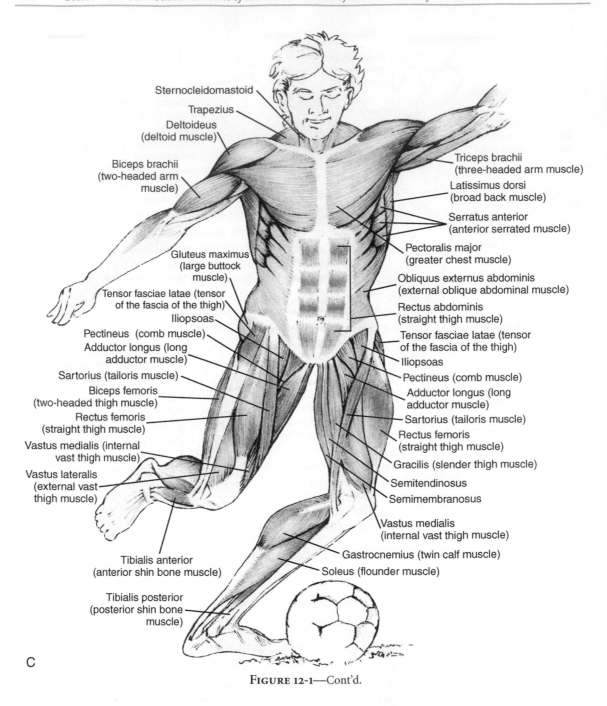

Sternocleidomastoid

Trapezius

Deltoideus
(deltoid muscle)

Biceps brachii
(two-headed arm
muscle)

Gluteus maximus
(large buttock
muscle)

Tensor fasciae latae (tensor
of the fascia of the thigh)

Iliopsoas

Pectineus (comb muscle)

Adductor longus (long
adductor muscle)

Sartorius (tailoris muscle)

Biceps femoris
(two-headed thigh muscle)

Rectus femoris
(straight thigh muscle)

Vastus medialis (internal
vast thigh muscle)

Vastus lateralis
(external vast
thigh muscle)

Tibialis anterior
(anterior shin bone muscle)

Tibialis posterior
(posterior shin bone
muscle)

Triceps brachii
(three-headed arm muscle)

Latissimus dorsi
(broad back muscle)

Serratus anterior
(anterior serrated muscle)

Pectoralis major
(greater chest muscle)

Obliquus externus abdominis
(external oblique abdominal muscle)

Rectus abdominis
(straight thigh muscle)

Tensor fasciae latae (tensor
of the fascia of the thigh)

Iliopsoas

Pectineus (comb muscle)

Adductor longus (long
adductor muscle)

Sartorius (tailoris muscle)

Rectus femoris
(straight thigh muscle)

Gracilis (slender thigh muscle)

Semitendinosus

Semimembranosus

Vastus medialis
(internal vast thigh muscle)

Gastrocnemius (twin calf muscle)

Soleus (flounder muscle)

C

FIGURE 12-1—Cont'd.

(hip extension) is performed by the muscles that originate from the ischial tuberosity, as well as by the gluteus maximus. All these muscles are inserted into the lower leg, which means that they flex the knee joint.

The Hip Adductor Muscles

These adductor muscles swing the leg medially. All these muscles originate mainly from the pubis and are inserted into the posterior surface of the femur via the roughened ridge that extends along

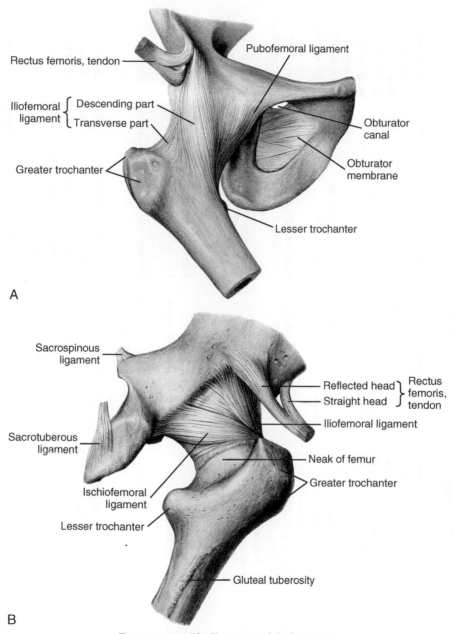

FIGURE 12-2 The ligaments of the hip joint.

the length of its shaft, the linea aspera. These muscles work powerfully when, in running, the foot leaves the ground and begins to swing forward. During the forward swing, the leg rotates laterally in relation to the hip. This can be accomplished because the adductor muscles are inserted into the

posterior surface of the femur. Overexertion that occurs in forceful movements such as wide sideways kicking in soccer, bringing the free leg forward in skating, or tough sprint training leads to groin injuries, causing discomfort in the muscle's area of origin.

TABLE 12–1 THE MAIN MUSCLES PRODUCING HIP MOVEMENT

Function	Muscles	Proximal Attachment	Distal Attachment	Innervation	Action
Flexors	Iliopsoas				
	Psoas major	Transverse processes, bodies and intervertebral discs of T12 and L1–L5 vertebrae	Lesser trochanter of femur	Ventral rami of lumbar nerves (L1–L3)	Acts jointly in flexing thigh at hip joint; stabilizes hip joint
	Iliacus	Iliac crest, iliac fossa, ala of sacrum, anterior sacroiliac ligaments	Inferior to lesser trochanter of femur	Femoral nerve (L2–L3)	Acts jointly in flexing thigh at hip joint; stabilizes hip joint
Abductors	Gluteus medius	External surface of ilium between anterior and posterior gluteal lines	Lateral surface of greater trochanter of femur	Superior gluteal nerve (L5 and S1)	Abducts and medially rotates thigh; stabilizes pelvis
	Gluteus minimus	External surface of ilium between anterior and inferior gluteal lines	Anterior surface of greater trochanter of femur	Superior gluteal nerve (L5 and S1)	Abducts and medially rotates thigh; stabilizes pelvis
	Gluteus maximus	See extensors	See extensors	See extensors	Abducts and adducts hip depending on which muscle fibers are activated
Adductors	Pectineus	Pectineal line of pubis	Pectineal line of femur	Femoral nerve (L2 and L3)	Adducts and flexes thigh
	Adductor longus	Body of pubis, inferior to pubic crest	Middle third of linea aspera of femur	Obturator nerve (L2–L4)	Adducts thigh
	Adductor brevis	Body and inferior ramus of pubis	Pectineal line and proximal part of linea aspera of femur	Obturator nerve (L2–L4)	Adducts thigh
	Adductor magnus	Inferior ramus of pubis, ramus of ischium (adductor part) and ischial tuberosity	Gluteal tuberosity, linea aspera medial, supracondylar line (adductor part), and adductor tubercle of femur (hamstring part)	*Adductor part:* obturator n. (L2 – L4); *Hamstring part:* tibial portion of sciatic nerve (L4)	Adducts thigh; adductor part flexes thigh; hamstring part extends thigh
Extensors	Gluteus maximus	External surface of ala of ilium, iliac crest, dorsal surface of sacrum and coccyx, sacrotuberous ligament	Upper fibers end in iliotibial tract inserting into lateral condyle of tibia; lower fibers insert on gluteal tuberosity of femur	Inferior gluteal nerve (L5, S1, and S2)	Extends thigh and helps lateral rotation; stabilizes thigh and helps extension of trunk

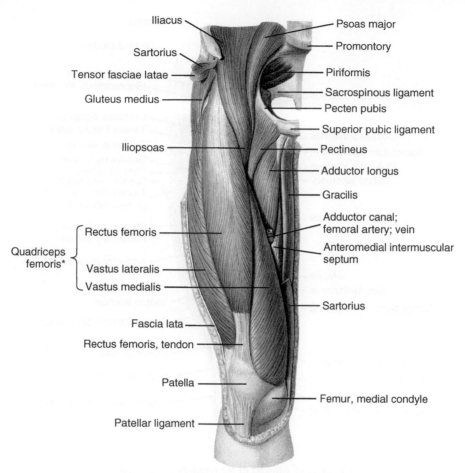

Iliacus

Sartorius

Tensor fasciae latae

Gluteus medius

Iliopsoas

Rectus femoris

Quadriceps femoris*

Vastus lateralis

Vastus medialis

Fascia lata

Rectus femoris, tendon

Patella

Patellar ligament

Psoas major

Promontory

Piriformis

Sacrospinous ligament

Pecten pubis

Superior pubic ligament

Pectineus

Adductor longus

Gracilis

Adductor canal; femoral artery; vein

Anteromedial intermuscular septum

Sartorius

Femur, medial condyle

FIGURE 12-3 Muscles of the thigh, anterior view.

Lateral rotation is accomplished by a number of small muscles that originate from the inner parts of the pelvis. They pass behind the femur and are inserted into its outer surface at the greater trochanter. They are used a great deal in activities such as ice-skating.

The Knee Joint

The very complicated knee joint is composed of the distal femur, proximal tibia, and patella. Although the fibula does not participate directly in the mechanics of the knee joint, some muscles that cross the knee attach to the fibula. The movements produced at the knee joint are flexing (bending), extending (straightening), and medial and lateral rotation of the lower leg in relation to the thigh.

The lateral rotation movement can occur when the knee is bent. The more the knee is bent, the easier it is to rotate the lower leg and the foot. During flexion, the femur rolls back on the tibia and then glides on the same spot on the tibia. The rolling movement continues until the anterior cruciate ligament is completely stretched, after which movement of gliding is initiated.

The anterior cruciate ligament thus prevents movement when the lower leg is moved forward in relation to the thigh. A common injury in soccer is rupture of the anterior cruciate ligaments, which can happen when a player's foot is blocked and the lower leg rotates medially. The posterior cruciate ligament is injured when the lower leg is pressed backward or when the knee is severely overstretched.

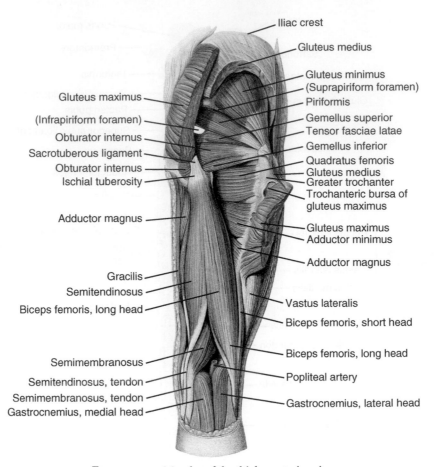

Iliac crest
Gluteus medius
Gluteus minimus
(Suprapiriform foramen)
Piriformis
Gemellus superior
Tensor fasciae latae
Gemellus inferior
Quadratus femoris
Gluteus medius
Greater trochanter
Trochanteric bursa of
gluteus maximus
Gluteus maximus
Adductor minimus
Adductor magnus

Gluteus maximus
(Infrapiriform foramen)
Obturator internus
Sacrotuberous ligament
Obturator internus
Ischial tuberosity

Adductor magnus

Gracilis
Semitendinosus
Biceps femoris, long head

Vastus lateralis
Biceps femoris, short head

Biceps femoris, long head

Semimembranosus
Semitendinosus, tendon
Semimembranosus, tendon
Gastrocnemius, medial head

Popliteal artery

Gastrocnemius, lateral head

FIGURE 12-4 Muscles of the thigh, posterior view.

The function of these two collateral ligaments is to prevent sideways bending of the knee. They are taut when the knee is stretched and slack when the knee is bent. This means, for example, that the lower leg can be rotated laterally until the ligaments are taut again. The lower leg usually cannot rotate as much medially as it can laterally because the cruciate ligaments in the joint twist around each other during medial rotation and thereby block the movement (Fig. 12-5).

The surface of the lower end of the femur is elliptical, and the upper extremity of the tibia is flat. Therefore there would be very little contact between their surfaces if the cartilage were not shaped to receive the end of the femur. The undersides of the menisci are plain, like the surface of the

tibia. As a consequence, the stress to which the knee is subjected can be distributed over a relatively large area. In flexion and extension of the knee joint, the menisci glide to suit the form of the condyles of the femur. Because the medial meniscus fuses with the medial collateral ligament, it is very easily injured by being subjected to excessive stress while in unusual positions.

Injury to the menisci resulting from rotational strain on a bent weight-bearing knee is very common. If there is a sudden pitching in the knee joint during lateral rotation of the lower leg, the medial ligament stretches and can thereby tear the meniscus, which is locked between the femur and tibia. Because of this, movements that strain the medial collateral ligament should be avoided.

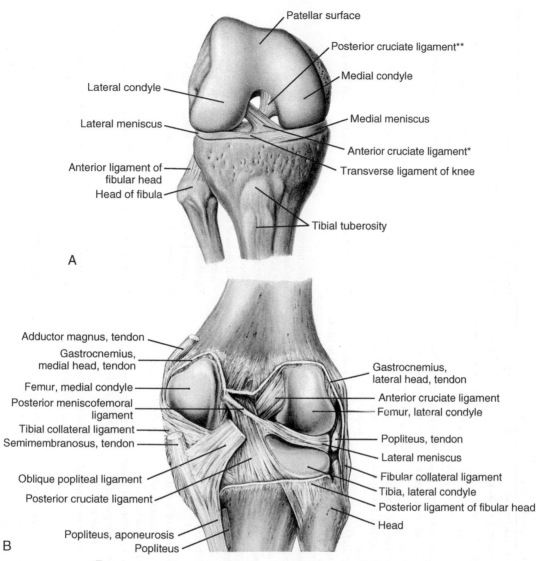

Patellar surface
Posterior cruciate ligament**
Medial condyle
Lateral condyle
Lateral meniscus
Medial meniscus
Anterior cruciate ligament*
Anterior ligament of fibular head
Transverse ligament of knee
Head of fibula
Tibial tuberosity

A

Adductor magnus, tendon
Gastrocnemius, medial head, tendon
Femur, medial condyle
Posterior meniscofemoral ligament
Tibial collateral ligament
Semimembranosus, tendon
Oblique popliteal ligament
Posterior cruciate ligament
Popliteus, aponeurosis
Popliteus

Gastrocnemius, lateral head, tendon
Anterior cruciate ligament
Femur, lateral condyle
Popliteus, tendon
Lateral meniscus
Fibular collateral ligament
Tibia, lateral condyle
Posterior ligament of fibular head
Head

B

Figure 12-5 Ligaments of the knee. **A,** Anterior view. **B,** Posterior view.

Muscles of the Knee Joint*

The Knee Extensor Muscles. The rectus femoris originates from the pelvis and flexes (bends) the hip joint. It is inserted into the patella and can straighten the knee with the help of the powerful tendon that extends from the patella to the tibia. Three other large extensor muscles, the vastus muscles, are inserted into the knee joint.

The Knee Flexor Muscles: The Hamstrings. All three hamstring muscles originate from the ischial tuberosity and run toward the knee. The biceps femoris muscle is inserted into the head of the fibula. It can rotate the lower leg so that the foot points laterally. The semitendinosus and semimembranosus muscles are inserted into the medial tibial condyle and can rotate the lower leg medially. The distance between the origin and insertion of these hip extensors and knee flexors varies greatly, depending on the angle of the hip and knee joint. Shortened hamstring muscles at the back of the thigh result in

*See Table 12-2.

TABLE 12-2   THE MAIN MUSCLES PRODUCING KNEE MOVEMENT

Function	Muscle	Proximal Attachment	Distal Attachment	Innervation	Action
Extensors	Rectus femoris	Anterior superior iliac spine and groove superior to acetabulum	Base of patella and via patella ligament to tibial tuberosity	Femoral nerve (L2–L4)	Extends leg at knee joint; also stabilizes hip joint and helps iliopsoas to flex thigh
	Vastus lateralis	Greater trochanter and lateral lip of linea aspera of femur	Base of patella and via patella ligament to tibial tuberosity	Femoral nerve (L2–L4)	Extends leg at knee joint
	Vastus medialis	Intertrochanteric line and medial lip of linea aspera of femur	Base of patella and via patella ligament to tibial tuberosity	Femoral nerve (L2–L4)	Extends leg at knee joint
	Vastus intermedius	Anterior and lateral surfaces of femur	Base of patella and via patella ligament to tibial tuberosity	Femoral nerve (L2–L4)	Extends leg at knee joint
Flexors	Biceps femoris	*Long head:* ischial tuberosity *Short head:* lateral lip of linea aspera and lateral supracondylar line	Lateral head of fibula; tendon is split at this site by fibular collateral ligament of knee joint	Sciatic nerve *Long head:* tibial division (L5–S2) *Short head:* common fibular division (L5–S2)	Flexes and rotates leg laterally; long head extends the thigh
	Semitendinosus	Ischial tuberosity	Medial surface of superior part of tibia	Tibial division of sciatic nerve (L5–S2)	Extends thigh; flexes and rotates leg medially
	Semimembranosus	Ischial tuberosity	Posterior part of medial condyle of tibia	Tibial division of sciatic nerve (L5–S2)	Extends thigh; flexes and rotates leg medially
	Popliteus	Lateral surface of lateral condyle of femur and lateral meniscus	Posterior surface of tibia, superior to soleal line	Tibial nerve (L4–S1)	Weakly flexes knee
Medial rotators	Sartorius	Anterior superior iliac spine and superior part of notch inferior to it	Superior part of medial surface of tibia	Femoral nerve (L2–L3)	Flexes, abducts, and laterally rotates thigh at hip joint
	Gracilis	Body and inferior ramus of pubis	Superior part of medial surface of tibia	Obturator nerve (L2 and L3)	Adducts thigh, flexes leg, and helps rotate leg medially
Lateral rotator	Tensor fasciae latae	Anterior superior iliac spine and anterior part of external lip of iliac crest	Superior part of medial surface of tibia	Superior gluteal nerve (L4–L5)	Abducts, medially rotates, and flexes thigh; helps keep knee extended; stabilizes trunk on thigh

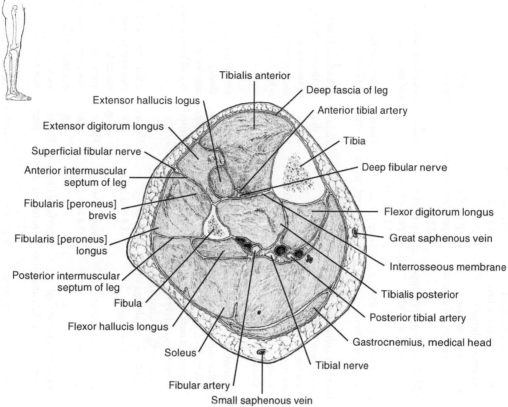

Tibialis anterior
Deep fascia of leg
Extensor hallucis logus
Anterior tibial artery
Extensor digitorum longus
Tibia
Superficial fibular nerve
Deep fibular nerve
Anterior intermuscular septum of leg
Flexor digitorum longus
Fibularis [peroneus] brevis
Great saphenous vein
Fibularis [peroneus] longus
Interrosseous membrane
Posterior intermuscular septum of leg
Tibialis posterior
Fibula
Posterior tibial artery
Flexor hallucis longus
Gastrocnemius, medical head
Soleus
Tibial nerve
Fibular artery
Small saphenous vein

FIGURE 12-6 Three compartments of the leg.

a stationary hip. When a person is unable to tip the pelvis forward, he or she will try to compensate for this by bending forward at the lumbar spine. Many back problems in athletes and other patients are caused by shortened hamstring muscles.

The Lower Leg and Foot

The musculature of the lower leg is arranged anatomically and functionally in three compartments (Fig. 12-6): anterior (extensor), lateral (fibular or peroneal), and posterior (flexor). The compartments are separated by fascial septa. The anterior compartment contains four flexor muscles. The lateral compartment includes two muscles. The posterior or flexor compartment contains muscles that are arranged in superficial and deep groups (Table 12-3). It is very important for practitioners to understand the structure of the compartments when treating compartment syndrome.

A muscle group that is very important for jumping and running is the triceps surae. This muscle has three parts: the gastrocnemius, with its two heads of origin (one from each of the femoral condyles), and the soleus. Together these three parts converge into the Achilles tendon, which is inserted into the calcaneus. The gastrocnemius flexes both the knee and the ankle so that the body can be raised on its toes (plantar flexion). The soleus muscle acts only on the ankle joint.

The Foot

A common problem, found in athletes and in other patients, is that when the calf muscle becomes tight and shortened, the foot tends to assume a position with downward-pointing toes. The muscles that hold the foot up—the foot flexors situated at the front of the lower leg between the tibia and fibula—are thus forced to work with constantly raised tension (tone)

TABLE 12-3	THE MAIN MUSCLES PRODUCING MOVEMENT OF THE ANKLE JOINT			
Function	Muscle	Proximal Attachment	Distal Attachment	Innervation	Action
Dorsiflexors	Anterior tibialis	Lateral condyle and superior half of the lateral surface of tibia	Medial and inferior surface of medial cuneiform bone and base of first metatarsal bone	Deep fibular (peroneal) nerve (L4 and L5)	Dorsiflexes and inverts foot
	Extensor hallucis longus	Middle part of anterior surface of fibula and interosseous membrane	Dorsal aspect of base of distal phalanx of great toe (hallux)	Deep fibular (peroneal) nerve (L5 and S1)	Extends great toe and dorsiflexes foot
	Extensor digitorum longus	Lateral condyle of tibia, superior three fourths of anterior surface of fibula, and interosseous membrane	Middle and distal phalanges of lateral four digits	Deep fibular (peroneal) nerve (L5 and S1)	Extends lateral four digits and dorsiflexes foot
	Fibularis (peroneus) tertius	Inferior third of anterior surface of fibular and interosseous membrane	Dorsum of base of fifth metatarsal bone	Deep fibular (peroneal) nerve (L5 and S1)	Dorsiflexes foot and helps eversion of foot
Superficial muscles of posterior compartment	Gastrocnemius	*Lateral head:* lateral condyle of femur *Medial head:* popliteal surface of femur, superior to medial condyle	Posterior surface of calcaneus via tendo calcaneus	Tibial nerve (S1 and S2)	Plantarflexes foot; raises heel during walking and during flexion of knee joint
	Soleus	Posterior head of fibula, superior fourth of posterior surface of fibula, soleal line, and medial border of tibia	Posterior surface of calcaneus via tendo calcaneus	Tibial nerve (S1 and S2)	Plantarflexes foot and stabilizes leg on foot
	Plantaris	Inferior end of lateral supracondylar line of femur and oblique popliteal ligament	Posterior surface of calcaneus via tendo calcaneus	Tibial nerve (S1 and S2)	Assists gastrocnemius in plantar flexing foot and flexing knee joint
Deep muscles of posterior compartment	Posterior tibialis	Interosseous membrane, posterior surface of tibia inferior to soleal line, posterior surface of fibula	Tuberosity of navicular, cuneiform, and cuboid bones and fourth metatarsal bone	Tibial nerve (L4 and L5)	Plantarflexes and inverts foot
	Flexor digitorum longus	Medial part of posterior surface of tibia, inferior to soleal line, and by a broad aponeurosis to tibia	Base of distal phalanges of lateral four digits	Tibial nerve (L4 and L5)	Flexes lateral four digits and plantarflexes foot; supports longitudinal arch of foot
	Flexor hallucis longus	Inferior two thirds of posterior surface of fibula and inferior part of interosseous membrane	Base of distal phalanx of great toe	Tibial nerve (L4 and L5)	Flexes great toe at all joints and plantarflexes foot; supports longitudinal arch of foot
Muscles of lateral compartment	Fibularis (peroneus) longus	Head and superior two thirds of lateral surface of fibula	Base of first metatarsal bone and medial cuneiform bone	Superficial fibular (peroneal) nerve (L5, S1, and S2)	Everts and weakly plantarflexes foot
	Fibularis (peroneus) brevis	Inferior two-thirds of lateral surface of fibula	Dorsal surface of tuberosity on lateral side of base of fifth metatarsal bone	Superficial fibular (peroneal) nerve (L5, S1, and S2)	Everts and weakly plantarflexes foot

in order to hold the foot in its normal position. Such tension may lie behind the pain that is experienced in the lower leg when an athlete trains too much in one session or runs on hard surfaces.

The foot can move along two axes: mediolateral for flexion and extension and anteroposterior for pronation and supination. Extension and flexion take place between the talus and both the tibia and the fibula at the ankle joint. Supination and pronation take place between the talus and both the navicular bone and the calcaneus at the subtalar joint. Supination and pronation take place simultaneously between several articulating surfaces that together form the subtalar joints. Movements of the ankle and subtalar joints are independent of each other. If the muscles that

control these two joints are unable to prevent movements that are too great or too sudden, the joint is still protected by the ligaments of the foot.

The ankle ligaments arise from the prominent lower ends of the tibia and fibula (the malleoli) and spread out down toward the articulating ankle bones. Thus the medial ligament of the ankle, the deltoid ligament (Fig. 12-7), arises from the medial malleolus of the tibia and is inserted into the calcaneus, talus, and navicular bones.

Three separate ligaments make up the lateral ligament. They all arise from the lateral malleolus of the fibula. One ligament extends forward and is inserted into the talus, the second passes downward to be attached to the calcaneus, and the third

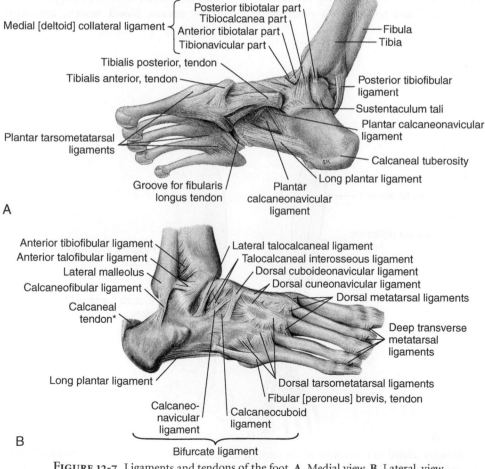

FIGURE 12-7 Ligaments and tendons of the foot. **A**, Medial view. **B**, Lateral, view.

extends backwards toward the posterior part of the talus. The origin of the deltoid (medial) ligament corresponds to the axis of motion of the ankle joint; thus it is always taut. The origin of the lateral ligament is situated below the axis of motion; thus its posterior part is taut when the foot points upward (dorsiflexion) and the anterior part is taut when the ankle is stretched (plantar flexion). When injured, the ligament is either partially ruptured or completely torn. In many cases, the ligament remains intact, but the malleolus is broken off.

Muscles of the Foot. Nine muscles control the major movement of the foot at two axes: mediolateral (flexion and extension) and anteroposterior (pronation and supination). The most important flexor is the triceps surae, although its movement is assisted by other muscles. The most important extensors are at the front of the leg between the tibia and fibula. Their tendons can easily be palpated on the top of the foot at the base of the tibia. Pronation is brought about by the two muscles whose tendons can be felt beneath the lateral malleolus of the tibia. Supination is produced mainly by the three muscles whose tendons pass behind and beneath the medial malleolus of the tibia (Fig. 12-8 and Table 12-3).

The Arches of the Foot. The articulated foot exhibits three distinct arches: a medial and a lateral longitudinal arch and a transverse arch. The medial longitudinal arch is formed by the calcaneus, talus, navicular, medial cuneiform, and first metatarsal bone. The lateral longitudinal arch consists of the calcaneus, cuboid, and fifth metatarsal bone (Fig. 12-9).

The transverse arch includes the cuboid and cuneiform bones and continues at the bases of the metatarsals.

The arches serve several purposes: They protect the nerves, blood vessels, and muscles on

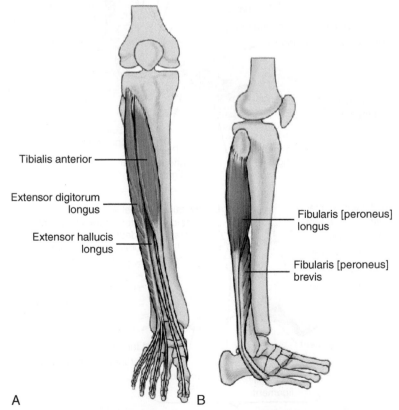

Tibialis anterior

Extensor digitorum
longus

Extensor hallucis
longus

Fibularis [peroneus]
longus

Fibularis [peroneus]
brevis

A   B

FIGURE 12-8. Muscles related to movement of the foot. **A,** Extensor muscles of the leg. **B,** Lateral (fibular) muscles. **C,** Triceps surae muscles. **D,** Deep flexor muscles.

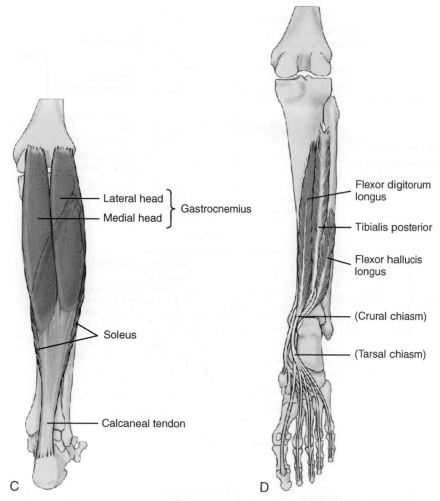

Lateral head
Medial head }
Gastrocnemius

Soleus

Calcaneal tendon

C

Flexor digitorum longus

Tibialis posterior

Flexor hallucis longus

(Crural chiasm)

(Tarsal chiasm)

D

FIGURE 12-8—Cont'd.

the plantar surface of the foot from compression during weight bearing; they help the foot absorb shock during impact with the ground; and they help store mechanical energy and release it to improve the efficiency of locomotion. Integrity of the arches depends primarily on ligamentous support, in addition to bone alignment and support from extrinsic muscles of the foot. The middle and lateral cuneiform bones are shaped and positioned to play the role of keystone in the transverse arch. Their wedge shape, wider dorsally than on their plantar surface, helps prevent their descent through the arch.

The plantar fascia, the long and short plantar ligaments, the spring ligament, the collateral liga-ments of the ankle, and the interosseous ligament of the subtalar joint all contribute important soft tissue support to the arches of the foot (Fig. 12-10). Research indicates that support of the arches depends on several structures; no single structure provides primary support.[1-3]

Abnormalities in arches in runners are associated with different injury patterns[4]: Runners with high arches report more ankle and bony injuries,[5] and those with low arches report more knee and soft tissue injuries. Deformed arches resulting from disruptions of the supporting ligaments and from weak and tight muscles lead to direct impairment of the arches.

Subtalar Neutral Position. The concept of the subtalar neutral position helps to illustrate postural

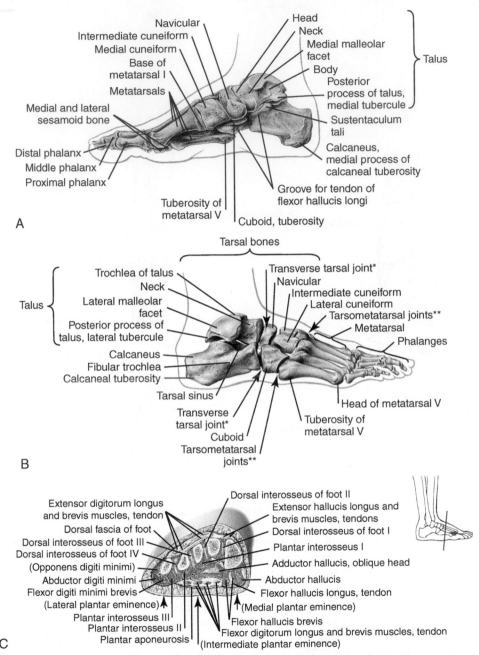

FIGURE 12-9 The three arches of the foot. **A,** Medial longitudinal arch. **B,** Lateral longitudinal arch. **C,** Transverse arch.

compensations in the foot. The neutral position of the subtalar joint is defined as neither pronated nor supinated.[6] Subtalar neutral position appears to maximize the area of contact between the talus and calcaneus. Movements away from the subtalar neutral position into pronation or supination decrease

the contact area.[7] Medial deviation of the calcaneus in relation to the leg constitutes a varus deformity; lateral deviation of the hindfoot on the leg is a valgus deformity (Fig. 12-11).

In upright stance with the tibias approximately vertical, a medially aligned hindfoot (i.e., a hindfoot

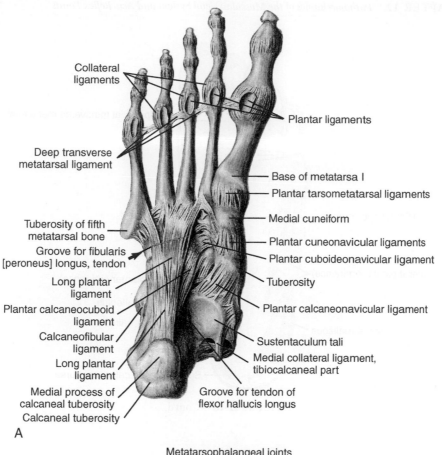

Collateral ligaments

Deep transverse metatarsal ligament

Plantar ligaments

Base of metatarsa I

Plantar tarsometatarsal ligaments

Medial cuneiform

Tuberosity of fifth metatarsal bone

Groove for fibularis [peroneus] longus, tendon

Long plantar ligament

Plantar calcaneocuboid ligament

Calcaneofibular ligament

Long plantar ligament

Medial process of calcaneal tuberosity

Calcaneal tuberosity

Plantar cuneonavicular ligaments

Plantar cuboideonavicular ligament

Tuberosity

Plantar calcaneonavicular ligament

Sustentaculum tali

Medial collateral ligament, tibiocalcaneal part

Groove for tendon of flexor hallucis longus

A

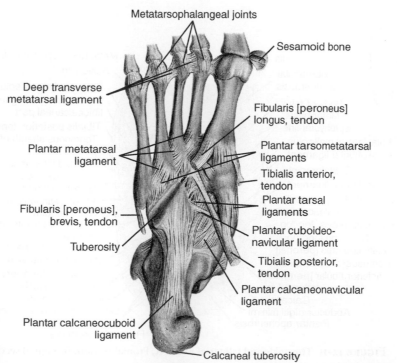

Metatarsophalangeal joints

Sesamoid bone

Deep transverse metatarsal ligament

Fibularis [peroneus] longus, tendon

Plantar metatarsal ligament

Plantar tarsometatarsal ligaments

Tibialis anterior, tendon

Plantar tarsal ligaments

Fibularis [peroneus], brevis, tendon

Tuberosity

Plantar cuboideo-navicular ligament

Tibialis posterior, tendon

Plantar calcaneonavicular ligament

Plantar calcaneocuboid ligament

Calcaneal tuberosity

B

FIGURE 12-10 Ligaments (A), tendons (B), and plantar aponeurosis (C) that support the arches of the foot.

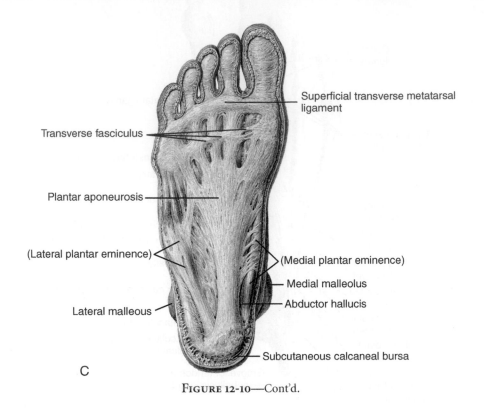

Superficial transverse metatarsal ligament

Transverse fasciculus

Plantar aponeurosis

(Lateral plantar eminence)

Lateral malleous

(Medial plantar eminence)

Medial malleolus

Abductor hallucis

Subcutaneous calcaneal bursa

C

Figure 12-10—Cont'd.

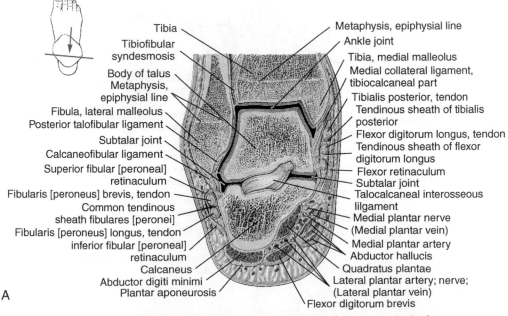

Tibia
Tibiofibular syndesmosis
Body of talus
Metaphysis, epiphysial line
Fibula, lateral malleolus
Posterior talofibular ligament
Subtalar joint
Calcaneofibular ligament
Superior fibular [peroneal] retinaculum
Fibularis [peroneus] brevis, tendon
Common tendinous sheath fibulares [peronei]
Fibularis [peroneus] longus, tendon
inferior fibular [peroneal] retinaculum
Calcaneus
Abductor digiti minimi
Plantar aponeurosis

Metaphysis, epiphysial line
Ankle joint
Tibia, medial malleolus
Medial collateral ligament, tibiocalcaneal part
Tibialis posterior, tendon
Tendinous sheath of tibialis posterior
Flexor digitorum longus, tendon
Tendinous sheath of flexor digitorum longus
Flexor retinaculum
Subtalar joint
Talocalcaneal interosseous liligament
Medial plantar nerve
(Medial plantar vein)
Medial plantar artery
Abductor hallucis
Quadratus plantae
Lateral plantar artery; nerve; (Lateral plantar vein)
Flexor digitorum brevis

A

Figure 12-11 The ankle and talotarsal joints. **A,** Frontal section. **B,** Sagittal section.

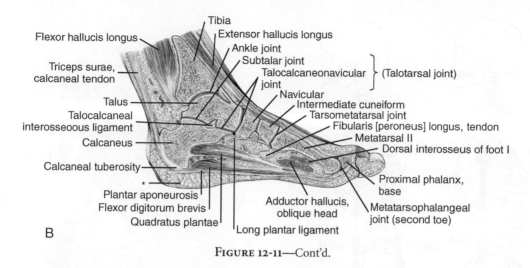

Tibia
Extensor hallucis longus
Ankle joint
Subtalar joint
Talocalcaneonavicular joint } (Talotarsal joint)
Navicular
Intermediate cuneiform
Tarsometatarsal joint
Fibularis [peroneus] longus, tendon
Metatarsal II
Dorsal interosseus of foot I
Proximal phalanx, base
Metatarsophalangeal joint (second toe)

Flexor hallucis longus
Triceps surae, calcaneal tendon
Talus
Talocalcaneal interosseoous ligament
Calcaneus
Calcaneal tuberosity
Plantar aponeurosis
Flexor digitorum brevis
Quadratus plantae
Long plantar ligament
Adductor hallucis, oblique head

B

FIGURE 12-11—Cont'd.

with a varus deformity) must be pronated excessively to contact the ground fully. The greater the varus deformity is, the more pronation is needed to contact the ground. Thus an individual with a varus hindfoot may pronate excessively or for an excessively prolonged period during the gait cycle.[8] Conversely, supination provides compensation for a lateral deviation (valgus deformity) of the hindfoot. Compensatory movements resulting from foot deformities are sources of pain in the foot, knee, thigh, and hip (Tables 12-3, 12-4).

FUNCTIONAL ANATOMY AND BIOMECHANICS OF THE TRUNK

The spinal column and its accessory structures are essentially involved in movements of the limbs. Athletes with back pain, for example, cannot move

the hip, knee, or shoulder quickly and smoothly. Excessive or uneven stress on the spine, or quick movement while in an unfavorable position, often causes back pain in athletes. For nonathletes, back pain is often related to poorly trained muscles of the back and possibly of the legs and abdomen. Behavior-related back pain is often caused by the wear and tear of lifting weights with poor technique or by sitting or working continually in a position in which the body is tilted forward.

When a person is standing, an imaginary line from the center of gravity to the ground passes about 5 cm in front of the center of disc L3. The back muscles are about 5 cm behind this line (Fig. 12-12). For a person weighing 80 kg, about 40 kg is on the center of gravity in front of L3; therefore, the muscle force *(F)* must equal 40 kg × 10 cm, or 400 N (newtons), in order to prevent the upper body from

TABLE 12-4	SUMMARY OF MUSCLES OF THE LOWER LIMB			
Muscles That Pass Across Hip Joint Only	**Muscles That Pass Across Both Hip and Knee Joints**	**Muscles That Pass Across Knee Joint Only**	**Muscles That Pass Across Both Knee Joint and Ankle**	**Muscles That Pass Ankle Only**
Gluteus maximus	Rectus femoris	Vastus medialis	Gastrocnemius	Soleus
Gluteus medius	Gracilis	Vastus intermedius		Tibialis anterior
Gluteus minimus	Tensor fascia latae	Vastus lateralis		Extensor hallucis longus
Pectineus	Biceps femoris	Popliteus		Extensor digitorum longus
Adductor brevis	Semitendinosus			Fibularis (peroneus) longus
Adductor magnus	Semimembranosus			Fibularis (peroneus) brevis
Psoas major	Sartorius			Flexor hallucis longus
Iliacus				Flexor digitorum longus
				Tibialis posterior

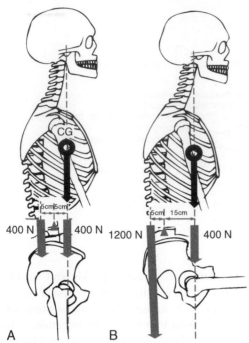

FIGURE 12-12 The lumbar biomechanics during standing (**A**) and sitting (**B**). The *dashed line* crosses the center of gravity (*CG*).

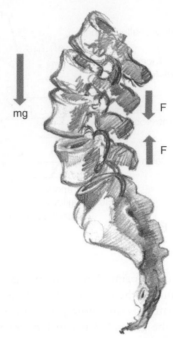

FIGURE 12-13 The disc pressure is the joint effect of the body weight (*mg*) and the muscular contraction forces (*F*).

falling forward. The total force acting on the disc is 400 N + 400 N, or 800 N. Sitting positions produce greater pressure on the disc than standing. When a person sits, the center of gravity is about 15 cm in front of L3, whereas the muscle's lever arm is still 5 cm behind, the same as when standing. Therefore, to maintain equilibrium and keep the body from falling, the back muscles need to exert a force of 1200 N:

$$F_{muscles} \times 5 \text{ cm} = 400 \text{ N} \times 15 \text{ cm}$$

$$F_{muscles} = 1200 \text{ N}$$

The force acting on the disc is 1200 N + 400 N, or 1600 N. Sitting in a chair with back support may reduce the distance of 15 cm, thereby diminishing the pressure on the disc. The back muscles must pull harder (static tension) when the body sits. Pressure on the disc is caused by the body weight (*mg*) acting on the disc from above and by the contraction force (*F*) of the surrounding muscles.

The total compressing force in Figure 12-13 is *mg* + *F*. The disc of a young person can withstand a stress of 800 kg, or 8000 N. The total area of the L3 vertebra in an adult is about 10 cm^2. That means the disc of a young adult can withstand a pressure of 8000 N/10 cm^2, or 800 N/cm^2. An elderly person can withstand half of this pressure.

Low back pain can have many different causes besides those related to tumor or infection. If the annulus fibrosus tears and the nucleus pulposus is pressed backward, the posterior longitudinal ligament, which runs posteriorly along the vertebral bodies, is stretched. When the ligament stretches, pain is produced through its sensory nerve endings. The disc itself harbors very few sensory nerve endings and so may not be the source of pain. This type of pain can be relieved if the patient prevents the back from stretching by avoiding certain activities, such as lifting heavy objects, leaning forward while working, or sitting still. If the nucleus pulposus bulges too far out, it can press against the nerve root, which passes through the intervertebral foramen. Pain is then felt in the muscles that are supplied by this nerve. For the same reason, pain can be felt in the shoulder when a cervical disc is injured. Tense muscles, small vertebra displacements, and worn-down intervertebral cartilage can put pressure on the nerves and cause pain. As another example, if the sciatic nerve is affected, the pain is felt in the leg muscles supplied by this nerve.

Some nerves (e.g., the lumbar plexus) that pass out from the intervertebral foramen and into a muscle can be drawn out a little farther by stretching of the back muscles. This can cause the nerves to be pressed against a protrusion on the disc, producing severe pain in the leg. The Lasègue test is used to confirm sciatica: The patient is placed on the back and lifts the painful leg so that the clinician can determine whether the sciatic nerve is irritated. This type of pain must not be confused with that felt by people with tight hamstrings.

Lifting something heavy and simultaneously twisting the trunk, which happens in shoveling snow, is very dangerous for people who suffer from back complaints because it creates the greatest pressure in the posterior part of the disc, which is not protected by extra ligaments (Fig. 12-14).

In the following example, a person who weighs 80 kg—of which 40 kg lies above the level of L3—lifts a 10-kg object. It is possible to calculate the stresses to which the spinal column is subjected in different postures. Distance is measured in centimeters and force in newtons.

A posture with flexed knees (Fig. 12-15, *A*) is the least stressful position. To do the specified work, the muscles of the back require the force (F_m) as follows:

$$F_m \times 5 \text{ cm} = (40 \text{ kg} + 10 \text{ kg}) \times 20 \text{ cm}$$

$$F_m = 200 \text{ kg} = 2000 \text{ N}$$

A posture with straight knees (see Fig. 12-15, *B*) requires

$$F_m = 300 \text{ kg} = 3000 \text{ N}$$

A posture in sitting position (see Fig. 12-15, *C*) requires

$$F_m = 400 \text{ kg} = 4000 \text{ N}$$

This calculation is purely mechanical. If a person has well-trained abdominal muscles and diaphragm, the mechanical stress of the back muscles can be reduced by about 40%. When lifting a weight, a person can build up pressure in the abdomen by tensing the diaphragm and abdominal muscles (Fig. 12-16), creating an up-and-down motion, which counteracts the tendency for abdominal collapse. The disc, which is a part of the abdominal cavity's back wall, is thus protected. This shows how important it is to have well-trained abdominal muscles, strong leg muscles, and correct posture in order to lift a weight correctly with support for the back. When practitioners consider any exercise that engages the back muscles, they must always account for the stabilizing effect of the abdominal muscles.

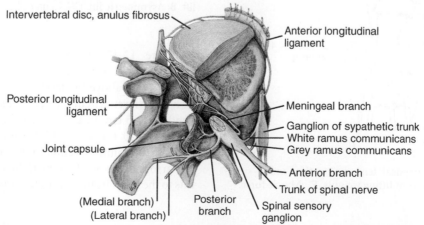

FIGURE 12-14 The nerves of the vertebral column and the posterior longitudinal ligament.

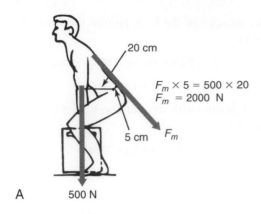

$$F_m \times 5 = 500 \times 20$$
$$F_m = 2000 \ N$$

20 cm

5 cm F_m

A   500 N

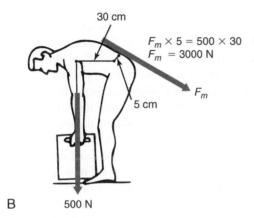

30 cm

$$F_m \times 5 = 500 \times 30$$
$$F_m = 3000 \ N$$

F_m

5 cm

B   500 N

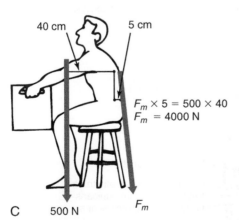

40 cm   5 cm

$$F_m \times 5 = 500 \times 40$$
$$F_m = 4000 \ N$$

C   500 N F_m

FIGURE 12-15 Physical tensions on the lumbar spine with different ways of lifting weights. F_m, Muscle force.

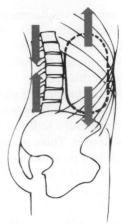

FIGURE 12-16. Well-trained abdominal muscles reduce tension of lumbar muscles.

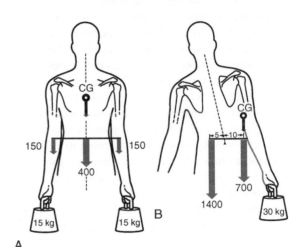

CG

150   150

400

15 kg   15 kg

A

CG

5   10

700

1400   30 kg

B

FIGURE 12-17 Weight-lifting techniques. **A,** Symmetric lift. **B,** Asymmetric lift. *CG*, Center of gravity.

Figure 12-17 shows the difference between symmetric and asymmetric lift. Suppose the body weighs 40 kg above the level of L3 and the load is 30 kg. The lever arm of the back muscles (for lateral bending) is 5 cm. In a symmetric lift, the total load is 700 N (150 + 150 + 400 N). For asymmetric lift, suppose the common center of the body plus load is 10 cm to the side of L3 on the right, even if the body tilts to the left. The back muscles must then contract with a force (F_m) of 1400 N ($F_m \times 5$ cm $= 700$ N $\times$ 10 cm), and so the total load on the disc is 700 N + 1400 N, or 2100 N. It is possible to calculate the forces that are necessary to swing a leg forward during running, jumping, hurdling, and other activities involving the legs and back. The weight and acceleration of the leg may cause the force of muscle contraction to reach about 4000 N. The iliopsoas is the major muscle responsible for this flexion.

Muscles of the Back (Erector Spinae)

From the perspective of functional anatomy, the muscles of the back can be classified into three groups:
1. Long back muscles that pass at least seven vertebrae (Table 12-5 and Fig. 12-18)
2. Back muscles of average length that pass two to six vertebrae (Table 12-6; see Fig. 12-18)
3. Short back muscles that pass only over the nearest vertebra (Table 12-7 and Fig. 12-19)

The muscles work together as a unit (Table 12-8). The most important muscles for turning the trunk are the rotators. A combination of bending and turning is important for all types of throwing.

It is believed that the most common cause of backache is cramp of the short muscles, particularly the rotators. If cramp occurs in one muscle, the muscles surrounding it contract to prevent movements that could tear it. This, in turn, cuts off the blood supply to the area, causing cramp in other muscles. Cramp may result from overexertion, unaccustomed movements, or minor vertebral displacements caused by sudden stress.

Abdominal Muscles

A well-functioning abdominal musculature unloads the back stress during lifting and stabilizes the spinal column, because the abdominal muscles are antagonists to the back muscles. The back muscles are always used during lifting, standing, and sitting. In the majority of people, abdominal muscles are weaker than back muscles. Strong abdominal muscles, hip flexors (iliopsoas, rectus femoris), and back extensors are very important for all sports. There are four abdominal muscles (Table 12-9 and Fig. 12-20).

TABLE 12-5	LONG BACK MUSCLES (INTERMEDIATE LAYER)*			
Erector Spinae	**Origin**	**Insertion**	**Innervation**	**Action**
Iliocostalis (lateral column): iliocostalis lumborum, iliocostalis thoracis. and iliocostalis cervicis	Broad tendons attached inferiorly to posterior iliac crest, posterior sacrum, sacroiliac ligaments, and sacral and inferior lumbar spinous processes	Angles of the ribs	Dorsal rami of spinal nerves of corresponding segments	Side bending and ipsilateral rotation when muscles contract unilaterally Trunk extension when muscles contract bilaterally
Longissimus (intermediate column)	A broad tendon attached inferiorly to posterior iliac crest, posterior sacrum, sacroiliac ligaments, and sacral and inferior lumbar spinous processes	Transverse processes of thoracic and cervical vertebrae and mastoid process of temporal bone	Dorsal rami of spinal nerves of corresponding segments	Side bending and ipsilateral rotation when muscles contract unilaterally Trunk extension when muscles contract bilaterally
Spinalis (medial column): spinalis thoracis, spinalis cervicis, spinalis capitis	Broad tendons attached inferiorly to posterior iliac crest, posterior sacrum, sacroiliac ligaments, and sacral and inferior lumbar spinous processes	Extend from spinous lumbar and thoracic processes	Dorsal rami of spinal nerves of corresponding segments	Side bending and ipsilateral rotation when muscles contract unilaterally Trunk extension when muscles contract bilaterally

*See Figure 12-18.

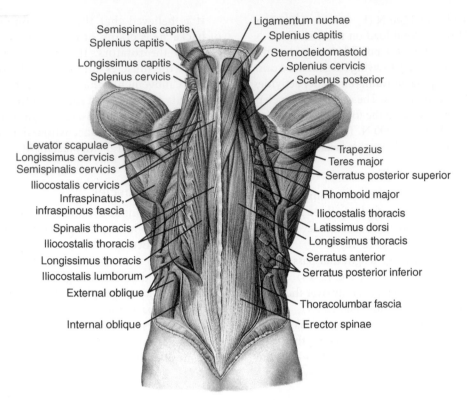

FIGURE 12-18 Muscles of the back.

TABLE 12-6   AVERAGE-LENGTH BACK MUSCLES (DEEP LAYER)

Muscles	Origin	Insertion	Innervation	Action
Semispinalis capitis	Transverse processes of T1–T6	Medial half between superior and inferior nuchal line	Dorsal rami of spinal nerves of corresponding segments	For corresponding region of spine: ipsilateral rotation when muscles contract unilaterally, extension when muscles contract bilaterally
Semispinalis cervicis	Transverse processes of T1–T6	Spinous processes of C2–C5	Dorsal rami of spinal nerves of corresponding segments	For corresponding region of spine: ipsilateral rotation when muscles contract unilaterally, extension when muscles contract bilaterally
Semispinalis thoracis	Transverse processes of thoracic vertebrae	Thoracic spinous processes	Dorsal rami of spinal nerves of corresponding segments	For corresponding region of spine: ipsilateral rotation when muscles contract unilaterally, extension when muscles contract bilaterally
Multifidus	Spinous processes and laminae from S4–C2 vertebrae	Spinous processes spanning one to three vertebrae	Dorsal rami of spinal nerves of corresponding segments	Side bending and ipsilateral rotation when muscles contract unilaterally Trunk extension when muscles contract bilaterally, stabilizing the spinal column

TABLE 12-7	SHORT BACK MUSCLES (DEEPEST LAYER)*			
Muscles	**Origin**	**Insertion**	**Innervation**	**Action**
Intertransversarii	Uniting spinous and transverse processes of consecutive vertebrae		Dorsal rami of spinal nerves of corresponding segments	Laterally flex superior vertebra; help extend vertebral column
Interspinalis	Uniting spinous and transverse processes of consecutive vertebrae		Dorsal rami of spinal nerves of corresponding segments	Help extend vertebral column
Rotatores	Transverse process of vertebra	Base of spinous process of superior vertebra	Dorsal rami of spinal nerves of corresponding segments	Rotate superior vertebra to the opposite side

*See Figure 12-19.

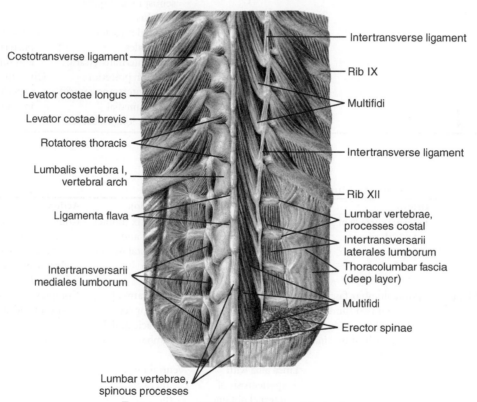

Costotransverse ligament
Levator costae longus
Levator costae brevis
Rotatores thoracis
Lumbalis vertebra I, vertebral arch
Ligamenta flava
Intertransversarii mediales lumborum
Lumbar vertebrae, spinous processes
Intertransverse ligament
Rib IX
Multifidi
Intertransverse ligament
Rib XII
Lumbar vertebrae, processes costal
Intertransversarii laterales lumborum
Thoracolumbar fascia (deep layer)
Multifidi
Erector spinae

FIGURE 12-19 Deep short muscles of the back.

Respiratory Muscles

The diaphragm is the most important muscle of respiration (Fig. 12-21). This muscle arises from the lumbar vertebrae, from the lower ribs, and from the xiphoid process. The diaphragm arches up like a dome into the chest cavity. When the muscle fibers contract, they become less arched and thus cause the central tendinous part of the dome to descend. During contraction, the volume of the chest cavity increases (inspiration) and the volume of the abdominal cavity decreases.

The diaphragm also assists the abdominal muscles in increasing intra-abdominal pressure to reduce stress on the back when a person is lifting

TABLE 12-8   LAYERS AND GROUPS IN THE EXTENSOR MUSCLES OF THE VERTEBRAL COLUMN

Muscle Group	Splenius Muscle	Erector Spinae	Transversospinalis Muscle	Suboccipital Muscle
Superficial layer	Splenius capitis Splenius cervicis	Iliocostalis lumborum, iliocostalis thoracis, iliocostalis cervicis Longissimus thoracis, longissimus cervicis, longissimus capitis Spinalis thoracis, spinalis cervicis, spinalis capitis	—	—
Intermediate layer	—	—	Semispinalis thoracis, semispinalis cervicis, semispinalis capitis Multifidus	—
Deep layer	—	—	Segmental muscles Interspinales Cervical intertransversarii: anterior, posterior Lumbar intertransversarii: lateral, medial Rotatores: longus, brevis	Rectus capitis posterior major and minor Obliquus capitis superior and inferior

TABLE 12-9   ABDOMINAL MUSCLES*

Muscles	Origin	Insertion	Innervation	Action
External oblique	External surface of 5th to 12th ribs	Linea alba, pubic tubercle, and anterior half of iliac crest	Interior six thoracic nerves and subcostal nerves	Compresses abdominal viscera and supports abdominal visceral flexion and rotation of trunk
Internal oblique	Thoracolumbar fascia, anterior two thirds of iliac crest, and lateral half of inguinal ligament	Inferior borders of 10th and 12th ribs, linea alba, and pubis via conjoint tendon	Ventral rami of inferior six thoracic and first lumbar nerves	Compresses abdominal viscera and supports abdominal visceral flexion and rotation of trunk
Transverse abdominis	Internal surfaces of 7th to 12th costal cartilages, thoracolumbar fascia, iliac crest, and lateral third of inguinal ligament	Linea alba with aponeurosis of internal oblique muscle, pubis crest, and pecten pubis via conjoint tendon	Ventral rami of inferior six thoracic and first lumbar nerves	Compresses and supports abdominal viscera
Rectus abdominis	Pubic symphysis and pubic crest	Xiphoid process and fifth to seventh costal cartilages	Ventral rami of inferior six thoracic nerves	Flexes trunk and compresses abdominal viscera

*See Figure 12-20.

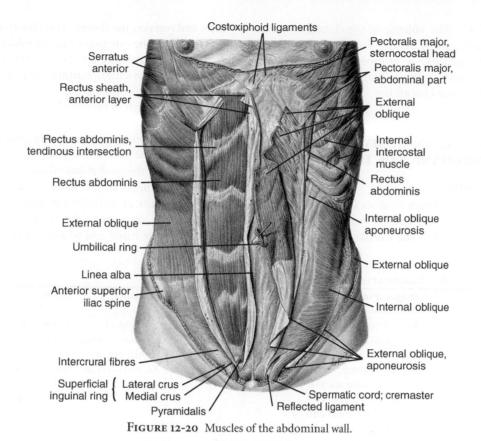

Costoxiphoid ligaments

Serratus anterior

Rectus sheath, anterior layer

Rectus abdominis, tendinous intersection

Rectus abdominis

External oblique

Umbilical ring

Linea alba

Anterior superior iliac spine

Intercrural fibres

Superficial inguinal ring { Lateral crus / Medial crus

Pyramidalis

Pectoralis major, sternocostal head

Pectoralis major, abdominal part

External oblique

Internal intercostal muscle

Rectus abdominis

Internal oblique aponeurosis

External oblique

Internal oblique

External oblique, aponeurosis

Spermatic cord; cremaster

Reflected ligament

FIGURE 12-20 Muscles of the abdominal wall.

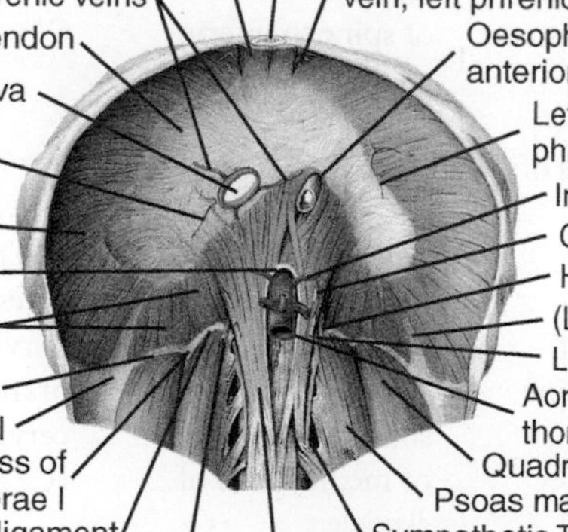

Xlphoid process

Sternal part

Inferior phrenic veins

Central tendon

Caval opening: inferior vena cava

Right phrenic nerve, phrenico-abdominal branch

Costal part

Median arcuate ligament

Lumbar part, right bundle, (lateral part)

Lateral arcuate ligament

Rib XII

Costal process of lumbar vertebrae I

Medial arcuate ligament

Azygos vein

(Sternocostal triangle): internal thoracic artery; vein, left phrenic nerve, phrenico-abdominal branch

Oesophageul hiatus: oesophagus; anterior and posterior vagal trunk

Left phrenic nerve, phrenico-abdominal branch

Inferior phrenic artery

Greater splanchnic nerve

Hemi-azgos vein

(Lumbocostal triangle)

Lesser splanchnic nerve

Aortic hiatus: abdominal aorta; thoracic duct

Quadratus lumborum

Psoas major

Sympathetic Trunk

Lumbalar part, right bundle, (medial part)

FIGURE 12-21 The diaphragm.

heavy objects. The volume of the chest cavity can also be increased by raising the ribs with external intercostal muscles. A number of muscles (e.g., back, chest, neck) may exert an influence on the rib cage during forced breathing.

FUNCTIONAL ANATOMY AND PATHOMECHANICS OF THE UPPER LIMB

The Shoulder

The shoulder complex consists of three bones: the clavicle, the scapula, and the humerus. The complex is connected to the axioskeleton via the ster-num and rests on the thorax. Thus the shape of the thorax affects the function of the shoulder.

The shoulder complex is composed of four joints: sternoclavicular, acromioclavicular, scapulothoracic, and glenohumeral.

The movements of the shoulder can be described as elevation and depression about the anterior-posterior axis, protraction and retraction about the superior-inferior axis, and upward and downward rotation about the medial-lateral axis.

The movements of the shoulder are controlled by three groups of muscles: the axioscapular plus axioclavicular muscles (Table 12-10), whose origins are on the trunk and whose insertions are on

TABLE 12-10 AXIOSCAPULAR AND AXIOCLAVICULAR MUSCLES*				
Muscles	Origin (Proximal Attachment)	Insertion (Distal Attachment)	Innervation	Action
Trapezius	Medial third of superior nuchal line, external occipital protuberance, ligamentum nuchae, spinous processes of C7–T12, lumbar and sacral processes	Lateral third of clavicle, acromion, and spine of scapula	Spinal root of accessory nerve, cranial nerve XI, and cervical nerves C3 and C4	*Superior fibers:* elevate *Middle fibers:* retract *Inferior fibers:* depress Superior and inferior fibers act together in superior rotation
Levator scapulae	Posterior tubercles of C1–C4 vertebrae	Superior part of medial border of scapula	Dorsal scapular nerve (C5) and cervical nerves C3 and C4	Elevate scapula and tilt glenoid cavity inferiorly by rotating scapula
Rhomboid minor and rhomboid major	*Rhomboid minor:* ligamentum nuchae and spinous processes of C7 and T1 *Rhomboid major:* spinous processes of T2–T5	Medial border of scapula from level of spine to inferior angle	Dorsal scapular nerve (C4 and C5)	Retract and rotate scapula to depress glenoid cavity; fix scapula to thoracic wall
Sternocleidomastoid	Lateral surface of mastoid process and lateral half of superior nuchal line of occipital bone	*Sternal head:* attached to anterior surface of manubrium *Clavicular head:* superior surface of medial third of clavicle	Spinal root of accessory nerve (XI) and branches of cervical nerve (C2 and C3)	*Acting alone:* tilts head to ipsilateral side, laterally flexes neck *Acting bilaterally:* flexes neck
Pectoralis minor	Third to fifth ribs near their costal cartilages	Medial border and superior surface of coracoid process of scapula	Medial pectoral nerve (C8 and T1)	Stabilizes scapula by drawing it inferiorly and anteriorly against thoracic wall

*See Figure 12-1.

the scapula; scapulohumeral muscles (Table 12-11), whose origins are on the scapula and whose insertions are into the humerus; and axiohumeral muscles (Table 12-12), whose origins are on the trunk and whose insertions are on the humerus.

The Elbow

The elbow joint consists of the articulations of the distal humerus, the proximal ulna, and the proximal radius. The movements of the elbow include flexion, extension, pronation, and supination. These

TABLE 12-11 SCAPULOHUMERAL MUSCLES*

Muscles	Origin (Proximal Attachment)	Insertion (Distal Attachment)	Innervation	Action
Deltoid	Lateral third of clavicle, acromion and spine of scapula	Deltoid tuberosity of humerus	Axillary nerve (C5 and C6)	*Anterior part:* flexes and medially rotates arm *Middle part:* abducts arm *Posterior part:* extends and laterally rotates arm
Supraspinatus	Supraspinous fossa of scapula	Superior facet on greater tubercle of humerus	Suprascapular nerve (C4–C6)	Helps deltoid abduct arm and acts with rotator cuff muscles
Infraspinatus	Infraspinous fossa of scapula	Middle facet on greater tubercle of humerus	Suprascapular nerve (C5 and C6)	Laterally rotates arm; helps hold humeral head in glenoid cavity of scapula
Teres minor	Superior part of lateral border of scapula	Inferior facet on greater tubercle of humerus	Axillary nerve (C5 and C6)	Laterally rotates arm; helps hold humeral head in glenoid cavity of scapula
Teres major	Dorsal surface of inferior angle of scapula	Medial lip of intertubercular groove of humerus	Lower scapular nerve (C6 and C7)	Adducts and medially rotates arm
Subscapularis	Subscapular fossa	Lesser tubercle of humerus	Upper and lower subscapular nerve (C5–C7)	Medially rotates and adducts arm; helps hold humeral head in glenoid cavity

*See Figure 12-1.

TABLE 12-12 AXIOHUMERAL MUSCLES*

Muscles	Origin (Proximal Attachment)	Insertion (Distal Attachment)	Innervation	Action
Pectoralis major	Clavicular head: anterior surface of the medial half of clavicle	Lateral lip of intertubercular groove of humerus	*Clavicular head:* lateral and medial pectoral nerve (C5 and C6)	Adducts and medially rotates humerus *Acting alone:* clavicular head flexes humerus, sternocostal head extends humerus
Latissimus dorsi	Spinous processes of inferior six thoracic vertebrae, thoracolumbar fascia, iliac crest, inferior three or four ribs	Floor of intertubercular groove of humerus	Thoracodorsal nerve	Extends, adducts, and medially rotates humerus
Serratus anterior	External surfaces of lateral parts of first to eighth ribs	Anterior surface of medial border of scapular nerve	Long thoracic nerve (C5–C7)	Protracts scapula and holds it against thoracic wall, rotates scapula

*See Figure 12-1.

movements occur at three separate joints: a hinge joint between the humerus and the ulna; a pivot joint between the ulna and the radius; and a ball-and-socket joint between the humerus and the radius. Women have a less prominent olecranon process and shallower corresponding fossa, which renders them more liable to overstretch the elbow joint.

Elbow flexor muscles are listed in Table 12-13 (Fig. 12-22). Biceps contribute greatly to the stability of the shoulder joint, in addition to functioning

TABLE 12-13 ELBOW FLEXOR MUSCLES*

Muscles	Origin (Proximal Attachment)	Insertion (Distal Attachment)	Innervation	Action
Biceps brachii	*Short head:* tip of coracoid process of scapula *Long head:* supraglenoid tubercle of scapula	Tuberosity of radius and fascia of forearm via bicipital aponeurosis	Musculocutaneous nerve (C5 and C6)	Flexes forearm when it is supine; supinates forearm
Brachialis	Distal half of anterior surface of humerus	Coronoid process and tuberosity of ulna	Musculocutaneous nerve (C5 and C6)	Flexes forearm
Brachioradialis	Proximal two thirds of lateral supracondylar ridge of humerus	Lateral surface of distal end of radius	Radial nerve (C5–C7)	Flexes forearm
Pronator teres	*Humeral head:* medial epicondyle of humerus *Ulnar head:* coronoid process of ulna	Middle of lateral surface of radius	Median nerve (C6 and C7)	Flexes and pronates forearm

*See Figure 12-22.

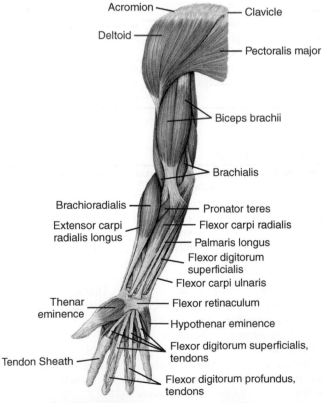

FIGURE 12-22 Elbow flexor muscles.

as the major elbow flexor. The major elbow extensor is triceps brachii (Table 12-14 and Fig. 12-23). The elbow supinator muscle is described in Table 12-15 and Figure 12-24.

The Forearm

Muscles of the forearm are described in Tables 12-16 to 12-18 and depicted in Figure 12-25.

TABLE 12-14 ELBOW EXTENSOR MUSCLES*

Muscles	Origin (Proximal Attachment)	Insertion (Distal Attachment)	Innervation	Action
Triceps brachii	*Long head:* infraglenoid tubercle of scapula *Lateral head:* posterior surface of humerus, superior to radial groove *Medial head:* posterior surface of humerus, inferior to radial groove	Proximal end of olecranon ulna and fascia of forearm	Radial nerve (C6–C8)	Extends forearm; long head stabilizes head of abducted humerus
Anconeus	Lateral epicondyle of humerus	Lateral surface of olecranon and superior part of posterior surface of ulna	Radial nerve (C7–T1)	Assists triceps in extending forearm; stabilizes elbow joint; abducts ulna during pronation

*See Figure 12-23.

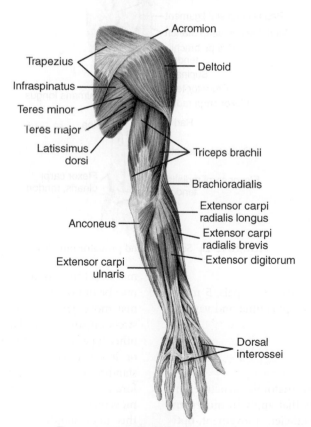

Acromion
Trapezius
Infraspinatus
Teres minor
Teres major
Latissimus dorsi
Anconeus
Extensor carpi ulnaris
Deltoid
Triceps brachii
Brachioradialis
Extensor carpi radialis longus
Extensor carpi radialis brevis
Extensor digitorum
Dorsal interossei

FIGURE 12-23 Elbow extensor muscles.

TABLE 12-15   **ELBOW SUPINATOR MUSCLE***

Muscles	Origin (Proximal Attachment)	Insertion (Distal Attachment)	Innervation	Action
Supinator	Lateral epicondyle of humerus, radial collateral and annular ligaments, supinator fossa, and crest of ulna	Lateral, posterior, and anterior surfaces of proximal third of radius	Deep branch of radial nerve (C5 and C6)	Supinates forearm (rotates radius to turn palm anteriorly)

*See Figure 12-24.

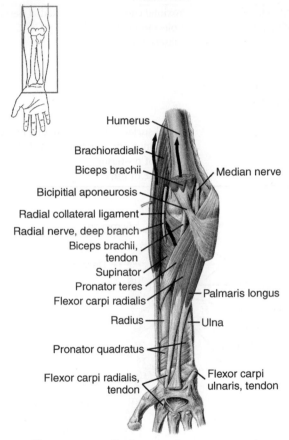

Humerus
Brachioradialis
Biceps brachii
Median nerve
Bicipital aponeurosis
Radial collateral ligament
Radial nerve, deep branch
Biceps brachii, tendon
Supinator
Pronator teres
Flexor carpi radialis
Palmaris longus
Radius
Ulna
Pronator quadratus
Flexor carpi radialis, tendon
Flexor carpi ulnaris, tendon

FIGURE 12-24 Supinator and pronator muscles.

The Wrist

The hand contains 27 bones—8 carpals, 5 metacarpals, and 14 phalanges—plus ulna and variable number of sesamoid bones.

SUMMARY

The relationship between anatomic structure and movement and the forces that apply in movement are complex. To achieve efficient movement, optimal structure is required. Musculoskeletal structure may be out of balance, causing impairment of normal movement, as a consequence of the physical stress on soft tissue that results from overtraining, other types of misuse of the body, external injuries, or internal pathologic processes. A basic understanding of normal functional anatomy is therefore a vital prerequisite for attempting to improve movement by restoring normal structure. With this understanding, a clinician can identify any

TABLE 12-16   MUSCLES OF THE ANTERIOR FASCIAL COMPARTMENT OF THE FOREARM

Muscles	Origin (Proximal Attachment)	Insertion (Distal Attachment)	Innervation	Action
Pronator teres	*Humeral head:* medial epicondyle of humerus *Ulnar head:* coronoid process of ulna	Middle of lateral surface of radius	Median nerve (C6 and C7)	Flexes and pronates forearm
Flexor carpi radialis	Medial epicondyle of humerus	Bases of second and third metacarpal bones	Median nerve (C7 and C8)	Flexes and abducts hand at wrist joint
Palmaris longus	Medial epicondyle of humerus	Flexor retinaculum and palmar aponeurosis	Median nerve (C7 and C8)	Flexes hand
Flexor carpi ulnaris	*Humeral head:* medial epicondyle of humerus *Ulnar head:* medial aspect of olecranon process and posterior border of ulna	Pisiform bone, hook of the hamate, base of fifth metacarpal bone	Ulnar nerve (C7 and C8)	Flexes and abducts hand at wrist joint
Flexor digitorum superficialis	*Humeroulnar head:* medial epicondyle of humerus *Radial head:* oblique line on anterior surface of shaft of radius	Middle phalanx of medial four fingers	Median nerve (C7–T1)	Flexes middle phalanx of fingers and assists in flexing proximal phalanx and hand
Flexor pollicis longus	Anterior surface of shaft of radius	Distal phalanx of thumb	Anterior interosseous branch of median nerve (C8 and T1)	Flexes distal phalanx of thumb
Flexor digitorum profundus	Proximal 75% of medial and anterior surface of ulna and interosseous membrane	Base of distal phalanges of medial four digits	Ulnar and median nerves (C8 and T1)	Flexes distal phalanx of fingers; assists in flexion of middle and proximal phalanges and wrist
Pronator quadratus	Anterior surface of shaft of ulna	Anterior surface of shaft of radius	Anterior interosseous branch of median nerve (C8 and T1)	Pronates forearm

TABLE 12-17   MUSCLES OF THE LATERAL FASCIAL COMPARTMENT OF THE FOREARM*

Muscles	Origin (Proximal Attachment)	Insertion (Distal Attachment)	Innervation	Action
Brachioradialis	Proximal two thirds of lateral supracondylar ridge of humerus	Lateral surface of distal end of radius	Radial nerve (C5–C7)	Flexes forearm at elbow joint; rotates forearm to midprone position
Extensor carpi radialis longus	Lateral supracondylar ridge of humerus	Posterior surface of base of second metacarpal bone	Radial nerve (C6 and C7)	Extends and abducts hand at wrist joint

*See Figure 12-25.

TABLE 12-18	MUSCLES OF THE POSTERIOR FASCIAL COMPARTMENT OF THE FOREARM			
Muscles	Origin (Proximal Attachment)	Insertion (Distal Attachment)	Innervation	Action
Extensor carpi radialis brevis	Lateral epicondyle of humerus	Posterior surface of base of third metacarpal bone	Deep branch of radial nerve (C7–C8)	Extends and abducts hand at wrist joint
Extensor digitorum	Lateral epicondyle of humerus	Middle and distal phalanges of the medial four fingers	Posterior interosseous nerve (C7–C8); a branch of radial nerve	Extends fingers and hand
Extensor digitorum minimi	Lateral epicondyle of humerus	Extensor expansion of little finger	Posterior interosseous nerve (C7–C8); a branch of radial nerve	Extends metacarpal phalangeal joint of little finger
Extensor carpi ulnaris	Lateral epicondyle of humerus	Base of fifth metacarpal bone	Posterior interosseous nerve (C7–C8); a branch of radial nerve	Extends and adducts hand at wrist joint
Anconeus	Lateral epicondyle of humerus	Lateral surface of olecranon and superior part of posterior surface of ulna	Radial nerve (C7–T1)	Assists triceps in extending forearm, stabilizes elbow joint; abducts ulna during pronation
Supinator	Lateral epicondyle of humerus, radial collateral and annular ligaments, supinator fossa, and crest of ulna	Lateral, posterior, and anterior surfaces of proximal third of radius	Deep branch of radial nerve (C5 and C6)	Supinates forearm (rotates radius to turn palm anteriorly)
Abductor pollicis longus	Posterior surface of shafts of radius and ulna	Base of first metacarpal bone	Deep branch of radial nerve (C5–C7)	Abducts and extends thumb
Extensor pollicis brevis	Posterior surface of shaft of ulna	Base of distal phalanx of thumb	Deep branch of radial nerve (C5–C7)	Extends metacarpophalangeal joints of thumb
Extensor pollicis longus	Posterior surface of shaft of ulna	Base of distal phalanx of thumb	Deep branch of radial nerve (C5–C7)	Extends distal phalanx of thumb
Extensor indicis	Posterior surface of shaft of ulna	Extensor expansion of index finger	Deep branch of radial nerve (C5–C7)	Extends metacarpophalangeal joint of index finger

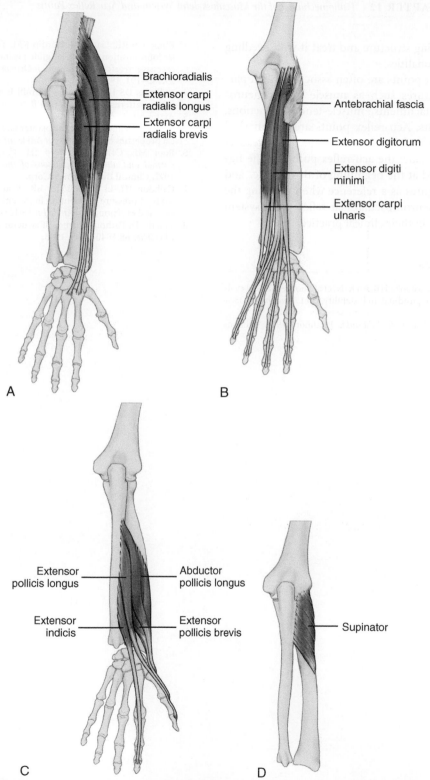

A

B

C

D

FIGURE 12-25 Muscles of the forearm. **A,** Radial muscles. **B,** Dorsal muscles: superficial layer. **C,** Dorsal muscles: middle layer. **D,** Dorsal muscles: deep layer.

Brachioradialis

Extensor carpi radialis longus

Extensor carpi radialis brevis

Antebrachial fascia

Extensor digitorum

Extensor digiti minimi

Extensor carpi ulnaris

Extensor pollicis longus

Abductor pollicis longus

Extensor indicis

Extensor pollicis brevis

Supinator

malfunctioning structure and treat it with needling and other modalities.

Acu-reflex points are often associated with particular structures such as muscle bellies, neuromuscular attachments, muscle-tendon junctions, and ligaments. Acu-reflex points are not marked on the muscle charts in this chapter, but readers may wish to label the acu-reflex points in the figures provided at the beginning of this chapter and use those figures as a reference when applying the integrative neuromuscular acu-reflex point system (INMARPS) in their clinical practice.

References

1. Huang C-K, Kitaoka HB, An K-N, et al: Biomechanical evaluation of longitudinal arch stability, *Foot Ankle Int* 14:353–357, 1993.
2. Inman VT: *The joints of the ankle*, Baltimore, 1976, Williams & Williams.
3. Klingman RE, Liaos SM, Hardin KM: The effect of subtalar joint position on patellar glide position in subjects with excessive rearfoot pronation, *J Orthop Sports Phys Ther* 25:185–191, 1997.
4. Williams DS III, McClay IS, Hamill J: Arch structure and injury patterns in runners, *Clin Biomech* 16:341–347, 2001.
5. Arangio GA, Chen C, Salathe EP: Effect of varying arch height with and without the plantar fascia on the mechanical properties of the foot, *Foot Ankle Int* 19:705–709, 1998.
6. Root ML, Orien WP, Weed JH: *Clinical biomechanics: normal and abnormal functions of the foot*, Los Angeles, 1977, Clinical Biomechanics Corp.
7. Calhoun JH, Li F, Ledbetter BR, et al: A comprehensive study of pressure distribution in the ankle joint with inversion and eversion, *Foot Ankle Int* 15:125–133, 1994.
8. Tiberio D: Pathomechanics of structural foot deformities, *Phys Ther* 68:1840–1849, 1988.

Using Dry Needling Acupuncture for Preventing Injury and Enhancing Athletic Performance

Preventive measures are the best way to decrease the incidence and severity of injury in sports, and many research programs and treatment methods have been developed for this purpose. However, the potential of dry needling acupuncture for *preventing* sports injuries has not yet been seriously recognized by sports medicine professionals.

Dry needling therapy is a specific modality for soft tissue dysfunction. Needling and needling-induced lesions activate built-in biologic self-regulatory mechanisms to normalize pathophysiology of soft tissues. Soft tissue accounts for about 50% of human body mass and is a part of every anatomic entity as either a structural or functional element; any pathologic insult, internal or external, can cause or be manifested as soft tissue dysfunction. Therefore dry needling acupuncture is a modality that can be used in almost every clinical condition that involves soft tissue dysfunction, ranging from postexercise syndrome, delayed-onset muscle soreness, precompetition stress, and myofascial pain to cancer in patients who are undergoing chemotherapy, radiotherapy, or both. If an injury necessitates surgical intervention, dry needling acupuncture can be used before and after surgery for improving rehabilitation.

The best practical way to prevent sports injury is to restore musculoskeletal homeostasis, which accelerates recovery from postexercise syndrome, delayed-onset muscle soreness, and soft tissue inflammation and rebalances musculoskeletal pathomechanics so as to enhance the efficiency and ease of movement.

INJURY PREVENTION: TREATING ASYMPTOMATIC ATHLETES

Preventing injury in asymptomatic athletes is of utmost importance. Injury prevention and performance enhancement are in fact the same issue.

Many injuries occur because the soft tissues—the muscles, fascia, tendons, and ligaments—are loaded with accumulated stress so that they are in a physical and physiologic state of "preinjury." Under these conditions, any overtraining, unusual movement or posture, or physical impact can cause an injury that would not happen, or would be less severe, in a healthy body. Examples of this would be different kinds of tendinitis, tendon avulsion, abnormal bone growth such as bone spurs caused by chronic muscle hypertension, and even bone breakage resulting from sudden contraction of tight muscles. All these conditions are caused by soft tissue dysfunction. If such dysfunctions were eliminated and if the chronic stress in the affected tissues were regularly treated, such injuries could be prevented.

In investigating the medical histories of several world-class athletes, the author has found that many of their injuries and surgical procedures could have been prevented if they had received proper regular preventive treatment to remove accumulated musculoskeletal stress or to alleviate hidden symptoms. In fact, he found that most athletes, professional and nonprofessional, have symptoms that are hidden to a greater or lesser degree. Even those who claimed to be symptom-free reported after treatment that they felt their musculoskeletal systems were much better coordinated and their muscles were stronger. Injuries resulting from musculoskeletal stress are often hidden, unknown in their early stages to both athletes and their physicians.

Many athletes and medical professionals understand the importance and necessity of injury prevention, and many programs have been developed for this purpose. The First World Congress on Sports Injury Prevention, which was convened in Oslo, Norway, in June 2005, is an example of the progress made in this field. Is it possible to prevent sports injuries? The answer is definitely "yes." Systematic research suggests that sports injuries can be reduced by 54% to 65%, depending on the type of sport and type of intervention (see later discussion in this chapter).

The use of dry needling acupuncture for sports injury prevention is a new approach that the author and colleagues have developed since the late 1990s. Their experience demonstrated that needling is very effective in restoring musculoskeletal homeostasis, which enhances efficiency of movement; accelerates recovery from postexercise syndrome, delayed-onset muscle soreness, and soft tissue inflammation; and rebalances musculoskeletal mechanics.

The author and colleagues have found that all healthy athletes benefit from a session of preventive dry needling acupuncture once a week, combined with a treatment 3 days before competition and another immediately after competition. This protocol enhances physical performance and prevents soft tissue injury by accelerating recovery from overtraining.

CLINICAL PROCEDURE FOR PREVENTING INJURY AND ENHANCING PERFORMANCE

A general procedure for asymptomatic athletes may follow these steps:
- Collection of an accurate history of sports career, including all injuries
- Recording of any current complaint
- A musculoskeletal screening examination
- Systemic or subsystemic treatment

A well-designed general musculoskeletal screening examination (Table 13-1) is suggested to identify possible pathology.[1] In this examination, asymmetry or mechanical imbalance can be identified. Any pathologic condition or imbalance that seems to be local can affect systemic physiology, function, or structure. In the author's experience, all athletes, professional

TABLE 13-1   MUSCULOSKELETAL SCREENING EXAMINATION

Instruction	Observation	Recording	
Handedness		R	L
Stand facing examiner	Acromioclavicular joints; general habitus		
Look at ceiling, floor, over both shoulders, touch ears to shoulders	Cervical spine motion		
Shrug shoulders (resistance)	Trapezius strength		
Abduct shoulders	Deltoid strength		
Full external rotation of arms	Shoulder motion		
Flex and extend elbows	Elbow motion		
Arms at sides, elbow at 90 degrees: flex, pronate, and supinate wrist	Elbow and wrist motion		
Spread fingers, make fist	Hand and finger motion, strength, deformities		
Tighten (contract) quadriceps; relax quadriceps	Symmetry of knee and ankle joints		
"Duck walk" away and toward examiner	Hip, knee, and ankle motions		
Stand with back to examiner	Symmetry: ear and shoulder levels, hips, popliteal creases, malleoli, scoliosis		
Knee straight, touch toes	Scoliosis, hip motion, tightness of lumbar muscles, hamstring and calf muscles		
Raise up on toes, heels	Calf symmetry, leg strength		
Arms at sides, anteroposterior positions of both arms and hips	Body rotation about superior-inferior axis		
Stand with side to examiner	Neck position and anterior-posterior skeletal alignment		

and amateur, are living with hidden musculoskeletal stress that can become symptomatic at any time during training or competition if it is not properly treated. The treatment should be provided in a systemic way with emphasis on any symptoms that have been revealed in the screening examination. There is a difference that should be noted between those with previous injuries and those without: Athletes with previous injuries are more vulnerable to recurring symptoms because their injuries or surgical procedures may have changed their anatomic structure to some degree, which can create an imbalance in their natural musculoskeletal biomechanics.

The following cases, from the author's own patients, serve as examples of preventive treatment for asymptomatic athletes or those with only minor musculoskeletal symptoms.

CASE STUDY I
An athlete without previous injuries

Ms. C, 26 years old, is a professional long-distance runner without previous history of injury. In the musculoskeletal screening examination, the author found that her right hamstring muscles were tight, her right hip was tilted posteriorly, and she had soreness on the left levator scapulae muscle. The following treatment was planned:
- Systemic approach: needling all 24 homeostatic acu-reflex points
- Symptomatic approach: needling sensitive areas of right hamstring on the biceps femoris, semitendinosus, and semimembranosus muscles

After treatment, Ms. C. felt that her right hamstring muscles were more relaxed, hip flexion was improved, and her left levator scapulae muscle was less sensitive.

However, her symptoms returned a few days later. Her history revealed that she had had these problems for the previous 2 years. Weekly treatment and special treatment 3 days before any big event were prescribed. The symptoms gradually subsided during the first 3 months, and after 6 months she felt no symptoms; in her running performance, she was achieving better times than she had 5 years previously.

CASE STUDY II
An athlete with previous injuries

Ms. D., 36 years old, was a professional long-distance runner. Five years ago she had surgery because of Achilles tendinitis in the left heel. It took 2 years for her to recover to the point of resuming training, but the muscles of her left leg had developed a tendency toward delayed-onset muscle soreness: She would feel pain in the lower left abdominal muscles just above the inguinal ligament while running downhill. The routine screening examination revealed that she felt this pain whenever she overextended the left leg. Further examination revealed sensitive and sore areas on the left quadriceps muscles. The treatment included systemic needling of the primary homeostatic acu-reflex points, as well as the symptomatic acu-reflex points on the lower back, hip abductor, and iliopsoas muscles to relieve hip stress. Symptomatic treatment focused on quadriceps, hamstring muscles, adductor muscles, the iliotibial band, and rectus abdominis muscles.

After treatment, there was no pain even during an overextension test. The author suggested to Ms. D. that she stop training for 2 days and and then resume training at a lower level for 1 week. Five days after the initial treatment, she received a second, similar treatment. In the following week, she gradually increased the intensity of her training. Ms. D. frequently felt some symptoms on the left leg, and she comes for screening examination and treatment regularly.

New frustration followed. Ms. D. resumed her training of 85 miles every week for 4 months without any symptoms, while maintaining weekly treatment. As winter came, she was training more in cold temperatures. One day she felt excruciating pain in the left lower abdominal region, but only when she ran downhill. Medical examination did not reveal any tissue problems, but postural screening demonstrated painful trigger points on the quadriceps femoris muscle and all adductor muscles. The left pubic tubercle was also very painful. In addition

(Continued)

CASE STUDY II
An athlete with previous injuries—Cont'd

to systemic treatment, special focus was given to the left pubic tubercle and trigger points. She was advised to stop training for 3 weeks and to train at reduced intensity after that. After six treatments on a weekly basis, she felt symptom-free and gradually resumed her normal training protocol.

EVIDENCE-BASED RESEARCH

The author emphasizes the systemic approach in treating both asymptomatic (no discernible symptoms) and symptomatic athletes, and this is well supported by his own clinical experience and equally by findings of evidence-based research in sports medicine. The purpose of the systemic approach is to adjust the biomechanical alignment and balance of the core structure, especially to release stress in the soft tissue of the spine to facilitate stability and strengthening of the core.

Since the late 1990s, core strengthening and stability has become the focus in sports rehabilitation and performance training. However, the concept of core strength was suggested as early as the 1920s by Joseph Pilates,[2] who noticed that developing a girdle of strength required recruitment of the deep trunk muscles. In addition, rehabilitation experts in various disciplines have historically taught the concept that stability of proximal segments is required for effective mobility of distal segments. For instance, a stable pelvis and trunk are needed for controlled movement at the knee and ankle.

Hodges and Richardson[2] revived the concept of core stability in the 1990s. They described the spine as inherently unstable and requiring active support from intra-abdominal pressure and tensioning of the thoracolumbar fascia and deep lumbar stabilizers. Core strength is thus considered to be the muscular support of the lumbar spine, which is necessary to achieve and maintain functional stability.[3] More recently, this concept has been expanded to include muscles of the hip[4] and the scapulothoracic musculature.[5] Properly developed core strength, providing sufficient core stability, has been suggested as a necessity for maintaining correct posture and alignment of lumbar and pelvic regions during all movement and particularly in sport because it enables powerful and coordinated extremity movements. Inadequate core strength results in poor core stability and may decrease biomechanical efficiency, as well as increasing the risk of injury.

Several studies have confirmed the relationship between core muscle weakness and the likelihood of injury. Some examples are mentioned here:

- Activation of the transversus abdominis muscle is significantly delayed among individuals with low back pain.[2]
- Activation of the obliquus internus abdominis, multifidus, and gluteus maximus muscles are similarly delayed on the symptomatic side of individuals with sacroiliac joint pain.[6]
- Trunk extensor isokinetic strength is significantly correlated with the disability level of low back pain among wrestlers without radiologic abnormalities in the lumbar region.[7]
- Hip muscle weakness and patellofemoral pain are positively correlated in female athletes.[8]
- Trunk muscle weakness is a risk factor for low back pain. Individuals who developed low back pain displayed an imbalance between trunk extensor and flexor strength.[9]
- A bilateral imbalance in isometric strength of the hip extensors is related to the development of low back pain.[10]
- Athletes with stronger hip abductors and external rotation are less likely to experience low back pain.[4]
- Persistent muscle atrophy is related to recurrence of low back pain. A recurrence rate of 30% was found in subjects receiving core stabilization therapy, in comparison with 84% for those who received only conventional medical management.[11]

SUMMARY

Biomechanically favorable extremity movement can exist only with a stable pelvis and spine. Core stabilization has been advocated for the treatment of such injuries as patellofemoral pain, iliotibial band syndrome, hamstring strain, and postoperative rehabilitation of ligamentous reconstruction. An unbalanced spine is also related to shoulder and neck problems. Thus a well-aligned and balanced musculoskeletal system is absolutely necessary for achieving effective movement in sports and daily life. Symptomatic treatment combined with a systemic approach can help patients attain maximal homeostasis of the musculoskeletal system, which not only prevents or reduces the risk of sports injury but also enhances physical performance because of the system's optimal alignment.

Dry needling acupuncture therapy offers its special value to athletes just as it does to many nonathlete patients. First, dry needling acupuncture, with its specific lesion mechanisms, accelerates the healing of soft tissue dysfunction, which is a major issue in all aspects of sports injury. Second, dry needling acupuncture helps to reduce the physical and psychologic stress that impair physical performance and increase the possibility of injuries. This chapter focused on the use of dry needling acupuncture as a preventive modality in sports medicine.

References

1. Gomez JE, Landry GL, Bernhardt DT: Critical evaluation of the 2-minute orthopedic screening examination, *Am J Dis Child* 1109–1113, 1993.
2. Hodges PW, Richardson CA: Inefficient muscular stabilization of the lumbar spine associated with low back pain: a motor control evaluation of transversus abdominis, *Spine* 21:2640–2650, 1996.
3. Akuthora V, Nadler SF: Core strengthening, *Arch Phys Med Rehabil* 85:S86–S92, 2004.
4. Leeturn DT, Ireland ML, Willson JD, et al: Core stability measures at-risk factors for lower extremity injury in athletes, *Med Sci Sports Exerc* 36:926–934, 2004.
5. Quinn E: *Sports medicine: core stability training. How to build a strong foundation.* Available at www.sportsmedicine.about.com/cs/conditioning/a/aa052002a.html.
6. Hungerford B, Gilleard W, Hodges P: Evidence of altered lumbopelvic muscle recruitment in the presence of sacroiliac joint pain, *Spine* 28:1593–1600, 2003.
7. Iwai K, Nakazato K, Irie K, et al: Trunk muscle strength and disability level of low back pain in collegiate wrestlers, *Med Sci Sports Exerc* 36:1296–1300, 2004.
8. Ireland ML, Willson JD, Ballantyne BT, et al: Hip strength in females with and without patellofemoral pain, *J Orthop Sports Phys Ther* 33:671–676, 2003.
9. Lee JH, Hoshino Y, Nakamura K, et al: Trunk muscle weakness as a risk factor for low back pain: a 5-year prospective study, *Spine* 24:54–57, 1999.
10. Nadler SF, Malagna GA, Feinberg JH, et al: Relationship between hip muscle imbalance and occurrence of low back pain in collegiate athletes: a prospective study, *Am J Phys Med Rehabil* 80:572–577, 2001.
11. Hides JA, Jull GA, Richardson CA: Long-term effects of specific stabilizing exercises for first-episode low back pain, *Spine (Phila Pa 1976)* 26:E243–E248, 2001.

CHAPTER 14

General Principles of Treating Soft Tissue Dysfunction in Sports Injuries

Previous chapters introduced the concept of dry needling acupuncture as a nonspecific modality for treating soft tissue dysfunction. Dysfunction of soft tissue is involved in all human pathophysiologic processes, and most sports injuries are typical soft tissue injuries. Every athlete, professional or non-professional, experiences injury. Many never completely recover, and their injuries become the root of chronic problems. In reality, these injuries can be prevented or completely healed in many cases if multidisciplinary approaches are combined organically and if athletes, their coaches, and their doctors fully understand the nature, the specific mechanisms, the effectiveness, and the limits of each modality.

Because of the nature of training and competition, most if not all athletes have certain kinds of physical and psychologic stress involving soft tissue dysfunction. Some of the stress is not manifested physiologically and is left unattended until it becomes severe enough to cause pathologic symptoms.

In dry needling acupuncture, fine needles are used to create lesions into particular spots in soft tissues, which activates the body's healing mechanisms to normalize soft tissue dysfunction. Dry needling acupuncture does not conflict with any other healing modality, whether biochemical or physical, and this is especially true when dealing with athletes. In fact, the available literature indicates that dry needling acupuncture is a good supplement to any other treatment modality, and in some cases, dry needling acupuncture alone provides effective results.

This chapter reviews common types of sports injury for which dry needling acupuncture can be helpful and effective as a supplementary modality with other medical procedures.

Dry needling acupuncture should be practiced only with a thorough understanding of human anatomy and the nature of pathophysiology. The purpose of this chapter is to describe the application of dry needling acupuncture to common sports injuries, and readers who need to review anatomy and pathophysiology for a particular injury may refer to the list of further reading at the end of this chapter.

SPORTS INJURIES OF THE SKIN

Dry needling acupuncture is very effective for the skin injuries described in the following discussions.

Sunburn

Sunburn is an inflammation of the skin, caused by ultraviolet radiation from the sun. All athletes practicing outdoor sports are vulnerable to sunburn, particularly those whose sport is practiced at higher altitudes, such as skiers and climbers. Sunburn can range from mild to severe. The skin is hot to the touch, with redness, pain, or blisters in severe cases.

The sunburned skin area should be treated once a day with needles that are 15 mm long and 0.18 to 0.25 mm in diameter. Needling density is about two to three needles per square centimeter. Before needling, the skin may be cleaned with cotton balls and cold water, but topical moisturizers should not be applied. After needles are removed, bleeding, if any, should be cleaned with cotton balls. Topical moisturizers can be applied 1 hour after treatment. To avoid potential infection, blisters should not be needled. However, if blisters are broken, proper procedures should be used to prevent infection.

Frostbite

Frostbite is caused by freezing of body tissue, which results in damage to the skin and subcutaneous layers. Skiers and mountaineers are prone to this injury in cold weather. Frostbite often affects exposed skin such as nose and ears but can affect any part that is subjected to sufficiently low temperatures. The symptoms may include white skin and numbness or a tingling sensation, and the skin appears loose and blackened when it is destroyed by frostbite.

The affected area should be treated once a day with needles that are 15 mm long and 0.18 mm diameter (the finest gauge). Needling density is about two to three needles per square centimeter.

Blisters

Blisters are formed where the skin encounters physical friction. Such friction can be caused by footwear during running or skating or by other sporting apparatus such as that used in gymnastics, baseball, or racket events. Physical friction causes separation of the epidermis from the dermal layer of skin or separation within the multiple layers of the epidermis itself. Serum, lymph, blood, or extracellular fluid fills the space between layers. The fluid in blisters is clear, but bleeding into the blister occasionally occurs and causes red or blue discoloration. The usual complaints are pain, stinging, and sensitivity at the injury site.

Treatment of blisters is the same as for sunburn. One treatment session should be provided every day.

Athlete's Foot

Athlete's foot is a skin infection that affects 70% of the population at various times. It is caused by a fungal infection produced by a class of parasites of the skin known as *dermatophytes*. The fungus thrives in the moist conditions produced by sweat. The site most commonly affected is between the fourth and fifth toes, where the fungus causes irritation, maceration, and fissures and scaling of the outer layer of skin. The symptoms are reddened, cracked, and peeling skin with itching, stinging, and burning sensation, and sometimes there is a noxious odor. The most common type of this condition is chronic interdigital athlete's foot.

Before treatment, the infected skin should be cleaned and dried. The affected skin is treated with needles in the same way as for sunburn. Any bleeding should be cleaned with cotton balls after the needles are removed. One treatment session a day should be provided.

SPORTS INJURIES OF THE HEAD AND NECK

Head Injuries

Traumas to the head are among the most serious injuries in sports; they can cause permanent symptoms and even fatality. Head injuries include concussion, contusion, hemorrhage, and skull fracture. Major signs and symptoms of these injuries include loss of consciousness, confusion, amnesia, and shock. All these injuries necessitate immediate medical attention.

Rehabilitation from head injuries varies widely, depending on the nature and extent of the injury. According to the author's experience, patients with a mild concussion may need months and sometimes years to recover from postconcussion syndrome.

The prognosis of head injuries may not be known for months or, in some patients, years. Patients may experience postconcussion symptoms, including headache, dizziness, amnesia, and musculoskeletal imbalance.

Dry needling acupuncture is a very helpful modality during rehabilitation for treating conditions caused by head injury. The treatment protocol consists of two parts: specific treatment, which focuses on the patient's complaint of local symptoms (e.g., stiff neck, nausea, tension in the trapezius and levator scapulae regions), and nonspecific treatment, in which the primary homeostatic acu-reflex points (ARPs) are needled for systemic symptoms such as headache, dizziness, or amnesia. Treatments should be provided twice per week for the first few weeks and then once per week until the patient feels maximal or complete recovery.

Neck Injuries: Strain, Contusion, and Fracture

Like head injuries, neck injuries can be very serious, even fatal, and necessitate immediate medical attention, particularly when vertebrae are broken or fractured. Neck injuries can be caused by sudden twisting, serious falls, and direct blows or physical impact from other athletes. The injuries may result in head, neck, and shoulder pain; a crackling sensation in the neck; loss of strength and mobility of the neck and shoulder; and even lower back symptoms. If not properly treated, long-term paralysis, loss of motion and coordination, and calcification and osteoporosis of the cervical spine may occur in severe cases.

Neck Strain

Neck strains are common and involve injuries to the muscles or tendons of the neck and shoulder area. Contusions are bruises to the skin and underlying tissue of the neck caused by direct physical force such as a blow. Dry needling acupuncture is the most effective modality for these conditions at all stages of the injury. Specific treatment includes needling the symptomatic ARPs on the neck and shoulder. Nonspecific treatment should include needling all the symptomatic ARPs. Treatment can be offered twice per week immediately after injury and then once per week after initial pain relief is achieved. In an area of contusion, needles 15 to 25 mm long and 0.18 to 0.20 mm in diameter can be used, in a density of two to three needles per square centimeter. Contusions or bruised skin can be treated once every day or every other day until complete recovery is achieved.

After neck surgery, dry needling acupuncture can be used for rehabilitation.

Cervical Nerve Stretch Syndrome

Blows to the head, shoulder, or ear may cause injury to the brachial plexus in contact sports such as hockey, football, and wrestling, Patients may experience severe, burning pain radiating from the neck to the arm and fingers; numbness, tingling sensation, pricking sensation, burning sensation, or creeping sensation of the skin; and muscle weakness. Chronic symptoms may develop, and the rate of recurrence may be high, if the initial injury is not properly treated to the point of complete recovery.

Dry needling acupuncture is very effective in treating this condition. Specific treatments include needling local homeostatic, symptomatic, and paravertebral ARPs on the neck, shoulder, and arm. Nonspecific treatment should be offered. Treatment should be administered twice per week immediately after injury and once per week during rehabilitation.

Whiplash (Neck Sprain)

Whiplash occurs when an athlete is struck from behind during a contact sport. The physical force causes sudden flexion or extension of the neck, or both, and the head is rapidly thrown both forward and backward. During the short duration of this motion, soft tissues of the neck such as discs, ligaments, cervical muscles, nerve roots, and intervertebral joints may be injured. The injured athlete may not feel any symptoms immediately after the accident, but they may follow soon.

According to the current understanding, the hip and trunk are the first body segments and joints to experience movement during whiplash. Forward motion in these structures is accompanied by upward motion, which acts to compress the cervical spine. This combined motion causes the head to revolve backward into extension, producing tension where the lower cervical segments extend and the upper cervical segments flex. With this rotation of the cervical vertebrae, the anterior structures of the cervical segments are separated, and posterior components, including facet joints, are severely compressed.

Whiplash symptoms may include pain and stiffness in the neck, in the shoulder, or between the shoulder blades, as well as loss of mobility of these joints. The patient may also experience ringing in the ears, dizziness, nausea, blurred vision, irritability, and fatigue.

Dry needling acupuncture is very helpful in treating whiplash symptoms. The treatment protocol is the same as for cervical nerve stretch syndrome. Again, both specific and nonspecific treatments are needed. Local and systemic treatments are equally important. The long-term prognosis for most whiplash injuries is good if proper care is received, although symptoms may persist and the neck may be prone to reinjury even many years later. To prevent this, long-term dry needling acupuncture is suggested as maintenance treatment even after complete recovery.

Acute Torticollis

Acute torticollis is a neck injury that can be caused by different mechanisms. Joint-related torticollis usually follows a sudden rotational movement of the head, such as that which occurs in many contact sports: a fall that causes a sudden torsion in the neck, or a direct blow to the head that causes sudden twisting. This sudden physical force causes a sprain in one of the joint facets and compresses the nerves in the neck, resulting in muscle spasms, pain, and loss of movement. There may be damage to the cervical vertebrae, cervical discs, or associated nerves. Slow-onset torticollis is disc-related and often arises spontaneously in the morning when the patient awakens. The cause of the injury must be determined. Severe cases necessitate surgery or other major medical intervention.

Typical symptoms include pain, with the neck frozen in one position, often rotated to one side and bent forward by the contraction of the cervical muscles. The neck and shoulder muscles may become stiff.

Treatment of the symptoms should include needling symptomatic ARPs in the neck and shoulder. Related symptoms on the arms and low back should be examined and treated. Dry needling acupuncture is very helpful, and full recovery can be expected in many cases. Dry needling acupuncture is also effective in rehabilitation for patients who require surgery. Two treatment sessions per week is suggested until the symptoms are reduced.

Cervical Disc Injury

Disc injury may be acute damage caused by sudden, forceful trauma to the cervical vertebrae. Daily repetitive stress, as in training, especially with excessive or improper lifting of weights, can also damage the discs. Chronic slow-onset injury is related to disc degeneration. Cervical discs are shock-absorbing pads that facilitate movement and provide support for the spinal column. They consist of a center region or nucleus pulposus and a surrounding annulus fibrosus separating each segmental vertebra between C2 and T1. (Only ligaments and joint capsules exist between C1 and C2.) Slipped discs occur when a gel-like substance leaks from the disc's interior, after a split or rupture of the disc (herniation). This substance can then exert pressure on the spinal cord or nerves of the cervical spine.

The symptoms are tingling sensation, weakness, and numbness or pain in the neck, shoulder, arm,

or hand. Motor and sensory dysfunction may also be present in the affected cervical area, and flexibility of the joints and muscles may be lost.

Dry needling acupuncture is very useful in relieving the symptoms. Treatment should be offered twice per week. Upper-body symptoms of the neck, shoulder, and arm, and lower symptoms on the low back and hip should be treated at the same time.

Cervical Radiculitis (Pinched Nerve)

The cervical plexus supplies innervation to the shoulder, arm, and hand. A pinched nerve, or cervical radiculitis, is inflammation or compression of one of these nerves. It occurs when a disc presses against the spinal nerves connecting to the spinal cord. The discopathy can be caused by repetitive stress from training or posture. Bone spurs or degenerating vertebrae can also impinge on a nerve. The affected nerves branch to numerous areas, and symptoms may radiate from the source along the nerves to the areas where the nerve travels or that the nerve supplies. Inflammation and pain associated with pinched nerves may continue or worsen if proper treatment is not received. The nerve may become permanently damaged through continued pressure and stress, and the condition may cause serious underlying injury to the vertebrae or spinal cord.

Pain may occur in the arm, chest, neck, or shoulders. Other complaints can include loss of movement in the neck, weak muscles in the arms and chest, and numb fingers.

With proper treatment, the prognosis of cervical radiculitis is generally good in mild and moderate cases. More serious or prolonged cases necessitate surgery to relieve compression of the nerve root. Nevertheless, dry needling acupuncture is a very helpful modality, although long-term treatment is needed for recovery in some cases, and the patients should be informed of this.

The treatment is the same as for other neck problems, including both symptomatic (specific) and systemic (nonspecific) treatments. Two sessions per week should be offered.

Cervical Spondylosis (Spur Formation)

Cervical spondylosis is a chronic degeneration of the vertebrae and discs of the neck. Bone spurs, or osteophytes, are bony projections that form along joints and are often associated with arthritis. Such spurs can rub against nearby nerves or occasionally on the spinal cord, causing pain and limitation in joint motion. The degeneration results from wear on the bones of the cervical spine over time.

Aging, repetitive stress on joints, reduced flexibility of ligaments, and tissue inflammation can cause discs to degenerate and become drier and less elastic. Such degeneration may cause discs to bulge and, in some cases, rupture. To adjust to the stress of excessive physical force, the vertebrae may develop bone spurs, which are new growths of bone along the margins of existing bones.

Typical complaints are neck pain radiating to shoulders and arms, loss of balance, tingling sensation, burning sensation, weakness or numbness in the arm or hands, and headaches radiating to the back of the head.

Cervical spondylosis is a common cause of spinal cord dysfunction in older adults. If the condition is not properly treated, the injury may progress and become permanent. Bone spurs and herniated discs can impinge and put pressure on the roots of one or more nerves of the cervical spinal cord.

Dry needling acupuncture is very helpful for cervical spondylosis in mild to moderate cases, although long-term treatment is required in many cases. Treatment follows the same protocol as for other neck problems and should consist of both specific and nonspecific approaches. Two treatment sessions per week should be sufficient.

Preventive treatment to reduce stress, pain, and inflammation in the neck is highly recommended for all athletes in order to avoid the development of cervical spondylosis. During the asymptomatic stage, one session per week is recommended.

SPORTS INJURIES OF THE UPPER LIMB

Shoulder and Upper Arm Injuries

The shoulder complex is composed of five joints: the sternoclavicular, the acromioclavicular, the coracoclavicular, the glenohumeral, and the scapulothoracic. The shoulder has developed extreme mobility at the expense of stability. Thus shoulder injuries are common in sports.

Fractures of the Clavicle and Humerus

A sudden blow to the clavicle resulting from the collision of two athletes (in sports such as football) or a fall on an outstretched arm can cause fractures of clavicle or humerus. Immediate medical care is needed, but dry needling acupuncture can be used to reduce swelling and pain immediately after the accident and before surgery. Dry needling acupuncture can be used in all phases of rehabilitation from the fracture, regardless of whether surgery is needed. Fine 15-mm-long needles should be used in the painful or swollen region. Special attention should be paid to safety practice so as to avoid injury to the lung below. The author recommends one session every day for swelling and two sessions per week for pain.

Dislocation of the Shoulder

Dislocation of the shoulder occurs when there is violent contact with another athlete or a solid object or when an athlete falls on an outstretched hand during abduction and external rotation of the shoulder.

Immediate medical attention is needed right after the injury. Dry needling acupuncture should be used at all phases of this injury for pain, swelling, restoration of mobility, and postsurgical rehabilitation. The dry needling acupuncture treatment should include neck and shoulder. Treatment involves needling the anterior shoulder capsule, the insertions of the middle and inferior glenohumeral ligaments, and the trapezius, deltoid, and other shoulder muscles, especially those originating on the scapula. One session every day for swelling and two sessions per week for pain of the soft tissues are recommended.

Shoulder Subluxation

Shoulder subluxation is a partial dislocation of the ball-and-socket joint of the shoulder. The humerus is held in the socket of the scapula by a group of ligaments. If these ligaments are torn, the ball of the humerus can slip partially out of the shoulder socket. An athlete who suffers from this injury may experience shoulder pain, looseness and weakness of the shoulder joint, or numbness in the shoulder or arm. Surgery is needed in some cases.

Shoulder subluxation can be caused by a direct blow to the shoulder in contact sports, a fall on an outstretched arm, or forcing of the arm into an awkward position.

Dry needling acupuncture treatment should be provided immediately after the injury for managing pain and reducing swelling and inflammation; other medical care, possibly including surgery, should also be sought immediately. Dry needling acupuncture is extremely helpful at all phases of treatment and rehabilitation for this injury. The author recommends one session every day for swelling and two sessions per week for pain symptoms.

Joint Separations of the Shoulder Girdle

Acromioclavicular and sternoclavicular separation can be caused by a direct blow to the shoulder or sternum, by a fall onto the shoulder or onto an outstretched hand, or by impact to the shoulder caused by another athlete landing on top of it.

Separation of the acromioclavicular joint ligaments usually happens during collision sports such as football and hockey; throwing sports such as javelin, hammer, and shotput; or during any training exercises that are designed to improve upper extremity strength. The athlete experiences pain, tenderness, and swelling at the acromioclavicular joint and pain or discomfort when the acromioclavicular joint is stretched during cross-body adduction (turning the injured arm medially). There may be palpable or observable joint deformity.

Sternoclavicular separation occurs when the sternoclavicular ligament is torn, which may happen when the shoulder forcefully strikes the ground or when another athlete lands upon it; when there is a direct blow to the shoulder; or when the person falls on an outstretched arm. The separation can happen in front of or behind the sternum. The symptoms are pain, tenderness, swelling at the joint, and possible displacement of the clavicle in front of or behind the sternum.

Dry needling acupuncture treatment is very effective in reducing pain, swelling and tenderness immediately after the injury and during all phases of healing and rehabilitation. Two or three needles should be inserted into the swollen ligaments and surrounding tissues. There should be one session every day for swelling and two sessions per week for pain.

Biceps Brachii Tendon Rupture

The biceps brachii muscles operate across three joints: the glenohumeral joint and the two elbow joints. A biceps brachii tendon rupture is the detachment of the tendon from the bone, and it usually happens at the proximal end of the tendon. The injury is caused by sudden trauma to the biceps brachii tendon during weightlifting or throwing activities. The injury can also be caused by weakness of the biceps brachii muscle or tears in the rotator cuff muscle caused by repetitive strain. It may also be connected to degenerative changes in the tendons in older people.

The injury produces sharp pain at the shoulder, inability to flex or extend the forearm, and a bulge or swelling in the upper arm.

Regardless of whether surgery is required, dry needling acupuncture treatment is helpful in reducing the symptoms immediately after the injury and during all phases of rehabilitation. One session every day for swelling and two sessions per week for pain are recommended.

Biceps Brachii Muscle Strain and Bruising

Muscle strain and bruising are among the most common sports injuries. Muscle strain is a tearing that is caused by the sudden extension of a joint beyond its normal range of function or by any other excessive physical demand made on the muscle. This type of injury to the biceps brachii or the pectoralis major and pectoralis minor can occur while the athlete wards off a check in hockey or tackling in football, during weight training, or as a consequence of sudden, violent torsion of the shoulder during throwing sports. The athlete may feel stiffness, tenderness, or pain in the affected muscles, and motion in the affected joints may be limited.

Other symptoms may include bruising of the muscles after a direct blow and tearing or rupture of the tendon.

Dry needling acupuncture is very helpful for muscle strains and bruising. Two to three needles per square centimeter can be applied every other day to the affected muscles where there is tenderness, pain, and discoloration. If the injury is on the chest area, the usual recommendations for safety should be followed to avoid puncturing the organs below.

Bicipital Tendinitis

Overuse of biceps brachii without proper relaxation or a sudden increase in the duration or intensity of training can stress bicipital tendons and result in tendinitis. This injury is common in athletes engaged in throwing sports and also in weightlifters, golfers, and rowers.

The injury produces pain and tenderness along the length of the tendon over the bicipital groove during resisted forearm supination and elbow flexion.

Dry needling acupuncture is very helpful in healing the tendinitis. Needles should be applied directly into the inflamed tendon, the surrounding tissues, the shoulder muscles, and the tender points in the biceps brachii. One session every day for swollen tissues and two sessions per week for pain are recommended.

Impingement Syndrome of the Shoulder

The major symptoms of impingement syndrome of the shoulder include shoulder pain during sleep when the patient rolls onto the injured arm, when the arm is rotated to reach the back, or when the arm is raised in the air. This injury is caused by a narrowing of the space between the rotator cuff and the acromion, and it impairs the joint movement.

The rotator cuff consists of four muscles—supraspinatus, infraspinatus, teres minor, and subscapularis—and includes their musculotendinous attachments. They work together to stabilize the glenohumeral joint. The subacromial bursa, the largest and most commonly injured bursa in the shoulder, provides the rotator cuff with lubrication for movement.

Damage and tears of the rotator cuff cause the humeral head to migrate from the normal position during elevation or rotation of the arm, which leads to impingement. Impingement syndrome is usually related to repetitive arm-overhead movements in tennis, swimming, golf, or weightlifting, and to throwing sports such as baseball. Impingement syndrome often becomes chronic.

In addition to conventional therapy, dry needling acupuncture is very helpful in relieving pain. Needles can be applied to all tender or painful areas including the area under the acromion.

Dry needling acupuncture should be offered immediately after surgery. One session every day for swelling and two sessions per week for pain and rehabilitation are recommended.

Rotator Cuff Tendonitis

Repetitive overhead arm motion, as in tennis, baseball, swimming, volleyball, and weightlifting, may create stress in the rotator cuff, which results in soft tissue inflammation and leads to rotator cuff tendonitis.

The rotator cuff aligns the head of the humerus in the scapula and stabilizes this ball-and-socket joint. After excessive repeated use of the rotator cuff, the rotator cuff muscles and tendons become tight, and the head of the humerus can pinch the cuff, which causes inflammation of the subacromial bursa that cushions the rotator cuff, acromion, and humerus. Symptoms may include weakness and pain during arm-overhead activities, pain in the shoulder when the patient lies on it, and a popping or cracking sensation in the shoulder.

As with other soft tissue pain, dry needling acupuncture can be used in all phases of this injury and when surgery is required. Treatment involves needling in the painful or tender area and its associated muscles and is provided usually twice per week for recovery and immediately after the surgery.

Regular weekly treatment of the shoulder with dry needling acupuncture can prevent this injury and improve the joint movement.

Shoulder Bursitis

Shoulder bursitis is often associated with rotator cuff tear, impingement syndrome, or regional soft tissue inflammation, and it is caused by overuse of the shoulder from the throwing motions of tennis, swimming, baseball, and weight training.

The tendons of the rotator cuff muscle rotate the humerus, raising the arm by pulling down the humeral head. At the same time, the deltoid muscle pulls up the arm. Through excessive repetitions of this action, the subacromial bursa that serves as cushion between the acromion and the rotator cuff may become irritated, which causes inflammation and accumulation of excess fluid in the bursa. Major symptoms are pain in the shoulder, especially when the arm is raised; weakness of the joint; limited motion of the shoulder joint; and pain when the patient sleeps on the injured joint.

Dry needling acupuncture is very effective in treating the pain of this injury. It can be applied at all phases of this injury and in patients with infection of the bursae. Tender, painful, and swelling areas and associated arm and shoulder muscles should be needled. Two sessions per week are recommended.

Frozen Shoulder (Adhesive Capsulitis)

Frozen shoulder is caused by scar tissue formed inside the space of the glenohumeral joint with reduced synovial fluid. This condition usually occurs after repeated tearing of soft tissue surrounding the joint, or it may be caused by scar tissue formed after shoulder injury or by adhesion after surgery. The joint capsule appears to be a major source of limitation of movement in this condition. A dull, aching pain is felt in the shoulder when the arm is lifted, and it often gets worse at night.

Accompanied by other therapies, dry needling acupuncture is a helpful modality for this injury, including cases in which surgery is required. Needling can be applied to all the tender and painful tissues and their associated musculature, twice per week.

Pectoral Muscle Tendinitis

The pectoralis major muscle forms the anterior wall of the axilla. It originates in the clavicle, sternum, and first six costal cartilages and inserts in the greater tubercle of the humerus. This muscle serves several functions, such as adduction and medial rotation of the humerus. Thus it is used in many sports when arms act to push away a weight or during climbing when one arm pulls the body up to the other arm, which is fixed.

Excessive force against the muscle from pushing by other athletes in contact sports or excessive load on the muscle during training may cause inflammation of the insertion tendon on the humerus. This injury may produce pain and weakness in the shoulder, and difficulty raising the arm.

Needling the pectoral insertion tendon, the muscle proper, and the associated shoulder muscles is very helpful for accelerating recovery. When needling the pectoral muscles, the practitioner must be careful to avoid pneumothorax. Two sessions per week are recommended.

SPORTS INJURIES OF THE ELBOW

The elbow is a hinge joint that consists of three bones: the humerus, the ulna, and the radius. The distal end of the humerus articulates with the ulna and the radius. The humerus and ulna are reinforced medially by the ulnar collateral ligament, which includes three strong bands: the anterior oblique, posterior oblique, and transverse. The capsule is reinforced laterally by the radial collateral ligament, a strong triangular ligament. All these ligaments connect the humerus to the ulna to stabilize the elbow joint. The annular ligament binds the head of the radius to the ulna, forming the proximal radioulnar joint.

The elbow is capable of flexion and extension, as well as pronation and supination.

Elbow injuries may occur in all kinds of training and sports as a result of overuse or trauma. Dry needling acupuncture can be used in all cases of elbow injury for accelerating soft tissue healing, especially as an adjunct to other treatment modalities ranging from physical therapy to surgery.

Elbow Fracture

Elbow fracture may be caused by a blunt force striking the elbow during contact sports, a fall directly onto the elbow, or torsion of the elbow beyond its normal range of motion. According to the location of the injury, the fracture can be classified as a distal humeral fracture, a radial fracture, or an ulnar fracture. The major symptoms are swelling and pain in the elbow region, loss of mobility, and deformity of the elbow.

Immediate medical care is needed. After emergency help, dry needling acupuncture can be used to reduce swelling and pain, and it accelerates healing in all cases. Needles can be applied to the painful, tender, and swollen tissues. In case of swelling, two to three needles per square centimeter may be used. Two treatment sessions per week should be offered.

Elbow Sprain

Elbow sprain is caused by overstretching or tearing of elbow ligaments. It is common in many sports with activities such as throwing or sudden twisting of the arm, or it can be caused by falling on an outstretched arm. The sprained elbow may be painful, with tenderness, swelling, or bruising around the elbow.

Dry needling acupuncture is a very effective modality for this condition and should be used immediately after the injury. Needles can be applied to the painful, tender, and swollen tissues. To reduce swelling, two to three needles per square centimeter may be used. One session every day for swelling and two sessions per week for pain are recommended.

Elbow Dislocation

Elbow dislocation is caused by a blow to the elbow, by violent contact between the elbow and another athlete (as in football), or by a fall on an outstretched arm. The trauma may affect the nerves or arteries of the arm, or both. The athlete who suffers from this injury may have severe pain, swelling, and loss of feeling in the hand.

Dry needling acupuncture can be used immediately after the accident to reduce swelling and pain. To reduce swelling, two to three needles per square centimeter may be used. One session every day for swelling and two sessions per week for pain are recommended.

Triceps Brachii Tendon Rupture

This relatively rare condition is also known as *tendon avulsion.* The triceps brachii tendon inserts into the back of the elbow. This location may be injured by falling or by the application of excessive force. Weightlifters and football linemen are at risk for this condition. The condition may also develop in nonathletes with hyperparathyroidism or diabetes mellitus.

Dry needling acupuncture is a very effective modality for athletes who suffer from this injury. To reduce pain, swelling, and muscle spasm, two dry needling acupuncture sessions per week should be provided. To reduce swelling, two to three needles per square centimeter in affected tissue may be used every day. Nonathletes with metabolic disorders may need more time for recovery.

Lateral Epicondylitis (Tennis Elbow)

This common injury is caused by strain from overuse of the extensor muscles of the hand or by direct impact to the elbow. Arthritis, rheumatism, or gout may cause the same symptoms. The inflamed tissues are painful and tender to the touch.

Various muscles attach to the lateral epicondyle of the humerus, including the extensor muscles of the hand, the anconeus, and supinator muscles. Thus the treatment should include needling both the inflamed tendon and the strained muscles. Dry needling acupuncture is very effective for this condition, but in some cases, recovery from the injury takes months because the inflamed tendon or tendons heal slowly. Dry needling acupuncture sessions may be offered twice per week. Application of moist heat to the tendon and muscles after needling is helpful.

Medial Epicondylitis (Golfer's Elbow)

The medial epicondyle is the insertion site of flexor muscles, and golfer's elbow is caused by repetitive overuse of these muscles—for example, forceful, repeated bending of the fingers and wrist, repeated stress on the arm during the acceleration phase of the throwing motion, and repeated tightening of the flexor muscles and tendons during a golf swing—or by trauma to the medial aspect of the elbow. Neck problems, arthritis, rheumatism, and gout may cause similar symptoms.

The symptoms are pain and tenderness at the medial epicondyle, particularly when the wrist is flexed or when objects are grasped or lifted. Extending the arm becomes difficult because of the pain.

As in lateral epicondylitis, dry needling acupuncture is very effective for this condition, but in some cases, recovery can take months because the inflamed tendon or tendons heal slowly. Dry needling acupuncture sessions may be offered twice per week; both the inflamed tendon and the strained muscles are needled. Application of moist heat to the tendon and muscles after needling is helpful. The neck should also be treated if it too is involved.

Thrower's Elbow

Repetitive strain from any throwing activity can cause this condition. Inflammation causes pain on both sides of the elbow, and additional complaints are numbness, stiffness, and weakness. Bone spurs and chips may develop from the chronic stress. This injury is found in athletes who throw repeatedly, such as pitchers in baseball and bowlers in cricket, and in those who throw javelin or play volleyball or tennis.

In addition to the three bones (humerus, ulna, and radius), the elbow includes three joints: the humeroulnar, humeroradial, and proximal radioulnar joints. A forceful throwing motion can damage these joints and their associated ligaments, tendons, and muscles. Throwing activity results simultaneously in compression of structures on the lateral elbow and stretching of structures on the medial elbow.

As with epicondylitis, dry needling acupuncture is very helpful for this condition, but recovery from this injury may take longer. Dry needling acupuncture treatment is similar to that of lateral and medial epicondylitis.

Elbow Bursitis

This injury is also known as *olecranon bursitis*. The olecranon bursa is located above the olecranon process, and it is the largest bursa in the elbow region. Noninflammatory bursitis is associated with repeated stress or acute trauma, whereas inflammatory bursitis is caused by such conditions as rheumatism and infection.

The symptoms include painful swelling, excessive fluid in the bursa, and reduced mobility of the elbow.

As with epicondylitis, dry needling acupuncture is very helpful for elbow bursitis, but recovery from this injury may take longer. Needles are applied directly into the swollen bursa at a density of two to three per square centimeter, both into affected tissue and into the tender area of the joint and associated ligaments, tendons, and muscles. Two dry needling acupuncture sessions per week should be offered.

SPORTS INJURIES OF THE WRIST AND FOREARM

Wrist Fracture

Wrist and forearm fracture may occur when an outstretched hand is used to break a fall. Such accidents happen in running, cycling, inline skating, skateboarding, and other sports.

The wrist complex includes the radiocarpal joint and intercarpal articulations. Most wrist movement occurs at the radiocarpal joint. Eight carpal bones are arranged in two rows: proximal and distal. The distal surface of the radius and the articular disc articulate with the proximal row of carpal bones: the scaphoid, lunate, and triquetrum. The intercarpal joints are a series of plane joints that have articulations between the two carpal rows (midcarpal joints), in addition to reticulations between each bone of the proximal carpal and distal carpal row. As a whole, the carpal bones form a convex dorsal arch. The arch is enclosed by a transverse ligament, the flexor retinaculum, to become a carpal tunnel.

The distal radioulnar joint is immediately adjacent to the radiocarpal joint. A cartilaginous disc separates the distal ulna and radius from the lunate and triquetral bones. Wrist fractures are breaks in one or more of these bones. Two common fractures are fracture of the end of the radius and scaphoid fracture, which involves the scaphoid or navicular bone, a small bone that joins the radius and is located on the thumb side of the wrist.

Dry needling acupuncture is very helpful in reducing pain and swelling and should be used immediately after the injury, regardless of whether surgery is needed. When surgery is necessary, dry needling acupuncture can be used immediately afterwards to accelerate healing during rehabilitation. Needles are applied to the tender tissues and the swollen issue at a density of about two to three per square centimeter. Two dry needling acupuncture sessions per week should be offered.

Wrist Sprain

Injury to ligaments of the wrist is common when the hand is extended to break a fall. Such accidents occur in ice skating, snowboarding, roller skating, cycling, soccer, football, baseball, and volleyball. An athlete with this injury may feel pain, swelling, and burning or tingling sensation, with bruising at the wrist.

Wrist sprains vary from moderate to severe. In severe cases, complete tearing of the ligaments may occur. Dry needling acupuncture is most effective if used immediately after the accident. Apply needles to the painful, swollen and bruised tissue at about two to three needles per square centimeter. Swelling can be treated once every day. Two sessions per week should be offered.

Wrist Dislocation

This injury is caused by falling on an outstretched hand. Most wrist dislocations involve the lunate bone of the proximal row of carpal bones and other bones. When the dislocation occurs, the affected bone is no longer properly articulating with adjoining bones. The injury affects the soft tissue surrounding the region of dislocation, including muscles, nerves, tendons, ligaments, and blood vessels. Thus numbness or paralysis below the dislocation may accompany the severe pain.

Dry needling acupuncture as an effective modality should be used immediately after the accident. Apply about two to three needles per square centimeter to the painful, numb, and bruised tissue in two sessions per week.

Carpal Tunnel Syndrome

This injury results from the compression of the median nerve in the carpal tunnel. As discussed previously, the carpal tunnel is a narrow, rigid structure composed of a transverse ligament and carpal bones at the base of the hand. The tunnel surrounds the median nerve, which enters the hand between the carpal bones and innervates the palm side of the thumb and fingers. Carpal tunnel syndrome is caused by excessive wrist movements such as repetitive flexion and extension of the wrist (as in cycling, throwing, racket sports, and gymnastics), which result in squeezing or compression of the median nerve in the tunnel at the wrist. Trauma or injury, including fracture or sprain, wrist swelling, arthritis, or hypertrophy of the bone, can also produce carpal tunnel syndrome.

Other symptoms of this injury include burning sensation, numbness, tingling sensation, itching in the palm of the hand and fingers, wrist swelling, decreased grip strength, and pain that can wake a person.

Dry needling is effective in relieving pain from this injury. The treatment should be started as early as possible. Needles are applied to the top of the ligament and into the carpal tunnel, the recurrent nerve point on the thenar muscles, and both the extensor and flexor muscles on the forearm. Two sessions per week should be offered.

Ulnar Nerve Injury

The ulnar nerve is susceptible to injury because it passes through the ulnar tunnel posteriorly at the elbow, between the medial epicondyle of the humerus and the olecranon of the ulna, and then across the wrist into the hand. Injuries at the elbow may affect the muscles innervated by the ulnar nerve in the forearm and hand, and injuries at the hand affect the intrinsic muscles supplied by this nerve in the hand. Overuse of muscles and tendons of the forearm or sudden trauma to the nerve within the ulnar tunnel at the elbow can cause the damage to the ulnar nerve.

The major symptoms of this injury may include tingling sensation on the ulnar side of the forearm, weakness and numbness on the ulnar side of the hand, and weakness and difficulty in grasping objects.

Dry needling acupuncture is very helpful for this injury. Needles can be applied to the ulnar tunnel area and to affected muscles and tendons on the forearm and hand. Two treatment sessions per week are recommended.

Wrist Tendinitis

The tendons of the wrist are encased in a tendon sheath, the tenosynovium. Tendon sheaths provide for smooth, friction-free sliding of the tendons. Overuse of the wrist in sports such as racquet sports, rowing, weightlifting, gymnastics, and any ball games and also repetitive stress from using a keyboard can cause inflammation, swelling, and thickening of the tendon sheath, which constricts the smooth movement of the tendons inside the sheath.

Dry needling acupuncture is a very effective modality for alleviating this condition. Two to three needles per square centimeter can be applied to the inflamed and swollen tissue and to the associated muscles. Two treatment sessions per week are recommended.

SPORTS INJURIES OF THE HAND AND FINGERS

Metacarpal Fracture

A direct blow to the hand, falling on the hand, or forceful strike with closed fist on a hard object can cause metacarpal fracture; these events happen in football, basketball, and other contact sports. A fracture of the neck of the fifth metacarpal is the most common type. Pain, swelling, and bruising occur locally, and bone deformity may be observed.

Immediate medical attention is warranted, and surgery is needed in some cases. Dry needling acupuncture can be used immediately after the emergency treatment. Needles can be applied to the tissue at the site of pain, swelling, and bruising. Needling may be needed in wrist tendons, wrist muscles, and associated tissue, along with the injured area.

Thumb and Finger Sprain

The ligaments of the thumb, which connect the metacarpal bone to the first phalanx at the base of the thumb, may be overstretched and torn. Repetitive overuse of the thumb with the index finger or other fingers may wear these ligaments and their muscles.

Blows to the hand and hyperextension of the finger joints when falling may damage the dorsal or palmar ligaments of the finger. Finger sprain is a common injury in many sports such as football, basketball, cricket, and handball and in all contact sports.

Dry needling acupuncture is effective in healing these conditions. Needles can be applied to the painful and swollen area, especially the base of the thumb on the radial, dorsal and palmar sides. The thenar muscles, other intrinsic muscles, and related flexor and extensor muscles should be examined and treated with needles. Two treatment sessions per week are recommended.

The same principle of treatment is applied to finger sprain. Needles can be applied to the painful, tender, and swollen tissues. The intrinsic muscles and flexor and extensor muscles should be examined.

Finger Dislocation

Fingers may become dislocated if they are struck by a football, baseball, or basketball or when the person falls onto the hand. Immediate medical care should be sought, and dry needling acupuncture can be used immediately after emergency treatment. Fine and short needles should be applied to the injured tissue to reduce pain and swelling. Two to three treatment sessions per week are recommended.

Hand and Finger Tendinitis

Tendons bear considerable mechanical stress when transmitting forces between muscles and bone. Overuse of the muscles causes inflammation of the tendons, tendon sheaths, and muscles.

Dry needling acupuncture is very effective in alleviating this condition. Fine needles can be applied to the inflamed tendon, and normal needles can be applied the related muscles. Treatment should be provided two to three times per week. The affected fingers should be properly cared for so as not to stress the inflamed tendons during recovery; otherwise, the condition may become chronic.

SPORTS INJURIES OF THE BACK AND SPINE

A healthy and well-balanced back is essential in all kinds of sports, as well as in daily life. Evidence-based research in sports medicine indicates that a stable core system is crucial for proper movement of the limbs.

Back injury is common in both sports and daily life, but fewer than 5% of back injuries necessitate surgery. Strength training of the back muscles is the best strategy for preventing back injury. Proper and regular maintenance of the back musculature is no less important than strength training. Dry needling acupuncture, with its unique mechanisms for treating soft tissue, is effective both for treating an injured back and for maintaining a balanced back. Even when the back is pain free, weekly dry needling acupuncture treatment is suggested for all athletes, especially those who are performing intensive training.

Muscle Strain of the Back

Back movements recruit extensors (including gluteal muscles), flexors (abdominal muscles and iliopsoas muscles), and oblique muscles (side muscles). Back strain often occurs in the lumbar region, although the thoracic region may also be involved.

Muscle strain can be caused by repetitive stress to the muscles or by sudden strain or torsion of the back muscles as a result of lifting or abrupt movements such as falling or colliding with another athlete. These injuries may happen in any sport and in daily activities.

Of all the medical modalities available, dry needling acupuncture is most effective in reducing pain and stiffness and in restoring the normal function of the spine. The core system affects all peripheral movement, which means that spinal disorder affects the movement of the limbs; therefore the treatment should be systemic. In addition to the lumbar region, the shoulders, neck, hips, iliotibial bands, hamstring muscles, and calf muscles should all be treated together. Two treatment sessions per week are recommended.

Ligament Sprain of the Back

Ligaments provide strong and flexible connections between bones. The spine is supported by several ligaments: The anterior and posterior longitudinal ligaments connect the vertebral bodies of the entire spine (cervical, thoracic, and lumbar). The causes of ligament sprain are the same as those of muscle sprain, and the injured soft tissue can be simultaneously both the muscles and the ligaments of the back.

Recovery from ligament sprain of the back takes longer than recovery from muscle sprain of the back. Dry needling acupuncture therapy is very helpful in alleviating this condition. Needles can be applied to the painful, tender, and swollen region. In most cases, direct needling of the ligament is impossible, and the treatment may focus on the sensitive area. When treating the condition, the practitioner should not ignore the neck, shoulders, hips, and lower limbs. Two treatment sessions per week are recommended.

Thoracic Contusion

Thoracic contusion may be caused by a collision on the back with another athlete, as in football; a blow from sports equipment, as in hockey or lacrosse; or a hard fall on the back. Bruising, swelling, pain, and tenderness may appear at the injured site.

Contusions are trauma to the subcutaneous tissue. The muscles are well vascularized, and blood flow in the tissue is likely to be high at a moment in sport when injury occurs. Blood seeps out from torn blood vessels and flows into the skin and subcutaneous tissues, forming ecchymoses. Capillaries are damaged by the physical force of impact, resulting in blood seepage into the surrounding tissue. Although most contusion injuries are minor, serious injuries such as fractures or internal bleeding may also be present.

Medical attention is needed immediately after the accident to rule out or confirm (and treat) severe injuries. Dry needling acupuncture is the most effective modality in alleviating the pain of this injury, both minor and severe. Two to three fine needles per square centimeter should be applied to the injured area every other day.

Disc Herniation

Intervertebral discs provide absorption from shock and allow for the smooth motion of the spine by preventing the bones from rubbing against each other. The spine is the first part of the body to start degenerating, and this can happen even in a person's early 20s; thus discopathy is a common problem in adults. The biomechanics of the spine is briefly introduced in Chapter 12. In addition to natural degeneration or age-related wear, disc herniation can be aggravated by improper lifting of weights, excessive strain on the spinal musculature, or physical trauma to the discs.

Pain can be felt in the back, neck, buttocks, legs, and feet, sometimes with numbness and tingling sensation. It may affect control of the bowels or bladder.

In addition to conventional medical approaches, dry needling acupuncture is very effective in alleviating pain in most cases of disc herniation, including those for which surgery is required. Systemic examination of the ARPs should be performed, and treatment in every case should be systemic. The treatment should include the neck, shoulder, upper and lower back, hips, legs, and even feet. Two treatment sessions per week are recommended.

For prevention of this injury, athletes should receive weekly systemic treatment to balance the musculoskeletal system.

Stress Fracture of the Vertebra

This common athletic injury occurs most often in gymnastics, weightlifting, and football. The injury is related to overuse, flexion, twisting, or hyperextension of the spine and most often is found in the fifth lumbar vertebra.

The symptoms include back pain and muscle stiffness or spasms, with tingling sensation in the thigh or lower leg.

Regardless of whether surgery is needed, dry needling acupuncture is very helpful in reducing the pain and tingling sensation and in restoring spine function. The treatment procedure is exactly the same as that for disc herniation, but the healing process in this injury may take a longer time. Two treatment sessions per week should be given.

This injury can be prevented by weekly dry needling acupuncture to reduce the stress on the musculature, tendons, and ligaments of the spine.

ABDOMINAL MUSCLE STRAIN

Spreading between the ribs and the pelvis, the anterior abdominal wall muscles encase the internal organs and hold them in place. These muscles also act to support the trunk and lower back and to assist movement. There are three layers of abdominal muscle. The deepest layer is the transversus abdominis, whose fibers run approximately horizontally. The middle layer is the internal oblique muscle, whose fibers are crossed by the outermost layer, the external oblique muscle. Overlying these three layers is the rectus abdominis muscle, which runs vertically on either side of the middle line of the abdomen.

Abdominal muscle strain is caused by overstretching or tearing of muscle fibers during sudden and violent movement of the trunk or trauma to the region. The symptoms include abdominal pain, lower back pain, and muscle spasms.

Immediate medical examination is needed to rule out or confirm (and treat) injuries of the internal organs or severe muscle injury.

As with all muscle strain, dry needling acupuncture is very effective in accelerating healing. Depending on the thickness of the abdominal wall, about one to three 25-mm- to 50-mm-long needles per square centimeter are applied to the strained muscles. Two treatment sessions per week are recommended.

SPORTS INJURIES OF THE HIPS, PELVIS, AND GROIN

Hip Flexor Strain

The iliopsoas and rectus femoris are the major hip flexors. Repetitive stress on the hip flexor muscles without adequate recovery is the major cause of muscle strain. Improper gait can also create this type of problem. This injury often occurs in running, in cycling, and in kicking and jumping activities. The symptoms include pain, tenderness, and inflammation in the groin area.

Dry needling acupuncture is very effective in treating this injury. Needles can be applied to the ARPs on the iliopsoas muscle, the adductor muscles, the rectus femoris muscle, and the iliotibial band. The hamstring muscles may need treatment, too. Two treatment sessions per week should be offered.

Hip Pointer

The iliac crest provides attachment for the hip flexors, the abdominal muscles, and the muscles that rotate the hip. Direct impact on the iliac crest can cause contusion, bruising, and inflammation of tissue or even bone fracture. Severe pain can be felt after the injury happens.

Dry needling acupuncture is very effective in treating this injury. Needles can be applied to the painful tissues with two to three needles per square centimeter, including the gluteal muscles, iliotibial band, and hip flexors. Two treatment sessions per week should be provided.

Avulsion Fracture

In an avulsion fracture, a tendon or ligament pulls away from the bone at its attachment, breaking the tendon or pulling a piece of the bone away with it. Forceful twisting, flexing, extending, or direct impact on a joint inducing forceful stretching can cause this injury.

Dry needling acupuncture is very effective for reducing pain, swelling, and inflammation. Needles can be applied to the ARPs on the injured area and associated muscles, in two treatment sessions per week.

To prevent avulsion, weekly treatment for reducing stress in the musculoskeletal system is highly recommended.

Groin Strain

Muscles involved in this problem include the pectineus, adductor brevis, adductor longus, adductor magnus, and gracilis. Groin strain often occurs in sports that require pivoting and quick changes of direction, such as soccer and hockey. The injury may range from mild pain in the adductor muscles to severe pain, tenderness, and inflammation in this area. Damage is usually localized to the musculotendinous junction, about 5 cm from the pubis.

Dry needling acupuncture is very effective in treating this injury. Needles can be applied to the symptomatic points on the iliopsoas muscle, the adductor muscles, the rectus femoris muscle, and the iliotibial band. The hamstring muscles need treatment, too. Two treatment sessions per week should be offered.

Osteitis Pubis

Inflammation of the pubic symphysis and the surrounding muscles may result from repetitive stress, or imbalance of the adductor muscles, iliotibial bands, or hip flexor muscles. Athletes who perform running, kicking, or rapid lateral movement, such as sprinters, soccer players, and hockey players, are more susceptible to this injury. Major symptoms include pain in the pubic symphysis, lower abdomen, and groin area.

Dry needling acupuncture is very effective in alleviating this condition, but healing may take a long time. Fine needles should be used directly on the pubic symphysis, and normal needles should be used on surrounding muscles, including the abdominal muscles, hip flexors, adductors, and iliotibial band. Two treatment sessions per week should be provided.

Stress Fracture

Stress fractures can occur in any bone but occur mostly in the bones of the foot, lower leg, and hip. This injury is mostly caused by repetitive stress or strength imbalance that results from muscle fatigue.

Fatigued muscles are tight and no longer able to absorb the shock of impact, and so the physical stress is transferred directly to the bone.

This injury creates generalized pain in the area, especially during weight bearing. The pain may be severe in the beginning and during running, and then it may subside but returns after running has finished.

Dry needling acupuncture is very effective in treating this injury. Needles can be applied to the symptomatic area. The treatment is used to balance the entire musculoskeletal system. Two treatment sessions per week should be provided.

Prevention of this injury is possible with weekly treatment for balancing the musculoskeletal system.

Piriformis Syndrome

The piriformis muscle originates at the internal surface of the sacrum and inserts at the superior border of the trochanter of the femur. It functions in helping lateral rotation of the hip joint, abducting the thigh when the hip is flexed, and assisting stability of the head of the femur in the acetabulum. Piriformis syndrome occurs when the piriformis muscle becomes tight and shortened and applies pressure on the sciatic nerve. It is caused by repetitive stress built up in the muscle, such as that engendered by incorrect gait during walking or jogging. The symptoms are similar to sciatica in that pain is felt along the sciatic nerve, triggered in walking up stairs, and increased after prolonged sitting.

Dry needling acupuncture is an effective treatment for this injury. Needles can be applied directly into the piriformis muscle on its belly, insertion, and origin area. In addition, as with any low back problems, the ARPs of the muscles in the thigh and leg that are innervated by the sciatic nerve should be needled also because these muscles are painful or inflamed, too. The treatment is used to balance the entire musculoskeletal system. Two treatment sessions per week should be provided.

Trochanteric Bursitis

The trochanteric bursa lies between the gluteus maximus and the posterolateral aspect of the greater trochanter. Several muscles cross this bursa and may rub across the trochanter when the muscles are tight and fatigued as a result of direct physical impact on the bone or repetitive stress, such as that which may affect the iliotibial band in running.

The symptoms include tenderness and swelling of the hip or thigh and pain in flexing or extending the hip.

Dry needling acupuncture is an effective treatment for this injury. Needles can be applied directly into the inflamed bursa and into related muscles on the hip, thigh, and lower leg. In addition, the treatment is used to balance the entire musculoskeletal system. Two treatment sessions per week should be provided.

SPORTS INJURIES OF THE THIGH

Femur Fracture

A hard impact on the femur—such as those that may happen in a motor vehicle accident, in a fall, or in football or hockey games—can cause femur fracture. This injury necessitates immediate medical attention. After emergency treatment, dry needling acupuncture can be applied to reduce pain, inflammation, and swelling before and after surgery and during rehabilitation. Two treatment sessions per week should be provided.

Quadriceps Strain

Four muscles make up the quadriceps: the vastus lateralis, vastus medialis, vastus intermedius, and rectus femoris. The quadriceps is involved in moving the hip and knee and supporting body weight. The rectus femoris is more susceptible to strain injury than the other three muscles. The injury can result from repetitive contraction without adequate relaxation or forceful contraction, which may occur in sprinting, jumping, football, hockey, and weight training.

Dry needling acupuncture is an effective treatment for this injury. Needles can be applied directly into the inflamed, tender, swollen, and painful area and also into related muscles on the hip, thigh, and lower leg. In addition, the treatment is used to balance the entire musculoskeletal system. Two treatment sessions per week should be provided.

Hamstring Strain

The hamstrings are composed of three separate muscles: the biceps femoris laterally and the semitendinosus and semimembranosus medially. The three muscles work together to extend the hip and flex the knee. During running, the hamstrings slow down the leg at the end of the forward swing phase and prevent flexion of the trunk at the hip joint.

Hamstring strain is a common injury in running and sprinting and is related to an imbalance in strength between the hamstrings and the quadriceps or to excessive overload on the muscles. The injury may involve both muscles and tendons.

Dry needling acupuncture is an effective treatment for this injury in cases where surgery is not required. Needles can be applied directly into the inflamed, tender, swollen, and painful area and into related muscles on the hip, thigh, and lower leg, such as the gluteal muscles, adductors, and abductors. In addition, the treatment is used to balance the entire musculoskeletal system. Two treatment sessions per week should be provided. If surgery is required, dry needling acupuncture can be used before and after surgery and during rehabilitation.

Thigh Contusion

A thigh contusion is a deep bruising of the muscles of the quadriceps or hamstrings near the femur. This common injury is caused by a strong impact to the muscles, as in football or hockey, or by a hard fall. This may cause bleeding in the muscles near the femur and results in the formation of scar tissue, which reduces muscular flexibility.

Dry needling acupuncture is an effective treatment for this injury. Needles can be applied directly into the inflamed, tender, swollen, and painful area and into related muscles in the hip, thigh, and lower leg. Two to three needles per square centimeter should be used. In addition, the treatment is used to balance the entire musculoskeletal system. Two treatment sessions per week should be provided. The area of contusion can be treated every other day.

Iliotibial Band Syndrome

The iliotibial band is a nonelastic collagen cord that stretches from the iliac crest, blends with the tensor fasciae latae and gluteus maximus muscles, and then descends to insert into the tubercle on the lateral proximal tibia. The tensor fasciae latae muscle flexes, abducts, and medially rotates the hip joint and stabilizes the knee.

Repetitive hip and knee flexion and extension while the tensor fasciae latae muscle is contracted creates tension and inflammation of the iliotibial band, leading to compression or friction of the band on the tissues below. The common symptoms are knee pain over the lateral condyle, especially during knee flexion and extension.

Dry needling acupuncture is an effective treatment for this injury. Needles can be applied directly into the inflamed, tender, swollen, and painful area on the iliotibial band and into related muscles on the hip, thigh, and lower leg. In addition, the treatment is used to balance the entire musculoskeletal system. Two treatment sessions per week should be provided.

SPORTS INJURIES OF THE KNEE

Ligament Sprains of the Knee

The knee has four supporting ligaments: the medial collateral, fibular collateral, anterior cruciate, and posterior cruciate. The medial collateral ligament spans from the medial epicondyle of the femur to the medial condyle of the tibia. This broad ligament holds the knee joint together on the medial side. Force applied to the lateral side may overstretch or tear this ligament partially or completely. A tearing of the medial meniscus may result from the sprain and necessitates surgical repair.

The anterior cruciate ligament spreads from the anterior intercondylar area of the tibia to the medial surface of the lateral femoral condyle. This ligament prevents posterior displacement of the femur on the tibia and helps check hyperextension of the knee. Sprain of the anterior cruciate ligament is another common injury. It can be caused by forceful twisting of the knee or by a direct blow on the knee.

Dry needling acupuncture is a helpful therapy for healing this type of injury. Needles can be applied directly into the inflamed, tender, swollen, and painful area and into related muscles on the thigh and lower leg. In addition, the treatment is used to balance the entire musculoskeletal system. Two treatment sessions per week should be provided. If surgery is required for repairing the ligament and the meniscus, dry needling acupuncture can be used before and after surgery to reduce pain and swelling.

Meniscal Tear

Meniscal tear is another common injury of the knee. The menisci help distribute the weight evenly through the joint, act as a shock absorber, and provide cushioning and protection for the ends of the femur and tibia.

This injury may be caused by forceful twisting of the knee joint and may accompany ligament strain as well.

Orthopedic surgery is necessary to repair this injury. Nevertheless, dry needling acupuncture is helpful before and after the surgery. Needles can be applied directly into the inflamed, tender, swollen, and painful area and into related muscles on the thigh and lower leg. In addition, the treatment is used to balance the entire musculoskeletal system. Two treatment sessions per week should be provided.

Knee Bursitis

The knee has five bursae: the suprapatellar, situated between the femur and the quadriceps femoris tendon; the subcutaneous prepatellar, situated between the skin and the anterior surface of the patella; the superficial infrapatellar, situated between the skin and the patellar tendon; the deep infrapatellar, situated between the tibial tuberosity and the patellar ligament; and the pes anserinus bursa, situated at the lower inside of the knee joint where the sartorius, gracilis, and semitendinosus muscles insert jointly as the pes anserinus tendon.

Repetitive pressure or trauma to the bursae or repetitive friction between bursa and tendon results in inflammation of the bursa, as well as of the tendon.

Dry needling acupuncture is an effective treatment for knee bursitis. Needles can be applied directly into the inflamed, tender, swelling, and painful area and into related muscles around the knee. Two to three needles per square centimeter can be applied to the swelling bursa. In addition, the treatment is used to balance the entire musculoskeletal system. Two treatment sessions per week should be provided.

Patellofemoral Pain Syndrome

Incorrect running gait, weak or tight quadriceps, chronic patellar stress, and improper shoes may cause this injury. The symptoms include pain in and under the patella and a dull, aching pain in the knee. The pain worsens after sitting for long time or walking down stairs.

Dry needling acupuncture is effective in treating this injury. Needles can be applied directly into the inflamed, tender, swollen, and painful area and into related muscles on the hip, thigh, and lower leg, especially the quadriceps. In addition, the treatment is used to balance the entire musculoskeletal system. Two treatment sessions per week should be provided.

Patellar Tendinitis

The patellar tendon is involved in extending the lower leg and is the area that experiences shock upon landing from a jump. When the quadriceps contracts to slow down the flexion of the knee, the tendon is forced to stretch. Repeated stress from flexion and extension may cause trauma to the patellar tendon.

Dry needling acupuncture is effective therapy for healing this injury. Needles can be applied directly into the inflamed, tender, swollen, and painful area and into related muscles on the thigh and lower leg. Two or three needles may be used directly on the tendon. In addition, the treatment is used to balance the entire musculoskeletal system. Two treatment sessions per week should be provided.

Chondromalacia Patellae (Runner's Knee)

This injury is characterized by pain in the knee that worsens after sitting for prolonged periods and is felt upon rising from a seated position or in ascending stairs. The injury is caused by repetitive microtrauma to the cartilage on the underside of the patella, by chronic misalignment of the patella, or by previous fracture or dislocation of the patella.

Dry needling acupuncture provides symptomatic relief. Needles can be applied directly into the inflamed, tender, swollen, and painful area and into related muscles on the thigh and lower leg. If surgery is required, dry needling acupuncture can be used before and after surgery. In addition, the treatment is used to balance the entire musculoskeletal system. Two treatment sessions per week should be provided.

Subluxation of the Patella

The patella is attached to the quadriceps tendon proximally and to the patellar tendon distally and articulates with the patellofemoral groove on the femur to form the patellofemoral joint. The patella slides over the groove during knee flexion. However, if the vastus lateralis is stronger than the vastus medialis, the imbalance forces the patella out of the groove. The same misalignment may occur if the side of the patella sustains a physical impact or if the knee twists strongly, which may happen upon landing from a jump.

This injury may cause pain and swelling or a feeling of pressure behind the patella, especially during knee flexion and extension.

Dry needling acupuncture is very effective for treating this injury. Needles can be applied directly into the inflamed, tender, swollen, and painful area. Needles can be applied to the quadriceps to balance the muscle tension on the patella. In addition, the treatment is used to balance the entire musculoskeletal system. Two treatment sessions per week should be provided.

The potential for this injury can be reduced by weekly balancing treatment.

SPORTS INJURIES BELOW THE KNEE

Fractures of the Tibia and Fibula

These fractures are caused by direct force on the bones, such that which occurs in landing from a high fall; by violent twisting when the foot is fixed; or by a rotational force on the bones, such as a tackle in football.

The symptoms include extreme pain, inability to move the leg or bear weight on the bones, swelling, and tenderness. Deformity may be observable.

Medical attention and emergency treatment should be obtained without delay. Dry needling acupuncture can be applied to the inflamed, tender, swollen, and painful area after emergency treatment and after surgery. In addition, the treatment is used to balance the entire musculoskeletal system. Two treatment sessions per week should be provided.

Calf Strain

Calf muscles, or triceps surae, include the gastrocnemius, soleus, and plantaris muscles. They insert into the foot through the Achilles tendon and are responsible for extending the foot and rising on the toes. When a person takes off from the ground or changes the direction of walking, the calf muscles must contract forcefully.

If the muscles are fatigued or not strong enough to manage situations in which forceful contraction is necessary, especially eccentric contraction (when contracting and stretching happen together, as in landing from a jump), tears in the muscle occur.

Dry needling acupuncture is an effective treatment for this injury. Needles can be applied directly into the inflamed, tender, swollen, and painful area. If surgery is needed, dry needling acupuncture is very helpful in rehabilitation. In addition, the treatment is used to balance the entire musculoskeletal system. Two treatment sessions per week should be provided.

Achilles Tendinitis

The Achilles tendon is the largest tendon in the human body, with a length of 15 cm and thickness of 2 cm. It originates from the musculotendinous junction of the calf muscles and inserts into the posterior base of the calcaneus. The force exerted by the Achilles tendon on the calcaneus can be 2.5 times body weight, and the compression force on the tibia is 3.5 times body weight during standing on the tiptoes of one foot.

Achilles tendinitis can be caused by fatigued calf muscles that results from repetitive stress from running and jumping, abnormal gait during running, untreated injuries to the calf or Achilles tendon, and improper footwear. This injury is often found in athletes who participate in sports such as running, basketball, volleyball, and jumping.

Symptoms are pain, swelling, and tenderness in the tendon and difficulty in running or jumping.

Dry needling acupuncture is an effective treatment for this injury. Needles can be applied directly into the inflamed, tender, swelling, and painful tendon and into the triceps surae muscle. In addition, the treatment is used to balance the entire musculoskeletal system. Two treatment sessions per week should be provided. Dry needling acupuncture is very helpful for rehabilitation if surgery is required for repair of the injury.

A weekly treatment to balance the musculoskeletal system may reduce the possibility of this injury.

Medial Tibial Pain Syndrome (Shin Splints)

This injury is common in running and jumping. The tibialis anterior muscle is the largest of the dorsiflexor muscles. It originates from the lateral condyle of the tibia and inserts into the medial and plantar surfaces of the medial cuneiform bone. The tibialis anterior muscle is responsible for ankle dorsiflexion and inversion of the foot. Its innervation is supplied by the deep peroneal nerve (L4 and L5).

Repetitive stress on the muscle causes inflammation, swelling, and a dull, aching pain on the medial side of the tibia.

Dry needling acupuncture is an effective treatment for this injury. Needles can be applied directly into the inflamed, tender, swollen, and painful area and into the origin and insertion of the muscle. In addition, the treatment is used to balance the entire musculoskeletal system. Two treatment sessions per week should be provided.

Stress Fracture

The tibia is a weight-bearing bone and sustains a large amount of impact, and so it is more likely to sustain stress fractures if it is exposed to repetitive stress, as in running and jumping sports. Fatigued leg muscles reduce the leg's ability to absorb shock, and this lessened ability, combined with training on hard surfaces, results in stress fracture. Bones are constantly repaired and rebuilt by movement of calcium from one area to another, and this process creates weak areas that are susceptible to stress fracture. Women are more susceptible to this injury because of deficiencies in bone density related to hormone changes and osteoporosis.

The symptoms may include pain in bearing weight, which is more severe in the early stages of activity, subsides in the middle, and returns at the end. Swollen tissue may be present.

Dry needling acupuncture is effective for treating this injury. Needles can be applied into the inflamed, tender, swelling, and painful area and into the origin and insertion of the muscle. In addition, the treatment is used to balance the entire musculoskeletal system. Two treatment sessions per week should be provided.

If an athlete receives weekly balancing treatment to reduce stress and muscle fatigue, the possibility of stress fracture can be reduced. Female athletes should pay special attention to their intake of calcium.

Anterior Compartment Syndrome

The tibia and fibula, the interosseous membrane, and the intermuscular fascial septa divide the leg into three compartments: anterior (extensor), lateral (fibular), and posterior (flexor). Each compartment performs a different function. However, the fascia that covers the muscles and encases the compartment and the bone is in the form of inflexible fibrous sleeves. When intramuscular swelling or inflammation occurs as a result of repetitive overuse of the muscles or acute trauma to the muscles that may cause intramuscular bleeding and edema, the intracompartmental pressure increases; this leads to deficiency of the blood flow and dysfunction of the tissues within the compartment.

The anterior compartment is more susceptible to this injury. The symptoms include pain and muscle tightness along the tibial and fibular bone, especially during exercise; decreased sensation on top of the foot over the second toe; and possible weakness and tightness of the foot muscles.

Dry needling acupuncture is the most effective therapy for this injury. Needles can be applied directly into the compartment and into the tissues. In addition, the treatment is used to balance the entire musculoskeletal system. Two treatment sessions per week should be provided. In cases of severe trauma, surgery may be required, but dry needling

acupuncture can be used before and after surgery to reduce the pain, inflammation, and swelling.

Prevention is possible if athletes receive regular dry needling acupuncture treatment to reduce chronic stress from overuse or to promote healing in the early stage of acute trauma.

Posterior Tibial Tendinitis

The posterior tibialis muscle is the deepest muscle of the posterior compartment and has both medial and lateral origins. The medial origin is on the posterior surface of the interosseous membrane and the lateral area of the posterior surface of the tibia. The lateral origin is on the upper two thirds of the posterior fibular surface, deep transverse fascia, and intermuscular septa. The muscle's insertion tendon runs from the calf muscle behind the medial malleolus to the navicular bone in the arch of the foot. This tendon supports the arch and assists inversion of the foot. If the navicular bone is misaligned, it causes stress on this tendon and results in tendinitis. The condition can be caused by improper running, ill-fitting footwear, or previous injury to the ankle.

The symptoms of this injury include pain and tenderness over the medial side of the tibia, ankle, and foot and swelling over the tendon.

Dry needling acupuncture is very effective for treating this injury. Needles can be applied directly into the inflamed, tender, swelling, and painful tendon and into the origin and belly of the muscle. In addition, the treatment is used to balance the entire musculoskeletal system. Two treatment sessions per week should be provided.

Ankle Sprain

Ankle sprain is a common injury in most sports, as well as in daily life. This injury involves the overstretching and tearing of the ankle ligaments when the foot is rolled medially or laterally, twisted forcefully, or twisted beyond its normal range. This can happen in running, jumping, sprinting, or walking on a surface that is uneven or unpredictable, and it can occur in the movements of basketball, football, and hockey.

All the ligaments of the ankle may suffer from this injury, but the lateral ligaments are more susceptible; in fact, lateral ankle sprain is the most common type. The injury happens when force is applied to the ankle during plantarflexion and inversion, injuring the anterior talofibular ligament. Medial ankle sprains are less common because the medial ligaments, the deltoid ligament, and the bony structure are very strong.

The symptoms are usually classified into three degrees. First-degree sprains are the mildest, with little pain and swelling, and third-degree sprains involve severe pain and swelling, inability to bear weight, and instability in the joint. The symptoms of second-degree sprain are of intermediate severity between those of first- and third-degree sprains.

Dry needling acupuncture is an effective treatment for this injury. Two to three needles per square centimeter can be applied directly into the inflamed, tender, swelling, and painful ligaments. The inflammation and swelling can be easily controlled if dry needling acupuncture is applied immediately after the injury. In addition, the treatment is used to balance the entire musculoskeletal system. Two treatment sessions per week should be provided. A daily treatment can be used to reduce severe swelling.

Ankle Fracture

This bone fracture can be caused by forceful twisting or rolling of the ankle or by impact on the medial or lateral ankle when the foot is planted on the ground.

Pain, swelling, and inability to bear weight may follow the injury, and deformity may be present.

Immediate medical attention and care are needed. Dry needling acupuncture can be used immediately after emergency treatment to reduce pain, inflammation, and swelling. After surgery, dry needling acupuncture can be used immediately to accelerate the healing and reduce the scar tissue.

Fibular (Peroneal) Tendinitis

The tendons of the peroneal longus and peroneal brevis muscles pass around the lateral malleolus and insert into the lateral side of the base of the first metatarsal bone and the lateral side of the base of the fifth metatarsal bone, respectively. These tendons

help stabilize the foot and assist eversion of the foot. Inversion of the foot causes these two tendons to stretch. Repeated stretching of these tendons, which may occur in running and jumping, causes irritation, swelling, inflammation, and pain in the tendon.

Dry needling acupuncture is an effective treatment for this injury. Needles can be applied directly into the inflamed, tender, swelling, and painful tendons. The origin and belly of the muscles should be needled along with their insertion. In addition, the treatment is used to balance the entire musculoskeletal system. Two treatment sessions per week should be provided.

Fracture of the Foot

Trauma to the bones of the foot or a fall, blow, collision or violent twisting can cause fracture in any of the 26 bones of the foot, but it is most common in the metatarsals. Female athletes with lower bone density are most susceptible to this injury. Severe pain, swelling, numbness, and possible deformity are associated with the injury.

Immediate medical attention and care are needed. Dry needling acupuncture can be used before and after emergency treatment and after surgery to reduce pain and promote healing. Needles can be applied directly into the inflamed, tender, swelling, and painful area. In addition, the treatment is used to balance the entire musculoskeletal system. Two treatment sessions per week should be provided.

Stress Fracture in the Foot

Stress fractures of the bones of the foot can be caused by repetitive stress from training that involves running and jumping on hard ground, by fatigued muscles that are no longer able to absorb shock and stress, by drastic changes to intensive training, or by improper footwear.

Stress fracture can occur in any of the bones of the foot, but it is most common in the metatarsals and the calcaneus. The symptoms may include pain and swelling at the fracture site, pain with weight bearing, and inability to walk.

Dry needling acupuncture is helpful therapy for healing this injury. Needles can be applied directly into the inflamed, tender, swollen, and painful tissue at the fracture site. In addition, the treatment is used to balance the entire musculoskeletal system. Two treatment sessions per week should be provided.

Stress fracture may be prevented if the muscles are regularly treated and the musculoskeletal system is routinely balanced to reduce stress.

Plantar Fasciitis

The plantar fascia, also know as the *plantar aponeurosis,* is a tough, fibrous tissue that originates from the tuberosity of the calcaneus and inserts into the metatarsal heads. This fascia supports the longitudinal arch of the foot. This fascia is under stress when the calf muscles are tight.

Repetitive ankle movements, tight calf muscles and Achilles tendon, running on hard ground, arch problems, hyperpronation, and improper shoes can all cause this injury. The symptoms include pain at the calcaneus bone, which may diminish during exercise and worsen afterwards.

Dry needling acupuncture is effective therapy for treating this injury. Needles can be applied directly into the inflamed, tender, and painful site. Good results can be achieved when needling is combined with vacuum therapy and electrical stimulation to reduce adhesion and improve blood circulation. In addition, the treatment is used to balance the entire musculoskeletal system. Two treatment sessions per week should be provided.

Heel Spur

When a section of bone becomes injured or irritated by chronic stress such as tight muscles or tendons, an abnormal calcium deposit or bone growth occurs. Athletes with previous injuries have a higher risk of bone spurs.

Dry needling acupuncture is a helpful therapy for this injury. Needles can be applied directly into the inflamed, tender, and painful tissue. In addition, use the treatment to balance the entire musculoskeletal system. Two treatment sessions per week should be provided. Dry needling acupuncture can be applied immediately if surgery is needed.

Prevention may be possible if regular balancing of the musculoskeletal system is performed to reduce the stress on the foot.

SUMMARY

This chapter has described a number of common sports injuries for which dry needling acupuncture can be applied to achieve recovery. As emphasized previously, dry needling acupuncture, as a nonspecific biologic modality, does not conflict with any other medical procedures and, in most cases, should be combined with other modalities to achieve the best results.

Additional Readings

Oatis CA: *Kinesiology: the mechanics & pathomechanics of human movement,* Philadelphia, 2004, Lippincott Williams & Wilkins.

This book provides excellent and detailed explanations of the mechanics and pathomechanics of human movement. It is an ideal textbook for understanding human functional anatomy.

Walker B: *The anatomy of sports injuries,* Berkeley, Calif., 2007, Lotus Publishing.

The author is a prominent Australian sports trainer with more than 20 years of experience in the health and fitness industry. This book provides concise and precise description of the sports injuries listed in this chapter with excellent, clear illustrations. In particular, it presents the appropriate medical treatment and prognosis for each injury. This is an excellent reference for athletes, coaches, and dry needling acupuncture practitioners.

Wirhed R: *Athletic ability and the anatomy of motion,* ed 3, Edinburgh, 2006, Elsevier.

This book provides an excellent explanation of the anatomy of athletic motion. It is a concise but very useful reference for both athletes and coaches.

CHAPTER 15

Preventive and Therapeutic Treatment of Injuries in Selected Sports

Dry needling acupuncture, with its unique physiologic mechanisms, can be used for preventing chronic injuries and injuries caused by overuse. It can also be used for enhancing physical performance because it promotes the coordination and smooth linkage of the musculoskeletal system, as well as treating soft tissue dysfunction and injury.

The same dry needling acupuncture therapy protocol can be used to both prevent and treat an injury in sports. Dry needling acupuncture therapy normalizes the mechanical and physiologic homeostasis of the musculoskeletal and other systems by means of various regulatory reflex systems. Some types of repetitive stress or overtraining fatigue develop silently in certain anatomic structures during intensive training and competition. These hidden problems impair musculoskeletal ability and reduce athletic performance but escape conscious recognition by the athletes, their coaches, and their physicians. Because of these hidden problems and declining capability of the body systems, there is more chance that these structures will suffer injury. At this stage, preventive treatment is most effective.

Because of the unique ability of dry needling acupuncture therapy to remove deep stress and fatigue of soft tissues, regular de-stressing treatment on a weekly basis is strongly suggested for all athletes. This treatment should focus on mechanical and physiologic homeostasis of the kinetics of the entire musculoskeletal system.

If an injury occurs, the same dry needling acupuncture treatment as was used for prevention can be used, in conjunction with other modalities, to accelerate recovery from the injury and heal the musculoskeletal dysfunction. The process of treating injuries has three phases: the acute phase, the rehabilitation phase, and the functional restoration phase.

In the acute phase, treatment focuses on the athlete's symptoms, and the injured tissues are given an opportunity to begin healing. Common conventional interventions include anti-inflammatory and analgesic medications, thermal modalities, and protection and relative rest of the injured body part. During the rehabilitation phase of care, the athlete's injured tissue continues to heal. Biomechanical alterations and consequent tissue overloads should be identified and treated with a program of progressive strengthening and conditioning, including flexibility and proprioceptive neuromuscular training throughout the kinetic chain. At the conclusion of the rehabilitation phase, the athlete is ready to progress to sport-specific functional exercises, culminating in a return to participation. During the functional restoration phase, the emphasis shifts from rehabilitation to systemic and specific reconditioning in order to achieve complete healing, to minimize the risk of repeating the injury, and to restore the previous functional ability.

Dry needling acupuncture therapy should be used in all three phases of injury management. In this chapter, common injuries in various sports are described for the purpose of detailing both prevention and treatment. A detailed discussion of the causes of the injuries is beyond the scope of this chapter, but a list of additional readings is provided for that information.

Because of the specificity of its mechanisms for passively normalizing soft tissue dysfunction, dry needling acupuncture therapy should be used first, before other modalities, as a routine preventive measure and during rehabilitation. Dry needling acupuncture therapy is a passive approach and does not involve any "active" procedure, such as stretching or joint mobilization. The passivity of dry needling acupuncture therapy, in fact, prepares tissues and joints for active or strengthening procedures and minimizes stress in the tissues.

Dry needling acupuncture therapy does not and cannot replace other preventive procedures such as strength-building exercises and other conventional medical examinations and procedures. Because it has no side effects, dry needling acupuncture therapy does not conflict with any other modalities.

RUNNING

The repetitive and cyclic nature of running often leads to an accumulation of mechanical stress that exceeds the adaptation threshold of the musculoskeletal system and results in a variety of injuries. The structures that commonly accumulate mechanical stress and tissue injury include the knee, ankle, shin, hamstring, Achilles tendon, calf muscle, and plantar fascia. This stress can be reduced and injuries prevented if regular de-stressing treatment protocols are adopted.

After examining 180 runners, James and Jones[1] reported 232 injuries at the knee (34%), posteromedial tibia (13%), Achilles tendon (11%), plantar fascia (7%), stress fractures (6%), and other sites (29%). Most of these injuries can be prevented and reduced if de-stressing and balancing is achieved through dry needling acupuncture treatment on a regular basis.

Patellofemoral Joint Pain

Hoke,[2] a physical therapist, provided a good analysis of the mechanical causes of patellofemoral joint pain: The knee extensor mechanism attenuates the shock, accepting body weight when the foot contacts the ground in running. This shock attenuation is accomplished through a smoothly controlled eccentric contraction of the knee extensors. The patellofemoral joint is a finely balanced system within the extensor mechanism, and multiple factors affect its alignment and function. The runner frequently experiences pain in the patellar region when this system lacks the necessary "balance of power" between medial and lateral forces. Excessive pronation of the foot also has been cited by multiple authors[3,4] as a contributory factor in the development of anterior knee pain. The early peak in knee flexion after foot contact coincides with the peak in rear-foot pronation, and if the pronation of the rear foot becomes excessive, there will be adverse stress on the knee in the sagittal plane (increased flexion) and frontal plane (increased tibial rotation).

This analysis clearly demonstrates the "balance of power" in the finely balanced alignment of the knee system. Regular treatment should include needling all the extensor muscles—lateral, medial, and frontal—of the knee.

Iliotibial Band Syndrome

The signs of iliotibial band syndrome are pain in the knee and in the trochanteric region. Several factors may contribute to the problems associated with the iliotibial band during running.[2] As the speed of forward ambulation increases, the base of the gait narrows. This is accompanied by increased adduction at the hip, which subjects the lateral hip musculature, including the iliotibial band, to increased tension. If other hip abductors become fatigued or weaker, as they often do, additional stress on the iliotibial band is created. As the contralateral hip drops inferiorly with the swinging limb, more hip adduction is created on the support limb, with more tension on the iliotibial band. The iliotibial band also plays a role in transverse plane rotation at the hip and lower leg. When the runner's rear foot pronates excessively as the lower leg internally rotates, stress is created on the iliotibial band. The increased internal rotation intensifies the stress and tightness on the external rotators of the hip.

To reduce the stress on the iliotibial band, homeostatic acu-reflex points on the lower back, hip, thigh, and leg should be all treated. In addition, hamstring and adductor muscles should be treated together.

Shin Pain

Shin pain may be a symptom of three conditions: stress fracture and stress reactions, exertional compartment syndromes, and musculoskeletal "shin splints."[2]

Stress fracture is common in the tibia (34%), fibula (24%), metatarsals (20%), and femur (20%); thus 58% occur in the shin.[5]

External compartment syndromes in the shin typically manifest as a feeling of pain, muscle tightness, or cramping brought on by exercise, and intracompartmental pressure is increased.

Musculoskeletal "shin splints" are related to the functions of the three leg compartments. The anterior compartment is responsible for two major movements. The primary movement is dorsiflexion of the ankle and foot to provide clearance of the swinging limb and the eccentric function of controlling plantarflexion of the ankle and digits. The secondary function of the anterior compartment is to decelerate rear-foot pronation by the anterior tibialis muscle. The lateral compartment controls rear-foot supination and provides balance for the strong inverter pull from the anterior and posterior compartments. The posterior compartment includes both the superficial and deep muscles. Of the deep posterior muscles, the posterior tibialis provides control of rear-foot pronation and prevents midfoot collapse during weight acceptance. The soleus fibers and the flexor hallucis longus also have been implicated in the symptoms of posteromedial shin splints.[2]

Dry needling acupuncture therapy is very effective in both preventing and treating shin pain. The three compartments should be treated together. The trigger points in the thigh and the core muscles should be needled as well.

Achilles Tendinitis

Many factors increase stress on the Achilles tendon. Tension in the tendon fibers is increased by intrinsic structural abnormalities such as tight gastrocnemius and soleus muscles, ankle equinus, and forefoot equinus. Excessive rear-foot pronation also increases stress across the fibers of the Achilles tendon. Because of its insertion medial to the subtalar joint axis, the Achilles tendon has a secondary role in the deceleration of subtalar pronation. Training also may play a role in excessive stress in this area. Increasing pace, uphill training, and running with primary contact on the forefoot all increase the stress on the Achilles tendon.

Treatment should include needling of the inflamed tendon and all the trigger points on the gastrocnemius and soleus muscles. Because of the hypovascularity of the tendon, the reparative process may require more time than for muscle injuries.

Regular de-stressing treatment of the calf muscle reduces the stress on the tendon and may prevent the injury.

Plantar Fasciitis

Plantar fasciitis can also have many causes. The plantar fascia plays an integral role in stabilization of the midfoot and forefoot during running. As the heel begins to rise, the fixed length of the plantar fascia places it under greater tension as it is "wound" around the metatarsal heads. This creates further stability for the late support phase, and this effect is commonly referred to as the *windlass mechanism*. When midfoot stability is lost under the initial loading of the foot, the plantar fascia may come under tension prematurely. As the heel rises in the unstable foot, the additional tension from metatarsophalangeal dorsiflexion may cause injury to the plantar fascia at its attachment to the medial calcaneal tuberosity. Midfoot and forefoot instability typically arise for one of two reasons: The midfoot may have inherently poor static support through the plantar ligamentous structures, or there may be a secondary loss of midtarsal stability as the rear foot moves beyond the normal range of pronation.[2]

Plantar fasciitis is a typical soft tissue dysfunction, and good therapeutic results can be achieved in most athletes by a combination of electrical dry needling acupuncture therapy with vacuum therapy. Electrical dry needling acupuncture relaxes the fascia, and vacuum therapy creates a negative pressure within the tissues while stretching the different tissue layers of the sole.

CYCLING

An understanding of the biomechanics of the cycle stroke helps clarify the injuries from cycling. There are two broad categories of injuries: (1) physical injuries from impact with an external object and (2) injuries resulting from overuse.[6]

Overuse injuries are the focus of this section, but dry needling acupuncture therapy can be used at all stages of most injuries. Among impact injuries, most are abrasions; others are contusions, lacerations, and fractures. Dry needling acupuncture therapy greatly accelerates tissue healing from abrasions, contusions and lacerations. It can improve healing after surgery, especially in reducing post-surgical pain and swelling.

Upper Extremities

Ulnar Nerve Neuropathy

The symptoms of ulnar nerve neuropathy include muscular weakness and loss of sensation along the area innervated by the ulnar nerve. The major mechanisms of this injury are prolonged pressure on the wrist and repetitive stress on the wrist and forearm.

Dry needling acupuncture therapy is very effective in treating this condition. The treatment should include both local de-stressing and core muscle adjustment.

Median Nerve Neuropathy

This condition is less common than ulnar nerve neuropathy. It is characterized by numbness along the median nerve as a result of repeated compression and pressure on the carpal tunnel.

Dry needling acupuncture is applied to the affected area, including the carpal tunnel. This treatment is usually very effective in treating this condition, and it is important not to ignore treatment of the core system.

de Quervain Tenosynovitis

This injury is characterized by pain on abduction and extension of the thumb as a result of inflammation of the extensor pollicis brevis and the abductor pollicis longus tendons. It can be caused by direct trauma, overuse, repetitive stress, excessive vibration, or movement involving sharp bending of the tendons.

Treatment should include the inflamed tendons and related muscles on the hand and forearm. Dry needling acupuncture accompanied with thermotherapy promotes satisfactory healing.

Lower Extremities

Chondromalacia Patella

The mechanism of this injury is excessive patellofemoral loading throughout the pedal stroke. The patellofemoral joint may be dynamically or statically misaligned. The symptoms include knee pain during uphill riding or during pedaling in high gear.

Dry needling acupuncture needling is applied to all the extensor and flexor muscles of the knee. This therapy provides good results but any misalignment, if detected, should be corrected through physical therapy.

Patellar Tendinitis

This injury is usually caused by excessive angular traction. Mechanical misalignment may include internal malleolar torsion or excessive subtalar joint pronation. The symptoms are characterized by patellar pain at the insertion of the tendon on the inferior patella pole during uphill riding or high-mileage rides.

Dry needling acupuncture therapy is very effective in treating this condition and should include both homeostatic and symptomatic acu-reflex points of the lower limb and the core system.

Quadriceps Tendinitis

Quadriceps tendinitis is characterized by pain at the suprapatellar area, either medial or lateral, and is caused by repetitive overload of the quadriceps muscles and their tendons. The pain can be felt during uphill riding, high-mileage riding, or riding into a head wind. The lower leg may exhibit excessive varus or valgus deformity.

Dry needling acupuncture therapy is very effective for reducing this pain by treating the quadriceps muscles and tendons. Nevertheless, other factors such as the alignment of the bicycle should be checked and corrected to avoid biomechanical misalignment.

Biceps Femoris Tendinitis

An overload of the biceps femoris manifests as posterolateral knee pain. Sensitive trigger points can be found at the insertion of the biceps femoris tendon into the fibular head. Knee varus may be detected.

Dry needling acupuncture therapy is very effective in treating this condition, and treatment should include all compartments of the thigh and lower leg.

Medial Patellofemoral Ligament Pain

The function of the medial patellofemoral ligament is to passively restrict patellar excursion. When the patella is pulled away laterally from the midline, the medial patella sustains the stress of the excessive traction, which results in internal tibial rotation, valgus knee, or excessive pronation. The cyclist feels the pain right on the tendon of the medial patellofemoral ligament and a popping sensation with each pedal stroke.

The treatment should include trigger points on both thigh and leg muscles, with trigger points on the patellofemoral ligament in addition to core muscles.

Achilles Tendinitis and Iliotibial Band Syndrome

This injury is described further in the previous section on running.

Spine

Microwhiplash Injury

The neck sustains cumulative microtrauma if it is held in a hyperextended position or when the cyclist uses overinflated tires. Multiple jarring motions are absorbed by the cervical tissues, which results in severe pain and an inability to hold the neck in an extended position.[7]

Dry needling acupuncture therapy is very effective in treating this injury, but the trigger points and the injured joints must be identified carefully. The practitioner must not ignore the trigger points in the shoulder and lower back.

BASKETBALL

Basketball requires strength, speed, power, and agility. Whereas year-round training is essential not only for good performance but also for the prevention of injury, the long season of competition in basketball, in addition to the regular training, fosters the accumulation of many intrinsic factors that lead to physical deficiency and predispose the athlete to injury.[8] Such factors may include muscle-strength imbalances, decreased neuromuscular activation pattern, muscle fatigue, musculoskeletal misalignment, and joint laxity.

Lower Extremity

Foot and Ankle Injuries

Ankle injuries are common in basketball. Basketball players with a history of ankle sprains exhibit a larger mean postural sway and have a larger sway area. Ankle sprains are often the result of landing on the lateral border of one foot and rolling the foot inward. The injury may involve the anterior talofibular ligament, the calcaneofibular ligament, and occasionally the posterior talofibular ligament.[9]

Medial ankle sprains are less common but also can occur from landing improperly or by pushing off from the outside of the foot, which causes the ankle to evert excessively.[9]

The deltoid ligament is very strong, and an avulsion fracture of the medial malleolus may be caused by a powerful force on the ligament. Ankle sprains are occasionally accompanied by the tearing of the interosseous membrane.

The distal tibiofibular ligament can also be sprained. This injury causes pain during excessive dorsiflexion or rotational movement.

Dry needling acupuncture therapy is very effective in reducing swelling, inflammation, and pain from ankle injuries. The treatment should be provided immediately after the injury, regardless of the nature of the injury; meanwhile, further examination can be conducted and other treatment modalities can also be used. It is very important that the muscles of the three compartments of the leg be treated together. The posture of the athlete should be examined so that any imbalance of the core system can be corrected.

Achilles Tendinitis

The forces that need to be attenuated during the contact phase of running and jumping are approximately eight times the body weight.[10]

This injury can be prevented by regular de-stressing treatment. Treatment of this injury is detailed in the previous section on running.

Shin Splints

Medial shin splints from the impact forces during repeated jumping and running are common in basketball. Excessive pronation can cause posterior tibialis tendinitis at the musculotendinous junction of the medial tibia. The posterior tibialis muscle concentrically supinates the foot and eccentrically controls pronation. Posterior tibialis tendinitis is usually associated with eccentric weakness of the posterior tibialis and weakness of the intrinsic foot muscles, the flexor digitorum longus, and the flexor hallucis longus.[11]

Shin splints can be effectively prevented if regular de-stressing treatment is applied to the three compartments of the leg. Dry needling acupuncture therapy is very effective in treating this condition, especially in the early stages. Once the symptoms appear, the treatment should include the three leg compartments, the thigh compartments, and the core system.

Knee Injuries

Knee injuries are the second most common injury in basketball, after ankle injuries.[12] They are the most common cause of missed games (66%)[13] and can be caused by contact, sudden changes in direction, or overuse. Overuse injuries are secondary to improper training or conditioning, excessive stress, or fatigue. The meniscus, ligaments, and patella can sustain acute injuries.[14]

Meniscal injuries are often caused by jumping, pivoting, and cutting. The player may complain of a locking sensation, joint tenderness, and limited knee extension.

Knee ligament injuries are often related to tibial and femoral rotation during cutting, pivoting, deceleration, landing off balance, or an external impact or force on the knee. A medial collateral ligament injury is caused by valgus stress, and a lateral collateral ligament injury by a varus stress. An injury to the anterior cruciate ligament can be caused by a combination of any of these movements.

Patellar tendinitis, or quadriceps tendinitis, is caused by microscopic tears resulting from the repeated stress of sprinting, deceleration, and jumping. The eccentric overload can result in mineralization of the fibrocartilage.[15]

Some of the knee injuries caused by chronic conditions can be effectively prevented by regular de-stressing treatment with dry needling acupuncture. Knee injuries should be treated immediately, regardless of the nature of the injury, because dry needling acupuncture can reduce swelling, inflammation, and pain; meanwhile, further diagnosis and other treatment should be performed. The treatment protocol includes dry needling trigger points on the muscles, tendons, and swollen tissues. Whenever possible, the core system should be treated.

Hamstring Strains

This injury can occur from large eccentric forces, especially if the muscles are already stressed or fatigued from overtraining. Most often the strain occurs at the proximal origin, but it may occur at the semimembranosus tendon, with pain along the posterior medial knee capsule.[16]

Regular de-stressing treatment can reduce the risk of this injury. Dry needling acupuncture is very effective in accelerating recovery during rehabilitation. The treatment should include not only the affected muscles but also the proximal and distal tendons, quadriceps muscles, and core system.

Thigh Contusions

A contusion results from the direct contact or impact from another player or object. Blood vessels are damaged, and some hemorrhaging occurs.

According to the author's experience, dry needling acupuncture is the most effective modality for healing this injury. The entire area of the contusion should be treated with dense needling.

Spine Injuries

Spine injuries in basketball are usually related to repeated trauma or falls, and the symptoms include contusion, sprains, and strains. Disc injuries may occur. The athlete may complain of muscle spasm in the back and of increased pain with hyperextension or rotation of the spine.[17]

Dry needling acupuncture is very effective in treating these soft tissue injuries. In addition to symptomatic treatment, the hip, neck, and shoulder should be treated at the same time.

Upper Extremity

Injuries to the upper extremity include sprains, contusions, bone fractures, and joint dislocations. Injuries most commonly occur in the fingers, wrist, hand, and shoulder.

Dry needling acupuncture is very effective in reducing swelling, inflammation, and pain in soft tissues and can be applied to all injuries, even if surgery is needed.

Heat Exhaustion

Heat exhaustion usually is related to a depletion of electrolytes and sodium. Water replacement is very important in sports.

When heat exhaustion happens, the homeostatic acu-reflex points can be needled, in addition to other medical procedures.

BASEBALL

Baseball is a sport enjoyed by young people as well as adult players. The act of throwing requires maximally accelerating and decelerating the arm within a short period of time. According to research of baseball injuries over a 3-year period among college baseball teams, 58% of the injuries were to the upper extremity, 27% to the lower extremity, and 15% to the trunk and back.[18]

The shoulder and elbow are the joints most vulnerable to injury in baseball players as a result of the high forces and torques, extremes of range of motion, and repetitions of throwing motion that they experience. Regular de-stressing treatment, in addition to other procedures such as strengthening and conditioning training, are recommended.

Shoulder

Rotator Cuff and Biceps Tendinitis

Inflammation of the rotator cuff tendons or the tendon of the long head of the biceps is a common injury. The injured muscles produce pain during examination of range of motion.

Dry needling acupuncture therapy is very effective in treating this injury. Treatment should focus on rotator cuff muscles, as well as associated conditions that contribute to impingement. When the shoulder is treated, the neck and back should be treated together as well.

Partial- or full-thickness rotator cuff tearing necessitates a surgical procedure, but dry needling acupuncture helps reduce swelling, inflammation, and pain before and after surgery.

Impingement

External impingement consists of bursa-sided rotator cuff irritation that results from any process that decreases the space between the rotator cuff and the acromion. These processes can be static or dynamic. Bursitis, tendinitis, and acromial spurring are all conditions that statically decrease the space available for the rotator cuff. When the rotator cuff

muscles are fatigued, precise rotator cuff control can be lost, and the humerus can become compressed against the glenoid. As a result, the humeral head migrates superiorly during glenohumeral elevation, which dynamically decreases the space available between the rotator cuff and the acromion.[19]

In internal impingement, rotator cuff fatigue lead to a cumulative effect of repetitive microtrauma to the anterior capsule and labrum, which results in stretching of these structures and consequent anterior translation of the humeral head. This anterior translation causes the undersurface of the posterior rotator cuff to be brought against the posterosuperior surface of the glenoid and labrum, which causes fraying and tearing.[19]

Dry needling acupuncture therapy is very effective in preventing and treating this injury. The treatment should include the symptomatic area and associated soft tissues. For local injuries, treatment of the musculoskeletal system is always beneficial.

Glenohumeral Instability

Instability is often found in the shoulders of overhead throwers as a result of repetitive stresses and extreme ranges of motion. When impingement or tendinitis is diagnosed, the underlying pathologic process is often actually instability that has been overlooked.[19] Dry needling acupuncture is helpful in conjunction with other medical procedures for healing this condition. This therapy is also helpful in all phases of rehabilitation.

Labral Injuries

Athletes with labral injury may complain of anterior shoulder pain, and a "click" is often associated with a certain range of motion.

Although further diagnosis and treatment (including surgery) may be needed, dry needling acupuncture is helpful in reducing swelling, inflammation, and pain during all phases of the treatment and rehabilitation.

Elbow

Overuse Injuries

Overuse injuries, usually involving the musculotendinous units, are among the most common injuries. Elbow tendinitis can involve the flexor pronator mass on the medial side, the extensor supinator mass on the lateral side, or the triceps posteriorly. Medial epicondylitis and triceps tendinitis are much more common because of the extreme valgus forces and elbow extension required for throwing. The medial musculotendinous structures can be injured either by microscopic tearing that results from the cumulative effect of repeated throwing or by macroscopic tearing that results from overly forceful muscular contraction. If this injury is treated improperly, the increased stress on the injured musculotendinous unit is passed on to the medially located ulnar collateral ligament and can result in attenuation or tearing of the ligament. If the ulnar collateral ligament is injured or becomes attenuated, the subtle instability that results has ramifications for all compartments of the elbow joint. Increased medial stress can subject the ulnar nerve to excessive traction. These compressive forces are also transferred to the radiocapitellar joint. Overload on the articular surface can lead to cartilage damage and loose bodies. Posteriorly, this overload is borne by the posteromedial olecranon. With continued throwing, osteophytes form and can give rise to intra-articular loose bodies.[19]

Dry needling acupuncture can be used in all phases for these conditions from prevention to rehabilitation in conjunction with other therapeutic modalities. It is very important that both the tendons and related muscles be treated at the same time.

Other Position-Specific Injuries

Outfielders are more likely to have musculotendinous injuries to the gastrocnemius-soleus complex and to the hamstring muscle group because they must accelerate rapidly from a stationary position to high speed. Infielders are subject to lower back injuries because they must perform unsupported forward flexion. Catchers are at risk for meniscal injuries of the knee because of the amount of time they spend in a deep squat.

All these athletes should undergo regular routine de-stressing treatment that focuses on specific muscles related to particular performance. Weekly de-stressing treatment is very efficient for preventing microscopic tearing of muscle and overuse fatigue.

GOLF

Professional golfers play and practice at least 10 months per year and hit hundreds of golf balls on a daily basis; thus they are susceptible to chronic overuse injuries. According to one survey of 226 professional golfers, 85% had been injured as a direct result of their profession, and each of the injured players had an average of two injuries during the course of their professional careers.[20] Of those players, 54% considered their injuries to be chronic. The relative proportions of chronic injuries were as follows: left wrist, 24%; low back, 23.7%; left hand and left shoulder, 7.1%; and left knee, 7%.

The lead upper extremity is the most important element of a healthy golf swing. However, a number of injuries are associated with the upper extremity requirements of the golf swing. Among these injuries are golfer's elbow, rotator cuff injury, fractures of the hook of the hamate, and de Quervain tenosynovitis.[21]

Shoulder

The function of the glenohumeral joint depends largely on the function of the scapulothoracic joint. Damage to the shoulder complex in golfers usually occurs in the lead shoulder (left shoulder for the right-handed golfer). Most of these injuries are of a chronic nature and may include rotator cuff strains and tendinitis, impingement syndrome, glenohumeral instability, bursitis, and snapping scapula syndrome. Acute damage can cause rotator cuff tears and glenohumeral subluxations.

Usually the injury starts with a low-grade ache and discomfort in the shoulder after playing or practicing. Symptoms increase during the backswing phase. With continued swing stress, the low-grade inflammation can turn into more serious disorder and dysfunction if left untreated, such as severe injuries to supraspinatus and infraspinatus muscles and full-thickness tears in the rotator cuff tendons or musculature.[22]

Older golfers and those with years of stressful practice are more vulnerable to the development of multidirectional instabilities of the lead glenohumeral joint and secondary shoulder impingement syndrome.[22]

Dry needling acupuncture therapy is very effective in preventing and treating the chronic soft tissue dysfunction of the shoulder musculature that develops into these injuries. Weekly de-stressing treatment is suggested for prevention, and two treatment sessions per week should be provided for treating the symptoms.

Elbows

The large amounts of pronation and supination involved in golf swings can cause elbow tendinitis and muscle strains because of the rolling-over effect of the muscles on the humeral epicondyles. Although both elbows can be affected, the lead elbow (left elbow in a right-handed golfer) is more prone to injury. Skilled golfers who swing on plane and have good overall swing mechanics tend to overstretch the left elbow extensor muscles during the late downswing. Less skilled golfers who swing over the top during the downswing tend to aggravate the medial flexor muscles in the right elbow.[22]

Dry needling acupuncture therapy is effective in treating these injuries, but complete recovery takes some time. Identifying the location of the inflamed tendons is critical, and both tendons and muscles should be treated simultaneously. Weekly de-stressing treatment is suggested for prevention, and two treatment sessions per week should be provided for treating the symptoms.

Spine

The torque and shear forces of the full swing motion put stress on the spine. Poor cervicothoracic posture, limited rotational mobility, and degenerative conditions can irritate preexisting spine disorders. Research evidence indicated that a large number of costal stress fractures in the lead-side rib cage of beginning golfers were misdiagnosed as "nonspecific back pain."[23] Pain and hypomobility in the lead (left) scapulothoracic area and paravertebral muscles are signs of vertebral and zygapophyseal joint dysfunction. Low back injuries ranging from lumbosacral sprains to herniated discs were reported in 48% of the respondents in one study.[21] The lumbar spine is prone to facet dysfunction and potential nerve-root irritation. Sacroiliac joint dysfunction and degeneration are also quite common in habitual golfers.[22]

Other spine problems may include spondylolysis (the breaking down of a vertebra) and spondylolisthesis (forward displacement of a vertebra over a lower segment, usually the L5 vertebra over the sacrum or the L4 over the L5).

Dry needling acupuncture therapy is very effective in reducing acute and chronic stress on the spine and in preventing further development of the spine symptoms. If injuries occur, dry needling acupuncture is very helpful for healing in conjunction with other modalities. Weekly de-stressing treatment is suggested for prevention, and two treatment sessions per week should be provided for treating the symptoms.

FOOTBALL

Football is a contact sport; it could even be described a collision sport. In a 1997 study by the National Collegiate Athletic Association (NCAA),[24] the injury rate among athletes was 3.8 per 1000 exposures in practice and 34.1 per 1000 exposures in games. Knees and ankles were the most common sites of injury, and sprains were the most common type.[24]

Muscle and Tendon Sprains

Dry needling acupuncture therapy is very effective in treating muscle and tendon sprains, whether the injury is caused by acute factors or by overuse. Weekly de-stressing treatment is suggested for prevention, and two treatment sessions per week should be provided for treating the symptoms. Dry needling acupuncture should be provided immediately after the injury.

Brachial Plexus Injuries

It has been reported that more than 50% of college football players have sustained brachial plexus injuries in the course of their playing careers.[25] Players with this injury may feel burning pain or weakness, or both, in the upper limb or paresthesia and temporary disruption of nerve function after a block or tackle. Recovery is usual, but in some cases in which symptoms persist for months, neural degeneration is confirmed by electromyography. These injuries may involve the spinal accessory, suprascapular, axillary, and long thoracic nerves.

Dry needling acupuncture is very effective in accelerating recovery in most cases. In severe injuries, dry needling acupuncture can be a helpful supplementary modality. Weekly de-stressing treatment is suggested for prevention, and two treatment sessions per week should be provided for treating the symptoms.

Achilles Tendon Rupture

This injury is common among quarterbacks and is the result of overuse or repeated injury. A quarterback may throw the football as many as 50 times in a game and a few hundred times during practice. Repeating the motion of dropping back to throw the football may cause inflammation of the tendon. This tendinitis weakens the tendon and makes it susceptible to tearing. The tendon also can tear as a result of the trauma of a one-time violent deceleration and planting motion, even in the absence of previous problems.[26]

Dry needling acupuncture is very effective in reducing the repetitive stress in both tendons and calf muscles if used regularly. In cases of acute rupture, dry needling acupuncture is very helpful in conjunction with other modalities, including surgery. Weekly de-stressing treatment is suggested for prevention, and two treatment sessions per week should be provided for treating the symptoms. Dry needling acupuncture should be provided immediately after the injury.

Injuries to the Shoulder, Back, and Knee

Dry needling acupuncture can be used for different purposes with these kinds of injury. In chronic or overuse conditions, dry needling acupuncture therapy can prevent soft tissue injury. For injuries, dry needling acupuncture can be used immediately to reduce pain and swelling and to accelerate recovery. After surgery, dry needling acupuncture is very helpful in rehabilitation.

Concussion

Concussion is a debilitating injury in sports. It is classified in three grades. Grade 1 concussion is characterized by confusion without amnesia and with no loss of consciousness; grade 2 is characterized by confusion with amnesia but no loss of consciousness; and grade 3 is characterized by loss of consciousness.

Dry needling acupuncture is very helpful in treating all three grades of concussion and postconcussion syndrome. The primary acu-reflex points and a few empirical points, including the median nerve points and the tips of the fingers, should be needled.

Heat Exhaustion

Heat exhaustion, caused by heat stress, can affect all football players because of the heavy equipment they wear. Football players are constantly changing posture, and the possible resulting rapid falls in blood pressure render them particularly susceptible to heat syncope.

Dry needling acupuncture can help restore homeostasis and reduce symptoms such as decreased skin blood flow, decreased or increased heart rate, gastric distress, and increased body temperature.

Other Common Injuries

Some football injuries are related to specific positions of the game. Offensive linemen are more prone to lumbar, knee ligament, and shoulder injuries. Wide receivers may have hamstring strains and tears of the anterior cruciate ligament. Defensive backs often have upper extremity injuries, including finger dislocations and hand and wrist sprains from defending or blocking their opponent's offensive players. Neck and shoulder sprains occur during tackling. Both field-goal kickers and punters develop overuse injuries.[3] Among kickers, the most common injuries are low back, hip flexor, and hamstring strains.

Dry needling acupuncture can be used for both prevention and treatment of all these soft tissue injuries.

SOCCER

Soccer is the most popular sport in the world and is considered to be relatively safe. The risk of injury is 85% for a high school football player, in contrast to 30% for a soccer player.[27] Of all injuries in soccer, 80% occur during physical contact between two players. Contact includes being kicked by and colliding with another player.[28] At higher levels of play, more injuries are caused by the mechanisms of running.[29]

Further research has demonstrated that 69% of injuries occur because of trauma, and 31% result from overuse. Between 84% and 88% of injuries in soccer occur in the lower extremities.[30] Most of these injuries are minor and result in little or no loss of playing time. The proportion of major injuries is from 8% to 10%; most occur in the lower extremities and include fractures, subluxations, and injuries to the ligaments of the knee. The principal site of major injury is the knee, which accounts for 50% of all severe injuries. It happens more often in female players than in male players: 31% versus 13%, respectively.[27]

Players aged 25 to 40 years have the highest injury rate (18%). This is because this group contains former college athletes with high skill levels and a more aggressive style of play. Younger players have lower injury rates and less severe injuries.[28]

Among all levels of injury, ankle sprain is the most common, followed by injury to the knee.[28,29] Skin lesions, contusions, muscle strains, and fractures constitute most of the remainder of injuries to the lower extremities. Less common injuries include shoulder dislocations, elbow fractures and dislocations, and injuries of the head and face, fingers, and groin and pubis.[28]

Lower Extremity Injuries

Ankle Sprains

Ankle sprains account for 36% of all injuries in soccer. The mechanism of this type of injury is most often running or tackling, and 80% of first-time ankle injuries occur during tackling. In cases in which the injury results from running, there is a high incidence of previous ankle injury.[29] An ankle sprain in many cases can be worse than a fracture in terms of the completeness of recovery.[31] Very often the injured athlete returns to the sport before he or she has regained sufficient strength and proprioception.

Inversion sprain is the most common type of ankle sprain. The injury involves the anterior talofibular ligament and calcaneofibular ligament. The less common eversion sprain involves the strong deltoid ligament on the medial side and often leads to an avulsion fracture of the tibia.[31]

Dry needling acupuncture is very effective in reducing pain and swelling. The treatment should be provided immediately after the injury. Injured ligaments should be identified and treated. The treatment should be delivered once every day or every other day during the first week after injury. In addition to the ankle area, muscles of the lower extremity and the core system should be treated twice a week. Even after the initial pain and swelling have been greatly reduced, the athlete should continue rehabilitation for some time before returning to the sport.

Shin Splints

In this book, *shin splints* refers to tendinitis in the anterior tibialis or posterior tibialis or to stress fracture syndrome. This injury is related to overuse. Medial shin splints are mostly caused by inflammation of the posterior tibialis tendon, whereas lateral shin splints are caused by inflammation of the anterior tibialis tendon or the extensor tendons of the digits.

Shin splints may result from the nature of the running surface; pes planus, genu varum or tibial varum; overuse; muscle fatigue; body chemical imbalance; and poor reciprocal coordination between the muscles of the anterior and posterior aspects of the lower extremity.[32]

Dry needling acupuncture is very effective in both preventing and treating these symptoms. As a preventive procedure, athletes should receive weekly de-stressing treatment. Once the symptoms appear, two treatment sessions should be provided. The protocol should include both the lower extremity and the core system.

Compartment Syndrome

In compartment syndrome, the fluid pressure in the tissue has exceeded normal levels and thereby places pressure on the muscles, tendons, blood vessels, and nerves. Ischemia follows this pressure increase and, in severe cases, can cause permanent damage to the extremity. Compartment syndrome can be acute or chronic; in severe cases, there is associated weakness of the dorsiflexors and toe extensors, as well as swelling on the dorsum of the foot.[32] Because of the symptoms, compartment syndrome is often confused with a stress fracture.

Dry needling acupuncture is very effective in preventing and treating compartment syndrome. Weekly de-stressing treatment can help prevent the injury, and two needling sessions per week can be used for treating the injury. The treatment should include dry needling acupuncture of all three compartments of the leg and thigh muscles. The core system should be included in de-stressing treatment.

Knee Injuries

Injury to the knee ligaments cause the longest absences from the sport, and nearly half of these occur during tackling.[29]

Knee injuries can be caused by different mechanisms. They may involve particular structures, as in rupture of the anterior cruciate ligament, tearing of the meniscus, or multiple injuries. Because of the complexity of the knee, readers are advised to read the available literature about the anatomy and mechanisms of knee injuries. Medical procedures to treat knee injuries differ according to the severity of the injury.

Dry needling acupuncture is very effective in decreasing inflammation, swelling, and pain and in restoring range of motion. Regular weekly de-stressing treatment reduces the potential risk of injury related to intrinsic factors such as muscle fatigue and joint misalignment. For tissue swelling, daily treatment is the most helpful. For pain and rehabilitation, two sessions per week should be delivered. The treatment should be provided immediately after injury, as well as after surgery.

Osteoarthritis

Osteoarthritis often occurs in athletes after a tear of the anterior cruciate ligament. This condition can be prevented or treated with dry needling acupuncture. The treatment should be used to thoroughly reduce stress on the knee by needling both flexors and extensors of the knee.

Thigh Injuries

Thigh injuries include muscle strains, contusions, and myositis ossificans. The quadriceps, hamstrings, and hip adductors are the most common sites of strains in soccer players. Symptoms of muscle strains include pain during activity or during an isometric muscle contraction, a feeling of muscle pulling during running or playing, and loss of function and the manifestation of increased tone.

Of soccer-related injuries, contusions have the highest incidence after knee and ankle injuries, and the quadriceps are the most commonly involved muscles. Symptoms of contusion include swelling, stiffness, and pain during muscle contraction. Acute care is more necessary than actual long-term rehabilitation in the management of contusions.[32]

Myositis ossificans is a complication of muscle contusion. The symptoms include pain, swelling, and the presence of a lump on palpation. Ectopic bone forms in the quadriceps muscle belly, and diagnosis is confirmed by radiographic examination.

Dry needling acupuncture is very effective in healing these thigh injuries. The treatment should be provided for two sessions per week. The treatment protocol should include both local treatment and the core system.

Groin Injuries

Groin injuries include adductor tendinitis, osteitis pubis, and muscle strains of the adductor muscles (adductor longus, adductor brevis, and gracilis). Inguinal hernias can be described as groin discomfort.

These symptoms can be caused by chronic conditions, such as muscle fatigue or overuse, or by acute injuries, such as a quick change in direction that occurs simultaneously with an associated external rotation or abduction movement.[33]

Regular weekly de-stressing treatment helps reduce chronic conditions such as muscle strains and tendinitis. Symptoms should be treated in two sessions per week. Both muscles and tendons should be treated, in addition to the core system.

Upper Extremity Injuries

Upper extremity injuries are more common in goalkeepers than in field players. Fractures of the elbows, fingers, and wrists as a result of falls or collisions are the most common types.

Common shoulder injuries include acromioclavicular sprains. Shoulder dislocations or acromioclavicular sprains are occasionally related to capsular laxity or violent collision.

These injuries should be treated by specialists, but dry needling acupuncture is very helpful in reducing pain and swelling if combined with conventional medical care. For swelling after injury, one treatment session every day can be provided, regardless of whether surgery is needed. In cases of surgery, two treatment sessions per week help reduce pain and swelling and accelerate recovery.

SKIING

Since the early 1980s, an enormous amount of research has been devoted to the forces and loads that bear on the human body during turns in skiing and to the muscle-phasic relationships that are needed to accomplish these tasks smoothly. These efforts have enabled the development of successful injury prevention and fitness training programs.[34] According to the database of one research group, 32% to 48% of all ski injuries are related to the knee; shoulder and back injuries account for another 15%.[35]

Large epidemiologic studies indicate that smaller, younger, lighter, and less experienced skiers have the highest risk of injury.[36] This research suggests that skill level seems to be the most important factor in determining the risk of injury for skiers. The likelihood of being injured is 33% among beginners, in contrast to 6.2% among skiers rated as intermediate or expert.

Knee

Knee injuries can be caused by several different mechanisms in skiing and may be in the form of isolated tears and ruptures of the anterior cruciate ligament, restraint damage such as injuries to the medial collateral or lateral collateral ligament, or bone bruising or chondral defects of the articular surface of the femoral condyles or tibial plateau.[34]

Dry needling acupuncture is helpful in reducing swelling, pain, and bruising and can be used in conjunction with other medical modalities for rehabilitation and before and immediately after surgery.

Shoulder

Anterior glenohumeral dislocation occurs from falling on an outstretched arm. Acromioclavicular separation may be caused by a direct blow to the shoulder that drives the acromion down in relation to the clavicle. "Skier's thumb," a common hand injury, occurs when the ulnar collateral ligament is subjected to forced abduction and hyperextension.

Dry needling acupuncture is very helpful in reducing pain and swelling when used in addition to conventional treatment.

ICE HOCKEY

Ice hockey is often described as the fastest team game, and because of the speed and style of play, it is regarded as a violent, aggressive sport with a high risk of many different types of injury.[37,38]

Injuries to the Head and Face

According to studies of elite Swedish ice hockey players, the risk of concussion during a career is about 20%.[39] Adult recreational players demonstrate even higher proportional risks of injuries to the head and neck (32%) and to the face (25%).[40]

Dry needling acupuncture therapy is very helpful in reducing pain and other symptoms after injuries to the head and face, including concussion. Treatment should be provided immediately after the injury while further examination and other medical procedures are being considered.

Upper Extremity Injuries

Upper extremity injuries are typically caused by collisions with other players. Injuries include severe trauma to the cervical spine (C1 to C7); fractures, separations, and dislocations; and contusions of soft tissue.

Dry needling acupuncture, in conjunction with conventional modalities, is helpful in treating all these injuries, specifically for soft tissue. Daily treatment should be provided to reduce swelling, and two sessions per week should be administered for pain and other symptoms.

Lower Extremity Injuries

The majority of lower extremity injuries are to the ligaments or menisci of the knee and ankle. Ankle sprain results from a severe dorsiflexion, eversion, and external rotation of the ankle. Knee injuries include damage to the collateral and anterior cruciate ligaments.

The condition of myositis ossificans traumatica is described as a sequela of severe contusion, hematoma, or fracture.[41]

In conjunction with other modalities, dry needling acupuncture is very helpful for healing all these injuries, especially in reducing swelling, pain, hematoma, and contusion. Daily treatment should be provided for swelling, hematoma, and contusion.

SWIMMING

Swimming has become one of the most popular sports. Injuries are common in competitive swimming and can limit the level of achievement and the length of a swimmer's career. According to one study, muscle activity increases with the onset of fatigue as the athlete tries to maintain speed in the water.[42] Muscle efficiency decreases as the rate of neural firing increases and the output of force decreases.[43]

Overtraining Syndrome

Overtraining is common among swimmers. Between 10% and 21% of swimmers experience signs of overtraining during the course of a competitive season.[44]

Early signs of overtraining may include recurring minor illnesses, changes in sleep patterns and nutritional habits, and overall mood instability. Female swimmers are often susceptible to the female athlete's triad: eating disorders, amenorrhea, and osteoporosis.[45]

Overtraining syndrome develops when training outpaces rest and recovery. The symptoms may include behavioral changes such as increased or decreased appetite, sleep disturbances, general fatigue, inability to concentrate, irritability, and loss of motivation. Other physiologic problems include nausea, diarrhea, changes in bowel habits, frequent colds or flu-like symptoms, and increased resting heart rate. Body weight may change according to the changes in eating habit. Musculoskeletal problems such as muscle strains, chronic muscle soreness, and minor ligamentous sprains may occur because of reduced muscle efficiency.[43,46]

Dry needling acupuncture is very effective for preventing and treating overtraining syndrome because it improves both musculoskeletal physiology and neuroendocrine physiology. Athletes should receive weekly de-stressing treatment before any signs develop. If symptoms appear, two treatment sessions should be provided. The treatment protocol should include restoration of homeostasis and symptomatic treatment. Other conventional modalities should be considered as well.

Overuse Injuries

The most common injuries in swimmers are related to overuse and cumulative trauma.[47] Cumulative, repetitive microtrauma can cause tissue damage that leads to overuse injuries. Early intervention is the key to preventing acute injuries from becoming chronic syndromes.

Inflammation is the primary acute symptom of microtrauma, and reducing inflammation is of the utmost importance in the treatment of overuse injuries.

Dry needling acupuncture therapy is very effective in healing overuse injuries. It can reduce or eliminate soft tissue stress, swelling, and edema. It can reduce inflammation and greatly accelerate the recovery and healing of microtrauma of soft tissue. Dry needling acupuncture can be a useful adjunct to other conventional treatment approaches.

Common Upper Extremity Injuries

An individual swimmer may move his or her upper extremities through 2 million strokes during the training of 1 year.[48] This amount of repetitive motion would itself be considered traumatic in comparison with normal wear and tear, and it often results in repeated microtrauma to the entire musculoskeletal structure: muscles, tendons, ligaments, and joints. The shoulder in particular is put through its maximal range of motion during each swimming stroke, which causes microtrauma, frequently leads to mechanical breakdown of the biomechanics of the shoulder complex, and results in various kinds of shoulder pain.[45]

Shoulder pain is the most common musculoskeletal injury among competitive swimmers. Numerous studies have demonstrated that basic impingement syndrome is the most common cause of shoulder pain in swimmers and that the underlying instability of the glenohumeral joint is a predisposition for inflammation of the subacromial bursa and tears of the glenoid labrum.[49]

Swimmer's Shoulder

Swimmer's shoulder is an overuse injury consisting of inflammation in the supraspinatus or biceps tendon, or both, and is usually caused by multidirectional glenohumeral instability or impingement of the tendons between the head of the humerus and the acromion process of the scapula. Local inflammation, swelling, ischemia caused by repetitive microtrauma, and tearing can alter the biomechanics of the shoulder joint. Clinical examination may reveal that the shoulder has a restricted pattern of movements in abduction and in external and internal rotation. Continuing practice while these symptoms are present causes significant alteration of the normal mechanics of the scapulae, neck, and trunk, resulting in secondary impingement and bursitis.[45]

Dry needling acupuncture is very effective in both preventing and treating swimmer's shoulder. Regular weekly de-stressing treatment can reduce overuse stress and restore normal physiology of soft tissue, thus preventing muscle inflammation and fatigue. Once shoulder pain appears, the athlete should receive two treatment sessions per week, including both local and systemic treatment.

Thoracic Outlet Syndrome

Thoracic outlet syndrome is a specific group of signs and symptoms resulting from compression of the subclavian artery, subclavian vein, and brachial plexus. The compression can occur at scalene muscle level, between the clavicle and the first rib, or in the area of the coracoid process. The structure being compressed can be the brachial plexus, an artery, or a vein.

The athlete may complain of muscle tightness and pain about the shoulder, neck, and clavicle at the position in the stroke in which the hand enters the water; pain in the lower face and ear; headache; radiating pain into the shoulder, thumb, and index and middle fingers; weakness and fatigue of the deltoid, biceps, triceps, or forearm muscles; loss of strength of the intrinsic muscles of the hand; and inability to control movement of the hand during the sculling motion of the pull-through phase.[45]

The diagnosis of thoracic outlet syndrome is not easy. Nevertheless, dry needling acupuncture is very effective in preventing and treating these symptoms. For prevention, the athlete should receive regular weekly de-stressing treatments. Treatment of the symptoms should include the neck, shoulders, upper limbs, upper and lower back, hips, and lower limbs. Two treatment sessions per week are required.

Elbow Injuries

Elbow injuries are injuries of overuse. Lateral epicondylitis is common, and the medial elbow is also susceptible to injury from strains of extensors or flexors. Triceps strains and synovitis can result from elbow stress. All these injuries decrease the efficiency of the stroke and increase the stresses on the shoulder and wrist, which result in inflammation.

Dry needling acupuncture is very effective in preventing and treating these injuries. For prevention, weekly de-stressing treatment should be administered to the neck, shoulders, upper limbs, core muscles, and lower limbs. Treatment of symptoms should follow the same protocol, with special attention to the inflamed tendons. If the tendons are inflamed, recovery will take longer.

Common Lower Extremity Injuries

Knee Injuries

The most common knee injury is a strain of the medial collateral ligament and is commonly referred to as *breaststroker's knee.* This is a chronic sprain of the medial collateral ligament that results from repetitive stress on this ligament.[50] Other knee injuries include patellofemoral pain, medial synovitis, and medial plica syndrome (medial synovitis).[51]

Dry needling acupuncture therapy is very effective in preventing and treating these knee injuries in swimmers. The protocol can be weekly de-stressing treatment for prevention and two sessions per week for treating symptoms.

Foot and Ankle Injuries

Tendinitis of the extensor tendons at the extensor retinaculum is the most common injury to the foot and ankle. Other problems include foot contusion, heel bruises, and ankle sprains from contact with the pool wall on flip turns or from slipping on a wet pool deck or ladder.[45]

Dry needling acupuncture is very effective in reducing pain, swelling, and inflammation of these injuries. The athlete should receive two sessions per week for treating these injuries in conjunction with other medical modalities.

Back Injuries

Low back injuries in swimmers are caused most often by repetitive stress during turns and the strain of poor head and body position in the water. Mechanical problems include spondylolysis, spondylolisthesis, and Scheuermann kyphosis, which is found in adolescent swimmers and results from repeated flexion of the thoracic spine.[52]

The typical swimmer's posture manifests as increased thoracic kyphosis, abducted or protracted scapulae, and a forward head position. These postural tendencies are further reinforced in swimmers who suffer from recurrent nasal and sinus problems caused by exposure to bacteria and chemicals in swimming pools.

Dry needling acupuncture is very effective in preventing and treating these back injuries. The same de-stressing protocol can be used for both prevention and treatment. For prevention, regular weekly treatment is needed. For treating symptoms, two sessions per week should be provided.

Neck Injuries

Freestyle swimming requires rotation of the head and neck, and this puts the cervical spine through rotation that repeats on every breathing cycle. Over time, these repetitive stresses overstretch the ligaments at one or more levels of the cervical spine,

which can result in a dysfunctional positioning of the vertebrae at the facet joint.[45] This causes neck pain, accompanied by muscle spasm.

Such pain can be effectively prevented or treated by dry needling acupuncture. De-stressing treatment should be provided once a week for prevention, and symptom-focused treatment should be provided twice a week to the injured athlete.

Spontaneous Pneumomediastinum

Spontaneous pneumomediastinum, also known as *mediastinal emphysema,* is relatively uncommon but well documented in athletes. The major symptoms include neck and chest pain, shoulder and back pain, abdominal pain, weakness, dyspnea, dysphagia, sore throat, and swollen neck. Some patients may experience shortness of breath and difficulty swallowing.

Subcutaneous emphysema is the most prevalent physical finding.[53] Spontaneous pneumomediastinum may be caused by several conditions that allow free air to enter the mediastinal tissues but may be caused in swimmers by frequent breath holding or performing the Valsalva maneuver.[45]

Dry needling acupuncture therapy is very effective in preventing and treating all the symptoms related to this condition. The usual weekly de-stressing treatment is used for prevention. Symptom-focused treatment should be provided to the athlete in two sessions per week. Other conventional modalities should be considered while dry needling acupuncture therapy is administered.

Other Medical Problems

Other medical problems related to swimming include chronic sinus infection, skin infection, and ear and eye infections. Dry needling acupuncture is helpful in improving sinus and skin infections. Even eye and ear infections are reported to have been ameliorated by dry needling acupuncture in traditional acupuncture literature.

TENNIS

Tennis players may have to move the body repeatedly in any direction, and poor flexibility of the key muscle groups often leads to injury. In addition to flexibility, proprioception and balance are vital to maintaining a player's center of gravity when the player changes directions. Because of the enormous physical demands of tennis, muscular strength and endurance also affect the risk of injury.[54]

Extrinsic factors also cause tennis injuries. Movement in tennis requires the musculoskeletal system to move with rhythm, timing, and a smooth sequential linkage from the ground upward. "Missing-link" syndrome occurs when a player hits an "all-arm" shot, in which the arm alone generates ball velocity during the forehand stroke and the more powerful links of the trunk and lower extremity are not used. As a result, the upper extremity is overstressed.[54] Detailed discussion of extrinsic factors of tennis injuries is beyond the scope of this chapter.

Wrist Injuries

The wrist is a distal link in the kinetic system. In addition to repeated motion of the wrist, compensatory movements often occur at the wrist joint to neutralize the adverse effects of movements of the preceding links during tennis strokes. This repeated action results in wrist injuries. Common examples include carpal tunnel syndrome and de Quervain tenosynovitis (inflammation of the extensor pollicis brevis and the abductor pollicis longus).[54]

The repeated twisting motions of the wrist can cause a tear at the ulnar side of the wrist, and other abnormal wrist motions cause tendinitis of the flexor carpi ulnaris and extensor carpi ulnaris.[55]

To reduce overload stresses on the wrist, the most distal link, tennis players need to learn efficient and effective movement and proper timing of the lower links.[56] Dry needling acupuncture provides de-stressing relief that reduces the possibility of overuse injuries. In addition, dry needling acupuncture promotes smooth coordination among the different links. For preventing and treating wrist injuries, the sensitive points in wrist area and in related muscles should be identified and treated. The athlete with wrist injuries should understand that pain relief is just a part of healing and that complete functional recovery of the wrist takes more time.

Elbow Injuries

Elbow injuries occur in 40% to 50% of average recreational tennis players who are more than 30 years of age. The most common injury is tennis elbow, or lateral epicondylitis, and the next most common is golfer's elbow, or medial epicondylitis.[57]

Dry needling acupuncture is effective in reducing overuse stresses and treating inflamed tissues. The tendinitis should be precisely located and treated, and trigger points in the related muscles should be identified and needled. As with wrist injuries, pain relief is just a part of healing of elbow injuries; complete functional recovery requires a longer time. De-stressing treatment should be provided once a week, before symptoms appear. Symptoms should be treated twice a week.

Shoulder Injuries

A common shoulder injury is impingement, in which the subacromial space narrows as the upper extremity is actively elevated overhead. Both the biceps tendon and the rotator cuff tendons lying in this space can be impinged. Causes of impingement include poor flexibility, muscle imbalance, decreased scapular stability, and poor stroke mechanics.[54] Researchers have demonstrated that anatomic adaptation occurs in the racket shoulder of the tennis player. This adaptation includes loss of active and passive range of motion in internal rotation and even a total loss of shoulder rotation, which results in overuse shoulder injuries.[58]

Dry needling acupuncture therapy is very effective in reducing overuse stress and treating inflamed tissues of shoulder injuries. The tender spots in the shoulder area should be precisely located and treated, and trigger points in the related muscles should be identified and needled. As with wrist injuries, relief of pain in shoulder injuries can be achieved in a few treatments, but this is only a part of the healing; complete functional recovery requires more time. De-stressing treatment should be provided once a week before symptoms appear, and symptoms should be treated twice a week.

Back Injuries

Low back strains and facet impingement syndromes are common injuries in tennis players. Several back injuries were found to be a result of high muscle and joint reaction force, especially during the cocking phase of the serve when the spine flexes laterally and hyperextends.[59]

Dry needling acupuncture therapy is very effective in reducing overuse stress and treating inflamed tissues. The trigger points on the shoulder, low back, hip, and lower extremity should be precisely located and needled. As with wrist injuries, relief of pain in back injuries can be achieved with a few treatments, but this is only a part of the healing; complete functional recovery requires more time. De-stressing treatment should be provided once a week, before symptoms appear. Symptoms should be treated twice a week.

Knee Injuries

Common knee injuries include patellofemoral tracking syndrome and patellar tendinitis. These are overuse knee injuries and are caused by the explosive, repetitive, and multidirectional movements in the sport.[60]

Patellofemoral tracking dysfunction may be caused by biomechanical imbalance, pronated feet, or a tight lateral retinaculum.[54]

Dry needling acupuncture is very effective for reducing overuse stresses in soft tissue. The trigger points on the low back, hip, and lower extremity, including the patellofemoral tendon, should be precisely located and needled. As with wrist injuries, relief of pain in knee injuries can be achieved in a few treatments, but this is only a part of the healing; complete functional recovery requires more time. De-stressing treatment should be provided once a week before symptoms appear. Symptoms should be treated twice a week. While the low back and the knee are treated, the neck and shoulder should also be examined and treated.

Ankle Injuries

Lateral ankle sprain is a common ankle injury.[61] Quick changes of directions and repeated stopping and starting motions are often the cause of this traumatic injury.

Dry needling acupuncture is very effective in reducing ankle swelling, pain, and inflammation. The treatment should be provided immediately after the injury. The location of the tender areas on both lateral and medial ankle ligaments should be treated once a day until swelling completely disappears and then twice a week. As with wrist injuries, relief of pain in ankle injuries can be achieved with a few treatments, but this is just a part of the healing; complete functional recovery requires more time. De-stressing treatment should be provided once a week.

VOLLEYBALL

Volleyball has become the world's most popular participation sport. Epidemiologic data suggest that jumping and forceful contact of the volleyball with the upper extremity in an overhead position (spiking and serving) carry the greatest risk for injury. It has been estimated that an elite volleyball athlete, practicing and competing 16 to 20 hours per week, performs approximately 40,000 spikes a year. This places enormous demands on the musculotendinous structure of the shoulders, knees, ankles, and low back. These structures are at significant risk for injuries in athletes.[62,63]

Blocking by players on the opposing team has been associated with the highest rate of injuries, especially ankle sprains.[62,63]

The injured athlete may experience pain, swelling, stiffness, erythema, or inability to perform at the usual level. A dysfunction in one structure places other tissues and structures under increased stress.

Dry needling acupuncture therapy is very effective in treating most common volleyball injuries.

Rotator Cuff Tendinopathy

Shoulder injuries account for 8% to 20% of volleyball injuries. The biceps and rotator cuff tendons are the tissues most commonly injured.[62] The shoulder girdle musculature does not generate very powerful torque in the upper limb. About 85% of the energy needed to spike or serve a volleyball is generated by the legs and back. After repetitive overload or acute trauma, the athlete begins to alter movement patterns in an effort to minimize symptoms and maintain performance.[64] This increases the risk of injury to other structures within the kinetic chain.

Typical symptoms of shoulder injury include pain, restricted range of motion, and muscle weakness and imbalance. Further examination may reveal that the scapulae are abducted and the musculature of the posterior shoulder girdle is tight, which limits internal rotation in the affected shoulder and thereby increases the risk for impingement of the supraspinatus muscle and attrition of the glenoid labrum.[64]

Dry needling acupuncture therapy is very effective for healing this injury. The location of the tender areas should be carefully identified and treated twice a week. De-stressing treatment once a week to reduce chronic stress of the girdle musculature and the entire kinetic chain is very effective both in preventing injuries and in enhancing performance ability.

Suprascapular Neuropathy

Suprascapular neuropathy (SSN) is an injury found in sports with overhead actions, such as volleyball. A study of 66 top-level German volleyball players revealed a 32% prevalence of this injury.[65] Suprascapular neuropathy is believed to occur as a result of the "floater" serve.[66] This is when the player stops the overhand follow-through immediately after striking the ball, which results in a forceful eccentric contraction of the infraspinatus muscle to decelerate the arm. This contraction is believed to cause traction from the myoneural junction to the spinoglenoid notch and consequent compression of the nerve. The symptom can be a weakness of the musculature without pain.

Dry needling acupuncture is very effective in healing suprascapular neuropathy. As usual, the location of the tender areas should be carefully identified and treated twice a week. Before any shoulder weakness is experienced, the injury can be effectively prevented by de-stressing treatment once a week to reduce chronic stress of the girdle musculature and the entire kinetic chain.

Hand Injuries

A variety of hand injuries may occur while an athlete attempts to block a spiked ball. A study of 226 volleyball players in the Netherlands revealed 235 injuries to the hand.[67] These injuries included sprains and strains (39%), fractures (25%), and contusions (16%). The remaining 20% were dislocations, mallet fingers, and open wounds. Of these hand injuries, 37% occurred during defense, 36% during blocking, 18% as a result of fall, and 8% while the athlete spiked the ball. The thumb and the little finger are the most vulnerable digits.

Another hand injury is antebrachial-palmar hammer syndrome, the symptoms of which are arm and hand pain, distal cyanosis, and pulselessness.

Dry needling acupuncture is very helpful in treating all kinds of hand injuries and at all phases of treatment. The location of the tender areas should be carefully identified and treated twice a week. Swelling and contusions should be treated every day.

Acute Knee Injuries

Acute knee injuries are rare but can require significant time for recovery before the athlete is able to return to play. Acute knee injury occurs most often when a player lands on another player's foot after jumping in the attack zone. Injury can involve the anterior cruciate ligament and menisci.[64] Other factors that may predispose the athlete to knee injury include overuse stresses of the musculoskeletal system, which can cause ligamentous laxity in women, and valgus angle at the knee.

Dry needling acupuncture is very helpful in reducing pain, swelling, and inflammation at all phases of treatment of acute knee injuries, including those for which surgery is required. The location of the tender areas should be carefully identified and treated twice a week. Swelling and contusions should be treated every day. Dry needling acupuncture can be applied immediately after the surgery.

Patellar Tendinitis

Patellar tendinitis, or "jumper's knee," is the most common overuse injury in volleyball.[63] The knee joint connects the body's two longest lever arms, the thigh and the lower leg, and it has to withstand high physical force, which renders it vulnerable to injury.

According to epidemiologic studies, patellar tendinopathy is related to repeated loading of the knee extensor mechanism.[63] This can result in partial microscopic tearing of the tendon and can eventually progress to complete rupture of the tendon if not properly treated.

Dry needling acupuncture is very effective in preventing and treating overuse-related patellar tendinopathy. For prevention, the athlete should receive weekly de-stressing treatment of the entire musculoskeletal system. For treatment of the injury, the location of the tender areas should be carefully identified and treated twice a week. Swelling and contusions should be treated once every day.

Ankle Sprain

Lateral ankle sprain accounts for 15% to 65% of all volleyball injuries.[63] In mild (grade 1) sprains, the anterior talofibular ligament may be stretched. In grade 2 sprains, one or two ligaments may be partially disrupted. Grade 3 sprains are characterized by complete tearing of one of more lateral ligaments. In early examination, the amount of swelling is typically correlated with the severity of the injury.

Of all known therapeutic modalities, dry needling acupuncture is most effective in reducing swelling of soft tissue. If treatment is provided immediately after the injury, the swelling is greatly limited, and the pain subsides when the swelling is reduced. Treatment of swelling should be provided once a day, and the entire musculoskeletal system should be treated twice a week. Meanwhile, further medical examination and other modalities should be considered even if dry needling acupuncture provides satisfactory result, because complete healing and functional recovery may take a long time for this type of injury.

INJURIES IN OTHER SPORTS

Injuries in other sports, such as martial arts or diving, can be caused by different mechanisms, but these injuries also manifest as soft tissue pain and dysfunction. The treatment, in principle and in practice, is exactly the same. For treating particular symptoms and anatomic locations, clinicians should consult this chapter and Chapter 14.

SUMMARY

Dry needling acupuncture is effective in treating many sports injuries and greatly accelerates healing and restoration of full function. What is unique about dry needling acupuncture therapy is that it passively reduces the physiologic stresses in deep soft tissue. It is passive because dry needling acupuncture procedure does not involve any stretching of tissue. Another unique feature is that dry needling acupuncture improves or restores the physical and physiologic homeostasis in deep soft tissue. Needling procedures work to smoothly coordinate the kinetic linkage of the entire musculoskeletal system, which improves the efficiency of the athlete's movement. In this way, the treatment enhances physical performance and prevents injuries caused by repetitive stress and by stress resulting from overuse.

Because of these unique mechanisms, dry needling acupuncture should be applied immediately after any injury and should be used in all phases of treatment and rehabilitation.

Prevention is the most economical procedure. Weekly de-stressing treatment not only prevents many overuse injuries but also enhances the physical performance and prolongs athletic careers, both professional and nonprofessional.

It is emphasized again that dry needling acupuncture adds value to conventional medical modalities, and it does not and should not replace them.

Additional Readings

Shamus E, Shamus J: *Sports injury prevention & rehabilitation*, New York, 2001, McGraw-Hill.

MacAuley D, Best T, editors: *Evidence-based sports medicine*, ed 2, Malden, Mass, 2007, Blackwell Publishing.

References

1. James SL, Jones DC: Biomechanical aspects of distance running injuries. In Cavanagh PR, editor: *Biomechanics of distance running*, Champaign, Ill, 1990, Human Kinetics.
2. Hoke BR: Running. In Shamus E, Shamus J, editors: *Sports injury: prevention & rehabilitation*, New York, 2001, McGraw-Hill, pp 241–266.
3. Grelsamer RP, McConnell J: *The patella: a team approach*, Gaithersburg, Md, 1998, Aspen.

4. Hoke BR, Lefever-Button SL: *When the feet hit the ground, everything changes. Level 2: Take the next step*, Toledo, Ohio, 1994, American Physical Rehabilitation Network.

5. Konradsen L, Berg Hansen E, Sondergaard L: Long distance running and osteoarthrosis, *Am J Sports Med* 18:379–381, 1990.

6. Powell B: Medical aspects of racing. In Burke ER, editor: *Science of Cycling*, Champaign, Ill, 1986, Human Kinetics, p 185.

7. Mellion MB: Neck and back pain in bicycling, *Clin Sports Med* 13:137–164, 1994.

8. Stone WJ, Steingard PM: Year-round conditioning for basketball, *Clin Sports Med* 12:173–192, 1993.

9. Nicholas J, Hershman E: In *The lower extremity and spine in sports medicine*, vol 1, St Louis, 1986, Mosby.

10. Traina SM, Yonezuka NY, Zinis YC: Achilles tendon injury in a professional basketball player, *Orthopedics* 22:625–626, 1999.

11. Hosea TM, Carey CC, Harrer MF: The gender issue: epidemiology of ankle injuries in athletes who participate in basketball, *Clin Orthop* (372):45–49, 2000.

12. Songzogni JJ, Gross ML: Assessment and treatment of basketball injuries, *Clin Sports Med* 12:221–237, 1993.

13. Molnar TJ, Fox JM: Overuse injuries of the knee in basketball, *Clin Sports Med* 12:349–362, 1993.

14. Peppart A: Knee rehabilitation. In Canavan P, editor: *Rehabilitation in sports medicine*, Stamford, Conn, 1988, Appleton & Lange, pp 320–321.

15. Roels J, Martens M, Mulier J, et al: Patellar tendinitis (jumper's knee), *Am J Sports Med* 6:363, 1978.

16. Ray J, Clancy L, Lemon R: Semimembranosus tendinitis: an overlooked cause of medial knee pain, *Am J Sports Med* 16:347, 1988.

17. Herskowitz A, Selesnik H: Back injuries in basketball players, *Clin Sports Med* 12:293–306, 1993.

18. McFarland EG, Wasik M: Epidemiology of collegiate baseball injuries, *Clin J Sport Med* 8:10–13, 1998.

19. Mohr K, Brewster CE: Baseball. In Shamus E, Shamus J, editors: *Sports injury: prevention & rehabilitation*, New York, 2001, McGraw-Hill, pp 28–29.

20. McCarroll JR, Gioe TJ: Professional golfers and the price they pay, *Phys Sports Med* 10(7):64–70, 1982.

21. Batt ME: A survey of golf injuries in amateur golfers, *Br J Sports Med* 26:63–65, 1992.

22. Geisler PR: Golf. In Shamus E, Shamus J, editors: *Sports Injury: Prevention & Rehabilitation*, New York, 2001, McGraw-Hill, pp 185–226.

23. Lord MJ, Ha KI, Song KS: Stress fractures of the ribs in golfers, *Am J Sports Med* 24:118–122, 1996.

24. National Collegiate Athletic Association: Injury Surveillance System: *Health and safety education outreach*, 1997, P.O. Box 6222, Indianapolis, Ind 46206.

25. Garrick J, Webb D: In *Sports Injuries: Diagnosis and Management*, ed 2, Philadelphia, 1999, WB Saunders, pp 198–202.

26. Vermillion RP: Football. In Shamus E, Shamus J, editors: *Sports injury: prevention & rehabilitation*, New York, 2001, McGraw-Hill, pp 311–338.

27. Metzl JD, Micheli LJ: Youth soccer: an epidemiologic perspective, *Clin Sports Med* 17:664–674, 1998.

28. Lindenfeld TN, Schmitt DJ, Hendy MP, et al: Incidence of injury in indoor soccer, *Am J Sports Med* 22:364–371, 1994.

29. Nielsen AB, Yde J: Epidemiology and traumatology of injuries in soccer, *Am J Sports Med* 17:803–807, 1989.

30. Ekstrand J, Gillquist J, Moller M, et al: Incidence of soccer injuries and their relation to training and team success, *Am J Sports Med* 11:63–67, 1983.

31. Arnheim DD, Prentice WE: *Principles of athletic training*, St Louis, 1993, Mosby.

32. Gassé S: Soccer. In Shamus E, Shamus J, editors: *Sports injury: prevention & rehabilitation*, New York, 2001, McGraw-Hill, pp 373–406.

33. Garrick JG, Webb DR: *Sports injuries: diagnosis and management*, ed 24, Philadelphia, 1999, WB Saunders.

34. Torry MR, Steadman JR: Alpine skiing. In Shamus E, Shamus J, editors: *Sports injury: prevention & rehabilitation*, New York, 2001, McGraw-Hill, pp 267–288.

35. Briggs KK, Steadman JR: *Pre-placement screening program for the ski resort industry: an 8-year study*, Vail, Colo, 1998, Vail Resorts Association Technical Report 8.

36. Shealy JE: Overall analysis of NSAA/ASTM data on skiing injuries for 1978 through 1981. In Johnson RJ, Mote CD, editors: *Skiing trauma and safety: 5th international symposium (ASTM STP-860)*, Philadelphia, 1985, American Society for Testing and Materials, pp 302–313.

37. Molsa J, Airaksinen O, Masman O, et al: Ice hockey injuries in Finland: a prospective epidemiologic study, *Am J Sports Med* 25:495–499, 1997.

38. Montelpare WJ, Pelletier R, Stark R: Ice hockey injuries. In Caine D, Caine C, Lindner K, editors: *Epidemiology of sports injuries*, Champaign, Ill, 1996, Human Kinetics, Chap 15.

39. Tegner Y, Lorentzon R: Concussion among Swedish elite ice hockey players, *Br J Sports Med* 30:251–255, 1996.

40. Voaklander DC, Saunders LD, Quinney HA, et al: Epidemiology of recreational and old-timer ice-hockey injuries, *Clin J Sport Med* 6:15–21, 1996.

41. Tredget T, Godberson C, Bose B: Myositis ossificans due to hockey injury, *CMAJ* 116:65–66, 1977.

42. Troup JP, Hollander AP, Bone M, et al: Performance-related differences in the anaerobic contribution of competitive freestyle swimmers, *J Sports Sci* 9:106–107, 1991.

43. Troup JP: The physiology and biomechanics of competitive swimming, *Clin Sports Med* 18:267–285, 1999.

44. Kammer CS, Young CC, Niedfeldt MW: Swimming injuries and illness, *Phys Sports Med* 27:51, 1999.

45. Shapiro C: Swimming. In Shamus E, Shamus J, editors: *Sports injury: prevention & rehabilitation*, New York, 2001, McGraw-Hill, pp 103–154.

46. Fry AC: Resistance exercise overtraining and overreaching, neuroendocrine responses, *Sports Med* 23:106–129, 1997.

47. Richardson AB: Injuries in competitive swimming, *Clin Sports Med* 18:287–291, 1999.

48. Richardson AB: Thoracic outlet syndrome in aquatic athletes, *Clin Sports Med* 18:361–378, 1999.

49. McMaster WC: Anterior glenoid labrum damage: a painful lesion in swimmers, *Am J Sports Med* 14:383–387, 1986.

50. Fowler PJ: Swimming. In Fu FH, Stone DA, editors: *Sports injuries: mechanisms, prevention, treatment*, Baltimore, 1994, Williams & Wilkins, pp 633–648.

51. Kenal KA, Knapp LD: Rehabilitation of injuries in competitive swimmers, *Sports Med* 22:337–347, 1996.
52. Fowler PJ, Webster-Bogart MS: Swimming. In Reider B, editor: *Sports medicine: the school-age athlete*, ed 2 Philadelphia, 1996, WB Saunders, pp 471–489.
53. Ferro RT, McKeag DB: Spontaneous pneumomediastinum presentation and return-to-play considerations. In Harmon KG, editor: *American Medical Society for Sports Medicine case report series*, 1999.
54. Jarosz-Hlis J: Tennis. In Shamus E, Shamus J, editors: *Sports Injury: Prevention & Rehabilitation*, New York, 2001, McGraw-Hill, pp 45–72.
55. Rettig AC: Wrist problems in tennis players, *Med Sci Sports Exerc* 26:1207–1212, 1994.
56. Werner S, Plancher K: Hand and wrist injuries, *Clin Sports Med* 17:407–421, 1998.
57. Leach R, Miller J: Lateral and medial epicondylitis of the elbow, *Clin Sports Med* 6:259–272, 1987.
58. Kibler WB, Chandler TJ, Livingston B, et al: Shoulder range of motion in elite tennis players, *Am J Sports Med* 24: 279–286, 1996.
59. Elliot BC: Biomechanics of the serve in tennis: a biomedical perspective, *Sports Med* 6:285–294, 1988.
60. Gecha SR, Torg E: Knee injuries in tennis, *Clin Sports Med* 7:435–452, 1988.
61. Hutchinson MR, Laparade RF, Burnett QM, et al: Injury survey at the USTA boys tennis championships: a six-year study, *Med Sci Sports Exerc* 27:826–830, 1995.
62. Briner WW, Cacmar L: Common injuries in volleyball: mechanisms of injury, prevention, and rehabilitation, *Sports Med* 24:65–71, 1997.
63. Pera CE, Briner WW: Volleyball injuries during the 1995 U.S. Olympic festival, *Med Sci Sports Exerc* 28(5S):738, 1996.
64. Drexler DM, Briner WW, Reeser JC: Volleyball. In Shamus E, Shamus J, editors: *Sports injury: prevention & rehabilitation*, New York, 2001, McGraw-Hill, pp 73–102.
65. Holzgraefe M, Kukowski B, Eggert S: Prevalence of latent and manifest suprascapular neuropathy in high-performance volleyball players, *Br J Sports Med* 28:177–179, 1994.
66. Ferretti A, Cerullo G, Russo G: Suprascapular neuropathy in volleyball players, *J Bone Joint Surg Am* 69:260–263, 1987.
67. Bhario NH, Nijsten MWN, van Dalen KC, et al: Hand injuries in volleyball, *Int J Sports Med* 13:351–354, 1992.

CHAPTER 16

Safety Issues in Dry Needling Acupuncture Practice

As with any medical procedure, the practice of dry needling acupuncture always entails some risk. Clinicians should be aware of this possibility and be well prepared for it in treating patients, beginning with the first session.

There are two kinds of safety issues in clinical practice: adverse reactions immediately after each treatment and the potential risk of each individual needling. Fortunately, any well-trained and careful clinician can bring the full benefit of dry needling therapy to the patient with minimal risk.

The research on safety issues in the field of dry needling is currently very limited, and the author used acupuncture literature that is applicable to dry needling practice.

SHORT-TERM REACTIONS AFTER TREATMENT

It is important for clinicians to be aware of short-term reactions after treatment. The majority of patients report positive outcomes after treatments; however, some normal but uncomfortable reactions can be experienced, and patients may interpret them as negative side effects (Table 16-1). These effects are harmless but may frighten some patients; therefore it is important that patients be informed of them before they receive the treatments. Most of these reactions disappear spontaneously without special care, or light massage or moist heat may be used to soothe the discomfort. According to clinical experience, reactive pain after treatment sometimes subsides in a few minutes if one or two needles are inserted in the reactive area.[1]

To avoid severe reactions such as syncope or fainting during treatment, all patients should be treated while lying on the bed in prone, supine, or side-lying positions. Some patients, such as middle-aged women with low blood pressure

or very healthy young men, are more susceptible to syncope during their first few sessions. Close attention should be paid to these patients during the first few sessions, and the needles should be removed immediately if patients show any sign of discomfort.

PREVENTION OF ADVERSE EFFECTS

Clinicians must understand what adverse effects may occur during treatment, how to prevent them, and how to manage them.

Table 16-2 lists the results of a survey of some of the acupuncture literature published in China.

PREVENTION OF NEEDLING ACCIDENTS

Understanding the Anatomy of Acu-Reflex Points

Each acu-reflex point (ARP) has specific anatomic features. ARPs on the limbs are relatively safe, but prolonged infection and swelling leading to muscular atrophy—mostly results of wet needling procedures—have been recorded. ARPs on the torso close to the internal viscera merit special caution for safe needling. The following areas must also be needled with caution:

1. Cervical area (posterior) from C1 to C2: This area contains vertebral arteries and the medulla oblongata.
2. Thoracic area from T1 to T12: The surface tissue is very close to the pleura and the lungs.
3. Lumbar area from L2 to L3: This area is near the lower part of the kidney.
4. Neck (lateral and front): This area is near big blood vessels and organs.
5. Chest: This area is near the lungs and heart.
6. Abdomen: This area is near the liver, spleen, and intestines.

TABLE 16-1	TYPES AND FREQUENCIES OF SHORT-TERM REACTIONS TO ACUPUNCTURE n = 9408	
Type of Reaction	**Number of Reported Reactions**	**Percentage**
Relaxation	7436	79.1
Feeling energized	3072	32.7
Other positive reaction	166	1.8
Tiredness	2295	24.4
Pain where needle was inserted	1154	12.3
Bruising	378	4.0
Pain other than at site of needling	373	4.0
Feeling faint or dizzy	248	2.6
Worsening of condition	165	1.8
Nausea	111	1.2
Sweating	79	0.8
Bleeding	66	0.7
Disorientation, anxiety, nervousness, insomnia, emotional lability	63	0.7
Ache or discomfort other than at site of needling	49	0.5
Itching, pins-and-needles sensation, tingling sensation, burning sensation	33	0.4
Irritation or ache at site of needling	24	0.3
Other negative reaction	33	0.4

Modified from MacPherson H, Thomas K. Short term reactions to acupuncture—a cross-sectional survey of patient reports, *Acupunct Med* 23:112-120, 2005.

TABLE 16-2	ACUPUNCTURE ACCIDENTS IN CHINA REPORTED FROM 1950 TO 2002*	
Types of Injuries	**Cases**	**Deaths**
Pneumothorax	172	16
Injuries of medulla oblongata	15	6
Heart injuries	6	5
Large-scale bleeding	12	4
Needling-induced infection	45	4
Cerebral bleeding	3	3
Liver injuries	3	3
Bleeding in subarachnoid space	40	2
Trachea injuries	3	2
Intestine injuries	15	2
Indirect reaction of unclear origin	10	2
Cerebellar injuries	1	1
Spinal cord injuries	4	1
Soft tissue injuries (atrophy)	412**	0
Syncope	183	0
Injuries of peripheral nerves	85	0
Allergic reactions	28	0
Gall bladder injuries	10	0
Vagus nerve injuries	9	0
Stomach injuries	8	0
Blood vessel inflammation	7	0
Spleen injuries	3	0
Kidney injuries	3	0
Urinary bladder injuries	2	0
Other unknown reactions of unknown origin	91	0
TOTAL	1170	51 (0.4%)

*Modified from Zhang Ren: *Prevention of acupuncture accidents*, Shanghai, 2004, Shanghai Science and Technology, p 17.
**Soft tissue injuries were caused mostly by wet needling.

Suggested Needle Sizes

Thick needles are more liable to cause internal bleeding and visceral injuries. The author suggests gauges of 32 to 34 (0.22- to 0.25-mm diameter) for longer needles (2 to 3 inches) and gauges of 36 to 38 (diameter ≤ 20 mm) for shorter needles (½ to 1 inch). Thicker needles (4 to 5 inches in length) may be used for needling the big muscles in the gluteal regions.

No Aggressive Needle Manipulation

Needles must not be manipulated strongly or aggressively (rotating or in a piston-like movement up and down). Needling efficacy does not depend on needle manipulation.

Proper Duration of Needling Time

In most cases, needles can be left in the ARPs from a few seconds to a few minutes. In cases of acute pain, a few seconds are sufficient for healing because the muscles may relax very quickly. In cases of chronic pain or internal disease, the needles should be retained longer to achieve more muscle relaxation, and this may cause the needle-induced lesions to stay longer and may reduce the swelling. In chronic cases, even 20-minute needling may not be sufficient to change the muscle physiology, and so a higher number of sessions is needed.

Using Electrical Percutaneous Stimulation

Practitioners must be aware of the following problems when using electrical percutaneous stimulation:

- Electrical percutaneous stimulation should not be used in neck and thoracic areas, so as to avoid interference with the brainstem, vagus nerve, or heartbeat rhythm.
- Muscle cramping caused by high-intensity or high-frequency stimulation can cause bone breakage.
- Electricity should never cross the spinal cord in cervical and thoracic areas.
- Stimulation should last no more than 10 minutes in each session. In most cases, 5 minutes is enough.
- High-intensity or high-frequency stimulation should not be used with patients who are weak or elderly.

Proper Body Positions for Treatment

The author suggests that patients assume the supine, prone, or side-lying position for all treatments. The sitting position, if unavoidable, should be properly arranged, and the patient should be closely supervised during the session.

Needles and Skin Cleaning

Only disposable needles should be used. The skin should be cleaned if necessary.

Patient Condition

Each patient has a different body size and a different pathologic condition. Before treatment, a practitioner should study the body and medical history of the patient in order to adjust correctly to every case.

Physiologic Conditions

Hunger, dehydration, physical exhaustion, low blood pressure, and other imbalances can cause syncope. A full urinary bladder should be emptied before treatment. Overeating or eating immediately before treatment may cause needle-induced vomiting, and so patients should wait at least 30 minutes after eating before they start treatment.

Pathologic Conditions

Hemophilic patients should never be treated with needling therapy.

Patients taking blood thinner medications must stop taking the drugs 2 days before the treatment.

Diseases of internal organs—such as those of the lung, heart, and stomach (emphysema, history of tuberculosis, fibroid lung tissue, or enlarged heart or stomach)—and spine diseases such as scoliosis and kyphosis may increase thoracic curvature, which renders the back muscles thin and loose. A smoker's lungs can collapse with tiny injuries. In these cases, needles can automatically advance into the thoracic cavity as the patient breathes. The liver and spleen may be closer to the surface when they become inflamed or swollen, forming a big mass in the abdominal area. In these circumstances, there is a risk of severe bleeding if the organs are punctured by needling.

UNDERSTANDING OF INCIDENTS IN NEEDLING THERAPY

Needling therapy is not free of side effects or danger, and its accidents can cause death. Acupuncture needling creates lesions in the body tissues. If the needle-induced lesions are created in the wrong locations, or in the correct locations but in the "wrong" person (e.g., patients with diseased or enlarged organs or thinner body walls), they may cause temporary or irreversible consequences.

To maximize medical benefit of needling therapy to patients, the author makes the following suggestions:

- Select patients carefully. Group D patients (those with more than 80 sensitive ARPs), very weak patients, and patients with very severe conditions should not undergo acupuncture treatment. These patients may use other safer modalities, from meditation to conventional procedures.
- Understand the patient's medical history. Genetically related diseases, inborn disorders, accidents, surgery, and other pathologic events

may all cause changes in the body's natural structure. For example, patients with scoliosis may have very thin muscles of the thoracic wall and back, and normal needling may cause pneumothorax.

- When using electrical stimulation, always start with mild intensity and low frequency. Never use electrical stimulation on the neck, chest, and upper back.

CASE ANALYSIS: PNEUMOTHORAX

In acupuncture, pneumothorax usually occurs in the following way: A needle punctures the lung tissue. Then the natural respiratory movement of the lung causes tearing at the injury and enlarges the puncture. The needling hole on the thoracic wall may become a one-directional valve such that air can be sucked only into the cavity and not the other way. If blood vessels are involved, both blood and air fill the cavity to form hemopneumothorax. All these conditions change negative pressure into positive pressure inside the cavity, especially in the diseased lungs of patients with emphysema, a history of smoking, and other respiratory disease.

Clinical Anatomy of Pneumothorax

According to anatomic data (Table 16-3), pneumothorax can be caused by improper needling in the following areas: (1) the back (from T10 up), (2) the side (from rib 9 and up), (3) the front (from rib 7 and up), (4) the supraclavicular fossa and upper border of sternal notch, and (5) the top of the shoulder. Table 16-3 lists the results from a study of acupuncture-induced pneumothorax conducted in China. These data are for reference only, inasmuch as the average body size among Chinese people is different from that of Westerners.

Signs of Pneumothorax

Mild signs include chest congestion, cough, and chest pain during movement.

Moderate signs include fast and shallow respiration and fast heartbeat; chest congestion; difficulty with respiration; stabbing pain in the costal area; strong and continuous cough; inability to lie down

TABLE 16-3	THICKNESS OF THE BODY WALL OF PARAVERTEBRAL ACU-REFLEX POINTS T1 TO L4*	
Level	Left (cm)	Right (cm)
T1	6.29 ± 1.11	6.01 ± 1.10
T2	4.99 ± 1.07	5.01 ± 1.04
T3	4.39 ± 0.85	4.30 ± 1.09
T4	4.01 ± 0.66	4.05 ± 0.33
T5	3.67 ± 0.85	3.77 ± 0.72
T6	3.54 ± 1.11	3.95 ± 0.86
T7	3.34 ± 1.73	3.65 ± 0.77
T8	No measurements	
T9	3.40 ± 0.72	3.56 ± 0.58
T10	3.33 ± 0.64	3.32 ± 0.97
T11	3.36 ± 0.72	3.25 ± 0.39
T12	3.42 ± 1.33	3.41 ± 0.45
L1	3.31 ± 0.88	3.77 ± 0.81
L2	3.58 ± 0.82	4.11 ± 1.17
L3	4.11 ± 1.10	4.61 ± 1.11
L4	4.03 ± 1.14	
L5	5.26 ± 0.88	5.93 ± 1.03

*Modified from Zhang Ren: *Prevention of acupuncture accidents*, Shanghai, 2004, Shanghai Science and Technology, p 143.

without pain; and dull pain and reduced range of motion in the shoulder and upper limbs.

Severe signs include fast and shallow respiration and fast heartbeat; strong stabbing pain on the injured side, radiating to the ipsilateral shoulder, upper limb, and abdominal area; severe difficulty with respiration; cold limbs; and sweating. The patient may lose consciousness.

CASE STUDY I
Pneumothorax

A 58-year-old woman had had lung and heart disease for 8 years, which was more severe during winter. The patient required acupuncture treatment for cough, shortness of breath, chest congestion, and excessive mucus.

Needling treatment: Points UB13 (acupoint at the level of T3) and UB15 (acupoint at T5) were needled to a depth of 1.5 cm. The patient felt chest and back pain and severe shortness of breath immediately after removal of the needles. Mouth respiration, sweating, and cold limbs were observed.

Continued

Examination: The patient's blood pressure was 110/80 mm Hg; pulse rate was 108/minute; heartbeat was 108/minute; respiration rate was 28/minute; temperature was 37.6° C. Dark-purple lips, right-sided convex chest, and increased distance between right ribs were noted. Clear and low respiratory sounds were heard in the right lung. The heart valve sounds were not clear. The white blood cell count was 19,800/mm^3, and the neutrophil count was 92%. Radiographs showed no lung tissue in the lateral and middle part of the right lung. Sixty percent of the right lung was compressed. Electrocardiography revealed sinus tachycardia and pulmonary P-wave.

Diagnosis: Severe right pneumothorax, secondary infection of chronic bronchitis, and complication of lung-heart disease with pulmonary cerebral disease.

Treatment: Oxygen was administered. Close drainage was performed at the second right intercostal muscles close to the sternum for 7 days. Antibiotics, steroids, and medication to excite the respiratory center were prescribed. The patient was discharged from the hospital after 13 days with complete recovery from pneumothorax.

INJURIES OF THE NERVOUS SYSTEM

When practiced without sufficient modern knowledge of anatomy, acupuncture needling may injure the central and peripheral nervous systems. It has been reported (see Table 16-2) that needle-induced injuries of the nervous system involve the cerebrum, cerebellum, brainstem, spinal cord, nerve trunks in the limbs and face, and visceral nerves. Of these injuries, subarachnoid-space bleeding is the most common.

Peripheral nerves, cranial nerves, and spinal nerves are the targets of acupuncture needling. Among injuries of the cranial nerves, the most common are injury to the facial nerve and injury to the trigeminal nerves. Reported injuries of spinal nerves have involved the sciatic, common peroneal, radial, median, ulnar, and diaphragmatic nerves.

CASE STUDY II
Pneumothorax

A 44-year-old male patient had had severe emphysema and rheumatoid heart disease for 5 years. Within the 2 months before hospital admission, severe cough with large volume of sputum and some blood had developed. The patient requested acupuncture treatment.

Examination: The patient's temperature was 36.2° C; pulse rate was 108/minute. Shortness of breath, atrophic left side of the chest, and enlarged right side of the chest (compensatory) were noted.

Needling treatment: Paravertebral points UB13 (T3 to T4), UB43 (T4 to T5), UB46 (T6 to T7), and UB47 (T7 to T8) were needled to a depth of 1.0 to 1.7 cm. Patient felt pain after insertion and asked for removal of the needles 6 minutes after insertion. The patient experienced very difficult respiration and sweating, and his lips became dark purple. Epinephrine (Adrenalin) was injected immediately, but the patient's heartbeat stopped in 10 minutes.

Autopsy: Findings were as follows: (1) right pneumothorax, needle holes in right inferior lobe, fibroid pleuritis and hemorrhage, and emphysema; (2) left severe fibroid tubercular pleuritis, pus in the thoracic cavity, shrunken lung lobes, emphysema, mild lobar pneumonia, and chronic bronchitis; and (3) chronic rheumatoid heart valve diseases (bicuspid, tricuspid, and aortic valves), interstitial connective tissue of the heart muscle, and fresh needle holes in right ventricle of the apex.

Analysis: The depth of needling was normal and within safety range, but both heart and lung were punctured as a result of deformation and enlargement and because the chest wall was thin. Chest and back ARPs should be avoided when such patients are treated.

CASE STUDY III
Stroke

A 59-year-old male patient had a history of high blood pressure and left hemiplegia. The patient was admitted to the hospital with cerebral stroke. After 3 weeks' hospital care, the condition was stable, and the patient requested acupuncture treatment.

Acupuncture treatment: The patient felt better after the first two sessions. On the third session, after Taiyang (temporalis muscle), Du 20 (Beihui, area between bregma and vertex on the skull), and UB10 (occipital area) were needled, the patient felt dizzy, with cold sweating and vomiting, and he lost consciousness after 1 hour, with incontinence of urine. The patient was readmitted to the hospital.

Examination: The patient's temperature was 39° C; blood pressure was 190/120 mm Hg; pulse rate was 92/minute. Deep coma, arrhythmia, left pupil diameter of 3 mm, right pupil diameter of 1.5 mm, bilateral positive Babinsky reflex, and blood in cerebrospinal fluid were noted.

Treatment: Intracranial drainage was performed; 25 mL of fresh blood was administered immediately, and another 10 mL was administered 5 hours later. Despite nasal feeding, antibiotics, and fluid infusion, no improvement occurred. The patient died on the fourth day.

Analysis: The cerebral hemorrhage in this case was not directly caused by needling. The patient had high blood pressure, and cardiovascular sclerosis was the major cause of the hemorrhage. However, acupuncture should be avoided if blood pressure is unstable. Fewer ARPs should be used for such patients.

INJURIES TO THE PERIPHERAL NERVES

From 1963 to 2002, 85 cases of peripheral nerve injury were reported in Chinese acupuncture journals (see Table 16-2). When the peripheral nerves are needled, the patient often feels an electric shock radiating to the distal part. When injury is present, the area innervated by the injured nerve may exhibit sensory deficiency, such as reduced sensitivity to touch or numbness, warmth, and pain. Motor deficiency may occur. In the face, the muscles of facial expression and of the eyelids may become unable to contract. In the arm, dropping wrist (radial nerve), involuntary thumb movement (median nerve), atrophy of the thenar muscles, and motion problems with the little and ring fingers (ulnar nerve) may occur. In the lower limb, stiff extension of the knee joint and weak gait (sciatic nerve) have been observed, as have difficulty in foot or toe extension, stepping on the heel, inability to stand on the toes, and dropping foot (common fibular nerve).

Most peripheral nerve injuries are caused by wet needling; a few, by dry needling. This type of injury is usually caused by three factors:

1. Needling of the following ARPs: SI17 (H2 greater auricular), GB34 (H24 common fibular), LI4 (superficial radial), and LI11(H9 lateral antebrachial cutaneous)
2. Aggressive manipulation of the needles (piston-like up-and-down movement, rotation)
3. Drug-induced toxicity in the nerves

Prevention of Peripheral Nerve Injuries

When wet needling is used, injection into large nerve trunks at these locations should be avoided.

Electrical stimulation should not be used on these ARPs; instead, the nearby muscle tissue can be needled. If electrical stimulation is used in the nerve trunk, the vibration of the needle can cause repeated injury.

Finer needles should always be used for therapy at peripheral nerves.

Treatment of Peripheral Nerve Injuries

Once injury is noticed, strong stimulation such as injection or strong electrical stimulation should be discontinued immediately. The following modalities are usually helpful in alleviating injury: light massage, local thermotherapy (with care not to burn the skin), vitamins, and physical therapy.

VISCERAL INJURIES

CASE STUDY IV
Kidney injury

A 37-year-old male patient had pain in the stomach and upper abdominal area and asked for acupuncture treatment. During the third session, both kidney areas were needled. The next day the patient felt pain and swelling in the right lumbar area and exhibited fever. Peripheral nephritis was diagnosed. Antibiotics were injected, and both fever and swelling were reduced. A week later, the patient experienced fever, lower back pain, and frequent urination. Nephrography revealed that the right kidney had shifted toward the lower right position. Kidney puncture was performed, and 200 mL of old blood was withdrawn. Two days later, the swelling reappeared. Surgical exploration revealed about 100 mL of blood under the kidney-covering capsule, a bloody swelling the size of a walnut on the upper kidney, and a horizontal cut about 6 cm wide and 1 cm deep on the posterior surface of the kidney. The kidney surface showed viscous necrosis. The kidney and surrounding tissues were surgically removed.

The kidneys are located between T11 and L3; the right kidney is 1 to 2 cm lower than the left one. The medial borders of the kidneys are about 3.5 cm from the midline. Respiration may move the kidneys up and down, but no more than the distance of one vertebra.

In case of light injury from acupuncture, the patient may feel slight pain in the lumbar area. When urine is examined under a microscope, a minor amount of red blood cells may be observed. This condition can be self-healing. Sometimes secondary bleeding is detected 2 to 3 weeks later. In case of severe injury, the patient may complain of lumbar pain, which may radiate to the shoulder, and of stiff lumbar muscles or swelling in the lumbar area, bloody urine, high fever, and feeling cold. In these cases, hemoglobin level decreases and the white blood cell count increases. Surgery may be needed for a severe condition if the patient experiences shock, bloody urine, increasing swelling, or infection.

SYNCOPE

Acupuncture-induced syncope happens mostly in young and very healthy men and in middle-aged women. Syncope is caused by a reflex of the vagus nerve. During this process, peripheral cardiovascular resistance decreases, and blood volume returning to the heart is low, which reduces the cardiac output and leads to low blood pressure and low perfusion to the brain. Syncope occurs in the following conditions:

- Lack of acupuncture experience (new patients are prone to syncope in the first one to three treatments; patients who have not have acupuncture treatment for more than 6 months should be regarded as new patients)
- Weakness, hunger, extreme dehydration (with sweating), and exhaustion, as well as alcohol consumption
- Strong, healthy, athletic young male patients
- Nervous, depressed, sentimental, melancholic, or highly emotional patients
- Middle-aged patients with blood pressure of 110/70 mm Hg or lower
- Environmental conditions such as extremely hot weather, low atmospheric pressure, or annoying noise
- Body position during treatment: The sitting position is associated with a higher risk, especially when the shoulders and neck are needled; of all cases of syncope, only 28% occur in a lying-down position, but those episodes usually last longer and produce more severe symptoms.

Syncope Symptoms

The presyncope stage may occur for only a few seconds. It is characterized by upper-body or whole-body discomfort, pale face, ringing in the ears, blurred vision, fast heartbeat, nausea, cold sweating, and excessive yawning.

The syncope stage is characterized by dizziness, chest congestion, nausea and desire to vomit, cold and flaccid limbs, loss of consciousness, blue lips and nails, profuse sweating, crossed eyes, incontinence of urine and solid waste, drop in blood pressure, and reduction of pulse rate to 40 to 50 per minute. A few patients exhibit seizure-like symptoms.

In the postsyncope stage, patients feel exhausted and sleepy and exhibit excessive sweating.

Some patients experience the syncope stage without presyncope; in mild cases, patients experience only presyncope and postsyncope stages.

Treatment involves lowering the head and raising the feet (as is done for patients in shock) and then needling the tips of the thumb, index, and middle fingers.

Prevention of Syncope

For new patients, the practitioner should explain the possible sensations of needling.

Patients with shy or depressed personality should be asked to focus on or stare at an object and try to calm themselves before needling.

Patients who are impatient or have unstable personality are asked to focus on performing simple math exercises so as to relax the body tissues.

Patients should rest or eat if they are exhausted or hungry.

Patients should soak both hands in warm water for 10 minutes, and then point PC6 (area posterior to wrist crease with median nerve below) is lightly needled.

Patients should look downward and close their eyes. The practitioner performs a light massage with his or her thumbs from the upper rim of the patient's ocular orbit to the median down for 30 seconds and then starts needling.

CASE STUDY V
Delayed syncope

A 38-year-old, healthy male patient with no cardiovascular problem and no history of syncope sought acupuncture treatment for lower back pain. The diagnosis was lumbar soft tissue injury, and three needles were inserted into ten-der points on each side of the lumbar area for 25 minutes. The patient experienced no discomfort. Just after the needles were removed, the patient complained of chest congestion and laid down. His face became pale, and sweat appeared on his forehead. The pulse was weak and thready, and heartbeat and respiration stopped. Sweating became profuse, and the patient's lips and nails turned blue. Epinephrine (Adrenalin) (1:1000), 1 mL, was injected, and heart massage was administered. After 3 minutes, the patient regained consciousness and vomited, and heartbeat and respiration returned to normal. An intravenous injection of hypertonic glucose, 40 mL, and an intravenous infusion of saline, 500 mL for 2 hours, were administered. The patient felt completely recovered afterward.

SUMMARY

Most accidents associated with needling therapy can be prevented if the clinician has good knowledge of human anatomy. Because of the uncertainty inherent in practicing medicine, clinicians may encounter some unexpected and unfavorable cases in their careers even if they are careful and have long professional experience. Clinicians must therefore know how to avoid technical mistakes and how to manage unexpected situations.

Needling therapy offers many unique medical benefits with very low risk. However, only with in-depth understanding of both physiologic mechanisms and potential risks can practitioners provide the best service to patients.

Reference

1. Filshie J, White A, editors: Adverse reactions to acupuncture. In *Medical acupuncture: a western scientific approach*, Edinburgh, 1998, Churchill Livingstone.

Additional Reading

White A, Cummings M, Filshie J: Safe needling. In *An introduction to Western medical acupuncture*, Edinburgh, 2008, Churchill Livingstone.

Credits List

CHAPTER 2

FIGURES 2-1, 2-2, 2-3 Adapted from Lovallo WR: *Stress and health: biological and psychological interactions,* ed 2, Thousand Oaks/London/ New Delhi, 2005, Sage Publications.
FIGURES 2-4 and 2-5 From Nolte J: *The human brain in photographs and diagrams,* ed 3, Philadelphia, 2007, Mosby.
FIGURE 2-6 Squires, LR: *Fundamental neuroscience,* ed 3, United Kingdom, 2008, Academic Press.
TABLE 2-1 From Lovallo WR: *Stress & health: biological and psychological interaction,* ed 2, Thousand Oaks, Calif, 2005, Sage Publications, p 58.

CHAPTER 3

FIGURE 3-1 Nolte, J: *The human brain: an introduction to its functional anatomy,* ed 5, St Louis, 2002, Mosby.
FIGURE 3-2 Squires, LR: *Fundamental neuroscience,* ed 3, United Kingdom, 2008, Academic Press.

CHAPTER 4

FIGURES 4-2, 4-7, 4-9 Wirhed R: *Athletic ability & the anatomy of motion,* ed 3, Edinburgh, 2006, Mosby.
FIGURES 4-3 AND 4-4 Adapted from Myers TW: *Anatomy trains: myofascial meridians for manual and movement therapists,* ed 2, 2009, Churchill Livingstone.
FIGURE 4-6 From Squire, LR et al: *Fundamental neuro-science,* ed 3, New York, 2008, Academic Press.
FIGURE 4-8 Nolte, J: *The human brain: an introduction to its functional anatomy,* ed 5, St Louis, 2002, Mosby.
FIGURE 4-8B Courtesy Dr. David Moran, University of Colorado Health Sciences Center. In Nolte, J: *The human brain: an introduction to its functional anatomy,* ed. 5, St Louis, 2002, Mosby.
FIGURE 4-8C Courtesy Dr. Nathaniel T. McMullen, Department of Cell Biology and Anatomy, University of Arizona College of Medicine. In Nolte, J: *The human brain: an introduction to its functional anatomy,* ed 5, St Louis, 2002, Mosby.

CHAPTER 5

FIGURES 5-1 AND 5-2 Thibodeau, GA: *Anatomy & physiology,* ed 6, St Louis, 2006, Mosby.
FIGURE 5-3 Adapted from Evans WJ and Cannon JG: The metabolic effects of exercise induced muscle damage, *Exercise and Sport Sciences Reviews* 19(1):99-125, 1991.
FIGURE 5-4 Adapted from Armstrong LE and VanHeest JL: The unknown mechanism of the overtraining syndrome, *Sports Medicine* 32:185-209, 2002.

TABLE 5-2 From Wilmore JH, Costill DI, Kenney WL: *Physiology of sports and exercise,* Champaign, IL: Human Kinetics, 2008, p 41.

CHAPTER 6

FIGURES 6-1, 6-5, 6-6, 6-7, 6-9, 6-10 Squires, LR: *Fundamental neuroscience,* ed 3, United Kingdom, 2008, Academic Press.
FIGURE 6-2 Courtesy of Dr. Zan Hee Cho.
FIGURES 6-3 AND 6-8 Ma, Y et al: *Biomedical acupuncture for pain management: an integrative approach,* St Louis, 2005, Churchill Livingstone.
FIGURE 6-4 Adapted from Mense S and Simons DG: *Muscle pain,* Baltimore/Philadelphia, 2001, Lippincott Williams & Wilkins.

CHAPTER 7

FIGURE 7-1 From Gunn CC: *Gunn approach to the treatment of chronic pain intramuscular stimulation for myofascial pain of radiculopathic origin,* ed 2, Edinburgh, 1996, Churchill Livingstone. IN Filshie J, White A: *Medical acupuncture a Western scientific approach,* New York, 1998, Churchill Livingstone.
FIGURE 7-2 Ma, Y et al: *Biomedical acupuncture for pain management: an integrative approach,* St Louis, 2005, Churchill Livingstone.
FIGURES 7-3, 7-4, 7-5, 7-6, 7-7 Sobotta: *Atlas of human anatomy,* Munich, 2006, Churchill Livingstone.

CHAPTER 8

FIGURES 8-1, 8-3, 8-4, 8-5, 8-6, 8-11, 8-14, 8-15, 8-16, 8-17, 8-18, 8-19, 8-20, 8-21, 8-22, 8-23, 8-24, 8-25, 8-26, 8-27, 8-28, 8-29, 8-30, 8-31, 8-32, 8-33 Sobotta: *Atlas of human anatomy,* Munich, 2006, Churchill Livingstone.
FIGURES 8-2, 8-12, 8-13, 8-34 Ma, Y et al: *Biomedical acupuncture for pain management: an integrative approach,* St Louis, 2005, Churchill Livingstone.
FIGURES 8-7 AND 8-8 Jenkins D: *Hollinshead's functional anatomy of the limbs and back,* ed 8, Philadelphia, 2002, WB Saunders.
FIGURES 8-9 AND 8-10 Ma Y et al.: *Biomedical acupuncture for pain management,* Elsevier, 2005. FitzGerald MJT, Folan-Curran J: *Clinical neuroanatomy and related neuroscience,* ed 4, Burlington, 2002, Saunders.
FIGURE 8-35 From Filshie J, White A: *Medical acupuncture,* Edinburg, 1998, Churchill Livingstone.
TABLE 8-7 Modified with permission from Devinsky O, Feldmann E: *Examination of the cranial and peripheral nerves,* New York, 1988, Churchill Livingstone.

CHAPTER 9

FIGURES 9-1, 9-2, 9-3, 9-4 Sobotta: *Atlas of human anatomy*, Munich, 2006, Churchill Livingstone.
FIGURE 9-5 From Putz R, Pabst R, Taylor AN, eds: *Sobotta atlas of human anatomy*, ed 14, St Louis, 2006, Churchill-Livingstone.
TABLE 9-1 Modified from Dung HC: *Anatomical acupuncture*, San Antonio, Tex, 1997, Antarctic Press, p. 145.
TABLE 9-7 Modified from Dung HC: *Anatomical Acupuncture*, San Antonio, Tex, 1997, Antarctic Press, p. 226.

CHAPTER 10

FIGURE 10-1 Chaitow L: *Muscle energy techniques*, ed 3, Edinburgh, 2007, Churchill Livingstone.
FIGURES 10-2, 10-3, 10-4, 10-5 Sobotta: *Atlas of human anatomy*, Munich, 2006, Churchill Livingstone.

CHAPTER 11

FIGURES 11-1 AND 11-2 Sobotta: *Atlas of human anatomy*, Munich, 2006, Churchill Livingstone.

CHAPTER 12

FIGURES 12-1, 12-12, 12-13, 12-15, 12-16, 12-17 Wirhed R: *Athletic ability & the anatomy of motion*, ed 3, Edinburgh, 2006, Mosby.
FIGURES 12-2, 12-3, 12-4, 12-5, 12-6, 12-7, 12-8, 12-9, 12-10, 12-11, 12-14, 12-18, 12-19, 12-20, 12-21, 12-22, 12-23, 12-24, 12-25 Sobotta: *Atlas of human anatomy*, Munich, 2006, Churchill Livingstone.

CHAPTER 16

TABLE 16-1 Modified from MacPherson H, Thomas K: Short term reactions to acupuncture – a cross-sectional survey of patient reports. *Acupunct Med* 23(3):112-120, 2005.
TABLES 16-2 AND 16-3 Modified from Zhang Ren: *Prevention of Acupuncture Accidents*, Shanghai, China, 2004, Shanghai Science and Technology Publisher, p. 17.

Index

Note: Page numbers followed by "*f*" refer to illustrations; page numbers followed by "*t*" refer to tables; page numbers followed by "*b*" refer to boxes.

Printed and bound by CPI Group (UK) Ltd, Croydon, CR0 4YY

03/10/2024

01040344-0002